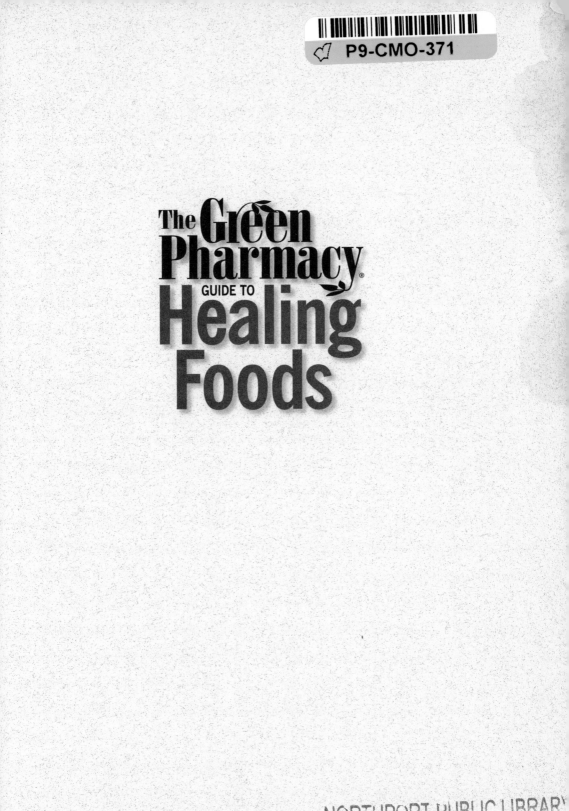

The Green Pharmacy®
GUIDE TO
Healing
Foods

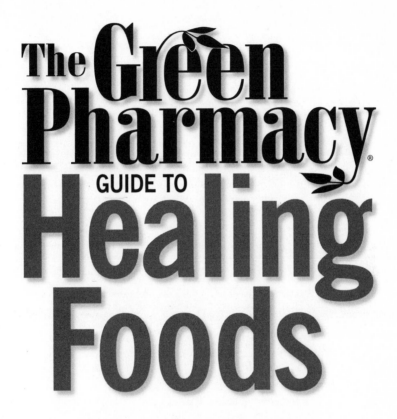

The Green Pharmacy GUIDE TO Healing Foods

Proven Natural Remedies to Treat and Prevent More Than 80 Common Health Concerns

James A. Duke, PhD

Author of the Million-Copy Bestseller *The Green Pharmacy*

RODALE

© 2008 by James A. Duke

Rodale books may be purchased for business or promotional use or for special sales. For information please write to: Special Markets Department, Rodale Inc., 733 Third Avenue, New York, NY 10017

Printed in the United States of America
Rodale Inc. makes every effort to use acid-free ⊗, recycled paper ♺.

Book design by Christina Gaugler

Library of Congress Cataloging-in-Publication Data

Duke, James A.
    The green pharmacy guide to healing foods : proven natural remedies to treat and prevent more than 80 common health concerns / James A. Duke.
        p.   cm.
    Includes index.
    ISBN-13 978–1–59486–712–5   hardcover
    ISBN-10 1-59486–712–7   hardcover
    ISBN-13 978–1–59486–713–2   paperback
    ISBN-10 1-59486–713–5   paperback
    1. Herbs—Therapeutic use.   2. Diet therapy.   I. Title.
RM666.H33.D8474   2008
615'.321—dc22   2008041588

Distributed to the trade by Macmillan

2 4 6 8 10 9 7 5 3   hardcover
2 4 6 8 10 9 7 5 3 1   paperback

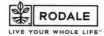

To the dedicated healers of the world, especially those who do no harm
and those who use foods as medicine when appropriate;

To the original researchers of the world,
who have painstakingly performed the necessary studies
that we authors eagerly digest and regurgitate;

To the staff of Rodale Books, who called many new ideas to my attention
in our efforts to select the most promising food "farmaceuticals";

To my family, friends, coworkers, and students, who often saw me grow
short-tempered as deadlines tightened like nooses around my neck;

And to you, my reader—I hope this book leads you
to new choices in healing that may spare you more expensive
and foreboding pharmaceuticals.

Contents

Part I Food as Medicine

Part II Food Remedies That Work

Introduction

Food for Thought . . . on Food

IT'S BEEN MORE THAN **10** YEARS since I wrote my book *The Green Pharmacy*. A lot has changed since then, especially as far as public perception of medicinal plants. Back then, they were something of a novelty, still on the fringes of legitimate medicine and science. Today, they're just short of mainstream. You can find their therapeutic compounds in products from cough drops to energy drinks.

Surely one of the reasons for the growing popularity of medicinal plants is the increase in legitimate research to support them. One of the most pervasive complaints about medicinal plants generally is that they're scientifically "unproven," even though many of them have been in use for hundreds if not thousands of years. Both the government and private institutions have been funding the investigation plants and their healing properties. The outcomes have been mixed for some, but others are faring quite well—even holding their own against prescription and over-the-counter pharmaceuticals.

Personally, I'll choose a plant over a pill any day. In fact, I've got dozens of these natural healers growing right behind my house, in my Green Farmacy Garden. They're laid out in plots by condition; from spring through summer and on into fall, I can harvest the plants as I need them—whether to treat an insect bite or to keep my gout from flaring up, which happens if I get careless.

So it shouldn't be a surprise that for my new book, *The Green Pharmacy Guide to Healing Foods*, I continue to favor the use of medicinal plants for minor complaints as well as for more serious chronic conditions, for which conventional treatments often are appropriate or necessary. In cases like these, medicinal plants may enhance the healing process and perhaps even reduce the need for medication. (Though I can't stress enough that you should never change any prescribed treatment plan without first consulting your doctor.)

For this book, I've expanded my usual definition of medicinal plants as herbs to include all plant-based foods—namely fruits, vegetables, beans, grains, and nuts and seeds. For the most part, they're remedies that you would easily find at your supermarket or farmer's market, or that you'd have other reason to keep on hand in your kitchen. I will admit to throwing in the occasional exotic, such as camu-camu, a fruit that I encountered on one of my numerous exploratory excursions to the Amazon. It is unmatched as a source of vitamin C. Right now it's available in only powdered form in the US. For my money, the actual fruit is a much better choice, because of all the other therapeutic compounds it contains.

This brings me to an important point: Though the conventional wisdom is to single out a particular nutrient in a particular food for its healing properties, I'm not entirely sold on this approach. Yes, our bodies require sufficient amounts of certain vitamins and minerals—the so-called essential nutrients—to carry out their basic biochemical functions. And nutritional deficiencies may contribute to the onset of certain diseases. That said, I'm convinced that no nutrient works in isolation. It's the synergistic effects of the nutrients and other compounds—especially phytochemicals—that give foods their healing potential. That's why foods are almost always a better choice than supplements, and whole, fresh foods are more beneficial than processed.

As you read this book, you're going to see an occasional reference to multiple activity menus, or MAMs. They're a product of the USDA Phytochemical Database, which I developed during my tenure with the USDA. Simply, a MAM identifies the phytochemicals in a particular medicinal plant, along with their respective therapeutic activities. Using this information, the MAM generates a "synergy score" that suggests how a plant might contribute to the prevention or treatment of a condition, relative to other plants. The MAMs aren't gold-standard research in and of themselves, but they can direct us to plants and plant-based foods that we may not have considered because they don't contain significant amounts of the essential vitamins and minerals.

Though this book is heavy on plant-based food remedies, you are also going to come across some animal products—mostly fish and dairy. Plant foods will always be my first choice, mainly because only they contain those all-important phyto-chemicals. Animal foods do not. Still, my editor and researchers persuaded me to include some animal products because they are they best available sources of certain nutrients. Calcium is a good example. You can get it in decent amounts from dark leafy greens, among other plant foods, but they rarely come close to dairy. Generally, I've tried to give plant-based alternatives to the animal-based remedies, so you can decide what's best for you.

I imagine that you're eager to jump to Part II of this book, where you'll find the remedies organized by condition. You're more than welcome to do so, but I would encourage you to sometime read through Part I. There you'll find helpful information on the science behind eating for good health, along with some suggestions for maximizing the nutritional "punch" of your own diet. You'll also find Duke's

Dozen, the 12 foods that I consider most beneficial for fighting disease, based on the nutrients and phytochemicals they contain.

In the condition chapters themselves, you'll notice that each remedy carries a rating of 1 to 3 stars. The ratings reflect a combination of scientific research, anecdotal evidence, and my own experience with particular remedies. They're entirely subjective, but I'm hoping that they may help prioritize your choices, as most conditions have a number of healing foods from which to choose.

A few other caveats to keep in mind:

1. If you're trying a food for the first time, proceed with caution—particularly if you have other known food allergies or sensitivities. Yes, foods are natural, an d generally, they're safe. But even they can cause trouble for some people. If you notice any sign of an adverse reaction, stop eating the food and see your doctor as soon as possible.

2. I mentioned this earlier, but it's important enough that I'll reiterate here: Please don't make changes to any prescribed treatment plan that you may be following without first consulting your doctor. Reducing the dosage of a medication without proper guidance can have serious consequences. Better to be safe than sorry, as the saying goes.

3. Whichever remedies you choose, be sure to give them adequate time to work. Some may produce results quickly, while others may take weeks to show their effects. Further, everyone responds differently to individual remedies. If one isn't doing the job for you—even after, say, 6 or so weeks—by all means try another one. You may need to do some experimenting to find what's right for you.

So are you ready to begin? Good. Let's explore together all of the amazing healing bounty that nature has to offer.

PART I

Food as Medicine

How Foods Heal

"Medicinal Foods" through the Ages— From Ancient to Modern Times

IF YOU'RE FAMILIAR WITH MY GREEN PHARMACY (or Farmacy, as I like to call it), you probably think that it's all about herbal remedies. That's partially true. Herbs have always been near and dear to my heart, and they still are. However, research over the past few decades has taken the Green Pharmacy in a new and interesting direction—away from the health food store and into the supermarket.

A growing body of literature indicates that a number of plant foods—fruits, vegetables, spices, and even beverages—offer many of the same healing powers that you'll find in herbal remedies. Foods, however, have a distinct advantage over their herbal cousins: Instead of depending on capsules, tinctures, and teas, you can incorporate foods into delicious, flavorful meals that are as satisfying as they are healing!

Of course, we all know that fruits and vegetables are healthful. That's why the government recently increased its recommendation from five servings to nine a day. But only now are we learning just how healthful they really are. To begin with, they're high in fiber, low in calories, and devoid of or low in harmful fats. But that's not all. Most have hundreds, if not thousands, of medicinal compounds, each of which has a specific impact on your health and well-being. As a result, you can choose to add various plants to your diet to treat certain ailments. For example, I eat celery almost every day to prevent the pain associated with gout, and garlic is part of my diet because I know it can benefit my heart and possibly even help control my chronic Lyme disease.

Over the next few pages, I'll give you some background on how plant foods heal, so you can gain a greater understanding of their role in your health. Then, in the chapters to come, I'll help you plan your own regimen to treat specific conditions with specific foods.

Food as a Historical Healer

The idea of "food as medicine" is hardly a new one. In fact, when you consider that ancient man lacked the technological capability of today's chemists, it only makes sense that their medicines came directly from nature.

In fact, evidence of using food to heal dates back thousands of years. Ayurveda, the traditional healing art of India, is a perfect example. It borrows many of its ideas from Hinduism, incorporating multiple therapies that include herbs, massage, and meditation. Ayurvedic practitioners may even go so far as to try a new diet to prevent or treat specific conditions. One medicinal food from Ayurveda may be familiar to you: turmeric, which often shows up as a spice in Asian cuisine. Aside from its unique flavor, turmeric may also prove a helpful treatment for people with arthritis, Alzheimer's disease, and some forms of cancer. Although the research evidence isn't yet conclusive, it's certainly highly suggestive, and my own experience using turmeric as an anti-inflammatory has been extraordinarily positive. (For more information on turmeric, see page 28.)

Ayurveda, also commonly referred to as Traditional Indian Medicine or Traditional Ayurvedic Medicine (TAM), shares this focus on food with another ancient form of medical practice, Traditional Chinese Medicine (TCM). TCM works from the concepts of "yin" and "yang," which in ancient Chinese philosophy refer to the two fundamental forces in the universe—the aggressive, hot, go-get-'em force (yang); and the passive, lie back and chill out force (yin). You get sick when these two forces fall out of balance in your body.

By now you're probably wondering what all of this has to do with food. In TCM, the foods you eat are seen as having yin properties—cooling and moistening—or yang properties—warming and drying. Depending on the condition you have, your practitioner will help you make food choices to restore balance between the two forces. For example, if you have a mucus-producing cough from a cold, your balance is skewed toward the yin, so you'll want to treat it with warming, drying foods like ginger tea and hot vegetable soups. As you can see, we borrow some of our ideas for treating illness from the Chinese, whether we're aware of it or not!

Better Living through Chemistry?

TAM and TCM are a far cry from Western medicine, which views food as the source of nutrition but ignores its healing properties almost entirely. That's not to say the American view of the diet—seeking a balance among protein, carbohydrates, and fat—doesn't make sense. It does. But it's limited—very limited.

The Chinese and Indian approaches basically say that the body will react in certain ways to certain foods. After all, we have co-evolved with and made use of the plants in our environment throughout the history of our species, so it only stands to reason that we would develop special relationships with some of them, as we have with members of the animal kingdom.

Now contrast that with our notion of modern medicine, which I like to call "better living through chemistry." Most synthetic drugs have been in use for only a few decades rather than a few thousand years, so the body just isn't used to handling them as it handles foods.

What's more, most plant foods contain thousands of bioactive compounds, each of which plays a unique role in the body. By contrast, the viewpoint of modern medicine is that we're looking for one "silver bullet," the so-called active ingredient—and all the other helpful compounds in any specific plant are tossed out and forgotten.

I'm not saying that all drugs are bad. In fact, quite the opposite is true: Drugs have saved the lives of many people. But it's tough to argue with the numbers: In 2005, pharmaceuticals killed at least 140,000 people in the United States—that we know of. The number may be even higher. As far back as 2002, the esteemed *Journal of the American Medical Association* recognized this problem, calling adverse drug reactions "a leading cause of death in the United States."

Now compare that with herbs and supplements. Altogether, they caused an estimated 29 deaths in 2005. The numbers speak for themselves.

The purpose of this book is not to scare you away from taking your medicines. After all, I need to take pharmaceuticals myself every now and then. Rather, what I'm hoping you'll do is "think outside the pillbox" and realize that by taking a different approach to what you eat, many conditions—and the medicines needed to treat them—can potentially be avoided completely.

The Supplement Scare

As you've already seen, supplements have proven safer than pharmaceuticals. However, this doesn't necessarily place vitamin supplements beyond criticism. Their effectiveness, most notably that of the "big three" antioxidants—vitamins A, C, and E—has come into question in recent years.

In the recent HOPE (Heart Outcomes Prevention Evaluation) study, more than 10,000 heart disease patients received either 400 IU of vitamin E or a placebo every day for six years. At the end of the trial, the researchers concluded that vitamin E really didn't do much better than the placebo at preventing death or other adverse outcomes from heart disease.

Vitamin C is generally considered safe even at high doses (though more than 1,200 milligrams can cause diarrhea in some people). But recently, the effectiveness of "megadosing" with vitamin C for illnesses like colds and flu has come under some fire. As the National Institutes of Health points out, more than 30 clinical trials with more than 10,000 participants have looked into the role of vitamin C in preventing colds, and no significant reduction has been noted. Vitamin C supplements may play a role in reducing the duration of colds, however.

Vitamin A (which exists in foods in the form of pre-vitamin A as well as carotenoids such as beta-carotene) has also been studied in supplement form, and it has shown some effectiveness for some conditions. The evidence indicates, however, that if you smoke or drink alcohol, you may want to steer clear of supplementing with pure beta-carotene, since it could actually increase your risk of lung damage, including even lung cancer.

Again, none of this is meant to scare you away from supplements. Quite the contrary; I take a number of them, and I think that multivitamins are a great means of getting a full complement of healthy nutrients in an economical way. I just find it interesting that when a single, specific bioactive compound is isolated, whether in a pharmaceutical or a supplement, the result is never as dramatic as people expect. That's because in nature, the compound works in combination with many others to bring healthful benefits to the body. Those combinations exist in only one place—whole foods!

The Food Renaissance

In recent years, you've probably noticed that you're hearing less about familiar nutrients, such as vitamins A, C, and E, in nutrition news and more about exotic-sounding ones, such as lycopene, quercetin, and resveratrol, to name a few. The reason is simple: Researchers are beginning to look beyond the macronutrients in foods, and they're discovering micronutrients and phytochemicals.

Some of the benefits these compounds offer stem from their antioxidant potential. In the simplest terms, antioxidants help your body by neutralizing free radicals, unstable oxygen molecules that the body can overproduce after exposure to toxins such as cigarette smoke, pollution, and even unhealthful foods. Beyond their antioxidant potential, many compounds help specific parts of the body remain healthy as well. Beta-carotene, lutein, and cryptoxanthin are good for your eyes. Phytoestrogens fight cancer. Capsaicin attacks arthritis pain. The list goes on and on.

The practical result of these new research discoveries is clear: Emphasis is shifting back to eating lots of healthful whole foods, particularly fruits and vegetables. And when the USDA plays along (which they did in 2005 by increasing their recommendation to nine servings of fruits and vegetables a day), you know we're making progress.

As I said earlier, I believe you can specifically tailor your diet to prevent or even reduce the symptoms related to a number of specific medical conditions—conditions as benign as a flaky scalp or as serious as a heart attack.

We'll have plenty of time to go over all these foods and the conditions they treat in the chapters ahead. First, though, let's look at an overview of some of the "heavy

Food vs. Pharma

If you think that pharmaceuticals are always more effective than food nutrients at treating medical conditions, you may be in for a surprise. For example, in studies, ginger has consistently beaten the drug Dramamine as a treatment for motion sickness. A pomegranate is so rich in phytoestrogens that a mere half a fruit can provide the equivalent of a daily dose of hormone replacement therapy (HRT) for menopause symptoms (though I wouldn't yet recommend it as a substitute for HRT). A flavonoid compound in blueberries, pterostilbene, lowered cholesterol as effectively as the commercial drug ciprofibrate (Lipanor) in clinical studies. And I know people who find turmeric, the root from which curry is derived, to be more effective than celecoxib (Celebrex) for treating arthritis pain because of its high levels of COX-2 inhibitors. Likewise, capsaicin, the hot ingredient in chile peppers, is much more potent as a COX-2 inhibitor than the now-banned drug Vioxx.

hitters" of the nutrition world as well as a rundown of some cutting-edge cures that we've only recently learned about.

What's Hot in Foods Now

When it comes to nutritional stars, it's funny how certain nutrients seem to go in and out of fashion. For a while, vitamins A, C, and E were hot. Now omega-3 fatty acids, lycopene, and vitamin D are getting all the attention. Next month, it may be something else.

However, just because a nutrient slips out of the limelight doesn't mean that it's no longer important to your health. Here's a quick look at some of the most important ones, from the old standbys to the new stars.

The Old Standbys

Though their reputation has taken a bit of a hit, it's still important to start any discussion of healing foods with the "big three" antioxidants—vitamins A, C, and E.

Arguably the most famous of the three is vitamin C, found in abundance in foods like bell peppers, papayas, strawberries, and oranges and other citrus fruits. Some exotic fruits, like acerola, camu-camu, and emblic, rarely available in North American supermarkets, may be richer in C. In studies, vitamin C has been linked to the prevention of a number of diseases—most notably heart disease but also some cancers. As a matter of fact, the USDA phytochemical database lists nearly 100 activities for vitamin C, and I could probably double that number in a few minutes of surfing the Web. Research has shown that vitamin C may work more quickly than other antioxidants, blocking free radicals before others even arrive on the scene.

Another significant heart helper is vitamin E, which has reduced the risk of heart disease in a number of studies. This nutrient, found in vegetable oil, sunflower seeds, nuts, and sweet potatoes, has also shown that it may help fight off lung and prostate cancer. Some evidence indicates that vitamin E is even more effective when consumed with vitamin C, reinforcing the idea that eating a variety of fruits and vegetables gives you the most benefits.

Finally, we can't overlook vitamin A. It has gotten its fair share of bad press in recent years, and some studies have even linked it to increased risks of heart disease and cancer. However, it's important to remember that these studies looked at high doses from supplements. The main source of this antioxidant available from foods is beta-carotene, which your body converts into vitamin A. When people stick to the amounts of beta-carotene present in orange and yellow foods such as carrots, squash, cantaloupe, and sweet potatoes, the antioxidant is considered quite healthful.

Naturally, these aren't the only important nutrients, and they're not the only ones I focus on in my own regimen. A lesser-known but equally important antioxidant is selenium (just three Brazil nuts supply a whopping 200 micrograms). The whole range of B vitamins may play a role in preventing the symptoms of neuropathy, a common nerve disorder, and some studies suggest they can treat or prevent Alzheimer's disease. And I focus on getting plenty of magnesium to prevent nighttime leg cramps.

Here again, it all comes back to focusing on a variety of foods to get a balanced intake of all the important nutrients! You can go to the USDA phytochemical database (www.pl.barc.usda.gov/usda_chem/achem_home.cfm) and search for the richest sources of thousands of nutrients and phytochemicals.

The Right Kinds of Fats

Aside from abundant amounts of antioxidant nutrients, the other thing that plant foods have going for them is that they're relatively devoid of the type of fat found in red meat and dairy products, which can harm your heart; and some have fats that are actually good for you. Certain nuts, olive oil, and avocados, for example, have monounsaturated fats, which seem to raise levels of "good" HDL cholesterol while leaving "bad" LDL and total cholesterol levels unchanged.

Another group of beneficial fats currently getting a lot of attention are the omega-3 fatty acids. Though fatty fish like salmon and tuna are usually cited as the best sources of omega-3's, the fish actually acquire them by eating primitive plant forms such as algae, which manufacture these acids.

There is a handful of rich plant sources that provide an omega-3 called alpha-linolenic acid (ALA), which can offer some but usually not all of the health benefits of the "fishy" omega-3's. Flaxseed and hempseed have omega-3's, specifically ALA, in abundance, but a tastier plant source is walnuts. (For more on walnuts, see page 29.)

Recently I learned that chia, of Chia Pet fame, is even richer in ALA. I'm having an Amazonian acquisition, called Inca peanut (*Plukenetia volubilis*, not related to the real peanut, *Arachis hypogaea*), analyzed as another contender. And in my Green Farmacy Garden, there's a weed that many Asians consume with sushi. It's called perilla, and it has more ALA than the better-known flaxseed.

The New Stars

For many of you, the information about vitamin C, vitamin E, and omega-3 fatty acids is old news. But how about lutein? Quercetin? Resveratrol? If they're familiar to you, pat yourself on the back—you're staying up to date with cutting-edge research on food. And they're not the only new stars in the healthful nutrition firmament. Among those causing the most excitement are flavonoids.

Flavonoids are a group of bioactive compounds found in plant foods. To date, more than 4,000 different flavonoids have been identified, and that may be just the tip of the proverbial iceberg (and I don't mean iceberg lettuce, which is much less likely to have them in abundance than more rustic leaf lettuces). Many of these compounds have been shown to have antioxidant as well as anti-inflammatory properties.

With so many potent flavonoids, it would be impossible to touch on all of them, but one you may have heard mentioned on the nightly news is resveratrol, a chemical in grape skins and grape leaves, peanuts, mulberries, and some less palatable weeds. Resveratrol may prevent clotting of the blood, and some researchers have even suggested it may retard the aging process at the cellular level.

Another is quercetin, found in onions and green and black tea, which may play a significant role in cancer prevention.

Beta-carotene may be the star of the carotenoid family, but other carotenoids, such as lycopene, lutein, and zeaxanthin, are also gaining attention. Lycopene, found in tomato products (and interestingly, in higher concentrations in tomato sauces and juices than in whole tomatoes), has gotten the most attention for prostate cancer prevention, though recent research has called its protective effects into question. Lutein and zeaxanthin, found in leafy greens, seem to be superstars when it comes to protecting the eyes from macular degeneration, a disease that affects a huge number of older adults.

So now that you've had a little taste of all the great things hiding in the produce aisles of your supermarket, are you interested in learning more? Read on!

CHAPTER 2

Eating for Optimal Health

Breaking Free from Our "White Bread" World

GETTING PEOPLE TO ADD HEALING FOODS TO THEIR DIETS can be challenging. And the low-quality foods typically available in American supermarkets certainly don't make that challenge any easier.

I've been wracking my brain trying to think of a delicate way to phrase this, but there's really no getting around it: The current state of the American diet is terrible. I think it's fair to say that our dietary choices are among the primary reasons that two-thirds of all Americans are overweight, and half of that number are obese. What's even more frightening is that our children are now paying the price for our poor eating habits. According to the Centers for Disease Control and Prevention, almost 20 percent of America's children are now overweight, and kids born in the year 2000 or later have a one in three chance of developing type 2 diabetes in their lifetimes.

This strongly suggests that the way we're eating today actually causes disease. Read on to see how this is happening and what you can do to change it.

The Problem with How America Eats

Consider this: Almost every edible item we buy comes with a label on it. The problem with a label, of course, is that it often indicates that the food is processed in some way, and often, the more processed it is, the more unhealthful it is. The implication is that we're surrounded by unhealthful foods—and, in fact, they're so pervasive in our supermarkets that unless you live on a farm, as I do, they're often difficult to avoid.

The first problem with processed foods comes down to simple vs. complex carbohydrates. By design, most of the processed breads and snack foods in the American diet are simple carbohydrates. You can often identify them by their color: white. White bread, white rice, white cookies, white cakes. This means they're easy to eat and easy to digest, and they have an immediate impact on your body's blood sugar. On the other hand, complex carbohydrates, found in fruits, vegetables, and whole grains, often take longer to chew and swallow, so you tend to eat less of them. Also, once they're in your body, you digest and metabolize them more slowly and less efficiently, so they affect your blood sugar more gradually and don't cause it to spike.

There's a fairly new tool called the glycemic index that makes choosing the right kinds of carbohydrates a whole lot easier. It ranks foods based on how drastically they affect your blood sugar level. Foods ranked low on the glycemic index are generally better choices, and foods ranked higher are poor choices. We Americans seem to rely on the glycemic index less than Europeans do, though I'm sure it's useful. (For more information, visit www.glycemicindex.com.)

Of course, carbohydrates aren't the only problem with processed foods; they're also often full of unhealthful fats. Granted, some whole foods, like red meat and dairy products, contain cholesterol-raising saturated fats, too. But many processed foods contain manmade trans fats, created by adding hydrogen to vegetable oil in a process called hydrogenation, which is why these fats are often listed on food labels as "partially hydrogenated."

Like saturated fats, trans fats elevate levels of "bad" LDL cholesterol and increase the risk of heart disease. Some studies even indicate that trans fats may lower levels of "good" HDL cholesterol, as well as contribute to smaller LDL particle size, which raises your risk even further.

Of course, when you get beyond all the science, there's a very simple reason that all these processed foods are bad for your health and well-being: They're taking up space on your dinner plate that should be occupied by healthful, nutrient-dense foods that are good for you.

The choice is plain and simple: Eat the right foods, and you can prevent disease. Eat the wrong ones, and you actually promote it.

Dieting Don'ts

It goes without saying that the glut of unhealthful foods in America has contributed to our obesity problems, so it's no surprise that everywhere you turn, there's a diet that promises dramatic overnight results in creating a new, thinner you. While many of these diet plans are not without merit, the most popular ones are far from perfect.

Low-carb diets such as the Atkins Diet gained traction for helping people lose a lot of pounds, but critics argued that they put too much emphasis on unhealthful saturated fats. It's also important to mention that carbohydrates are not inherently bad—they're essential components of any healthful diet. The key, of course, is to choose the right carbohydrates (whole fruits, vegetables, and whole grains instead of processed and refined carbs) instead of cutting them out entirely.

In contrast to the low-carb diet, a more time-tested approach to weight loss is the low-fat diet. Fat is incredibly calorie dense, so it makes good sense that restricting it from your diet would help you lose weight. But here again, there's more to the story than meets the eye. Just as with carbohydrates, it's the type of fat that can make a big difference in your health. For this reason, the American Heart Association recommends limiting overall fat intake to around 30 percent of your daily calories, with monounsaturated fats (found in nuts, seeds, olives, and avocados) making up 15 percent of total calories, and saturated fats (found in red meat and dairy foods) making up 7 to 10 percent.

Also, be wary of "low-fat" foods at the supermarket. While these may be better for your health than the full-fat versions, they're often poor substitutes for healthier choices like fruits, vegetables, nuts, and whole grains. And they're often full of sugar.

Considering my background in the area of plant research, you might think my dietary leanings would be more toward vegetarianism. The fact is, while I definitely emphasize plants heavily in my overall diet, I must admit that I'm not a strict vegetarian.

Studies have shown that when followed diligently, a vegetarian diet can have incredible health benefits, including significantly reduced rates of cancer and heart disease. However, what these studies don't take into account is just how difficult it is for the average person to adhere to a strict vegetarian or vegan lifestyle. Granted, if people are very skillful about making the right food choices, vegetarianism can be one of the most healthful diets you can follow. But many vegetarians don't make the right choices, and as a result, it's not uncommon for them to have dangerous deficiencies of vitamin B_{12} and protein.

For all of that, I'm far from being a meat-monger, though I do take a slightly different approach to vegetarianism, which I'll outline in greater detail below.

How to Eat Today

Moderation in all things: It may be a cliché, but there's really no better way to describe how we should tailor our diets to live healthfully and disease free.

In the pages that follow, you'll find a treasure trove of information about specific foods that will prevent and even treat a number of diseases. But first, it helps to have a handful of approaches that will help you incorporate more of these healthful foods into your everyday routine. Here's how to do exactly that.

Eat like your ancestors. Interestingly, of all the fad diets that have come and gone over the years, the one that has perhaps drawn the most criticism is the blood type diet devised by Peter J. D'Adamo, MD. Dr. D'Adamo's theory is that different blood types evolved based on whether our direct ancestors were hunters, gatherers, or farmers or took some other role in primitive society.

While I can't attest to the specific blood type theory, I think there's something to this concept of eating like your ancestors did—a "Paleolithic diet," if you will. In

Africa, Zulus live healthy lives subsisting almost entirely on animal products. Even their herbs are often taken as a milk tincture. Other tribal groups subsist almost entirely on plants and have for a long time.

This seems to suggest that different people do have different needs. If that's the case, then the best source of advice for what you should be eating is probably your own body. For the average person, this means that you shouldn't restrict meat if it's what you crave. Rather, make it part of a balanced diet with a good blend of fruits, vegetables, and healthful whole grains.

Be a Jeffersonian vegetarian. As I mentioned earlier, I'm not a strict vegetarian, but meat isn't a major part of my routine either. Instead, I consider myself more of a "Jeffersonian vegetarian." Let me explain.

While our third president, Thomas Jefferson, wasn't a strict vegetarian, his preference for vegetables over meat was well documented. As the president himself said in 1819, "I have lived temperately, eating little animal food, and that not as an aliment so much as a condiment for the vegetables, which constitute my principal diet."

I try to tailor my diet the same way, viewing meat more as flavoring for a vegetable-based dish than as the main course. If you'd like to restrict your meat intake in favor of more vegetables, I think this centuries-old approach is a great way to do it.

Stick to the S's. My approach to having a "Jeffersonian diet" leads me to my next tip for how to eat: Stick to the S's. And by S's, I mean soups, stews, and salads. All

Try an Amazonian Approach

With the emphasis on regions in a lot of popular diets (South Beach, Sonoma, Mediterranean), maybe it's time we tried an Amazon diet. No region in the world has more species, many as yet unknown to science, or so many native foods packed with great healing potential—avocados, blue corn, Brazil nuts, cocoa beans, hot peppers, peanuts, sweet potatoes; the list goes on. And many vegetal varieties that originated in the Amazon are now comfortably cultivated outside the tropics.

If Americans were to focus more on these healthful Amazonian foods and less on harmful meats and processed foods, I'm convinced this diet would do people at least as much good as the Mediterranean or other regional diets. And it's not as exotic as it sounds. Many of the Amazonian products I mentioned can now be grown closer to home, and depending on where you live, some may even be cultivated locally.

three are wonderful vehicles for incorporating as many healthful fruits, vegetables, and herbs as possible into a delicious, fulfilling meal. If you're someone who craves meat, these dishes allow you to take the Jeffersonian approach with ease: You can use meat as a smaller component to flavor the meal rather than as the main course.

Go grazing—in both senses of the word. My last approach to healthful eating is becoming increasingly more accepted in nutrition circles, and that is to graze. In other words, eating five or six small meals throughout the day may be a better approach than the traditional "three squares" a day. And studies seem to support that this practice may actually help you consume less food overall.

That's one definition of grazing, which I recommend. But here's another: To many wild-food enthusiasts, grazing means eating a lot of wild vegetables and fruits. Many of my readers aren't yet experienced in determining which wild foods are safe and which are dangerous, but I believe that we human grazers, in this latter, narrower sense, are more liable—like range-fed animal grazers—to have the right proportion of healthful fats in our diets.

I indulge in both senses of grazing. I incorporate healthful fruits, vegetables, and nuts into my diet by munching on them throughout the day. I take the same approach with healthful herbal teas, not just mint and ginger but dozens of different teas over time. Of course, Mrs. Duke certainly helps by keeping the house stocked with nuts and dried fruits instead of cookies and crackers. That way, when the urge to eat hits, the only grazing options are healthful ones. It's an approach that can help anyone.

Then, as I walk through my garden and woods, I indulge in that second way of grazing, consuming lots of weird wild things that my ancestors ate but my parents didn't—wild grape leaves and tendrils, green briar tendrils, dozens of edible weeds (some tasty, some pretty bad), and some wild fruits.

The Bountiful Buffet

Given the pace and pressures of modern life, taking the time to prepare and eat healthful meals may seem a praiseworthy but unrealistic goal. Not only are we surrounded by processed foods, but we often find ourselves eating in dining establishments, where we have no control over what's offered and what isn't. Well, I'm here to assure you that you do have control. In my experience, if you're resourceful and determined, you can have a healthful repast pretty much anywhere you go.

When Mrs. Duke and I are on the road and eating in restaurants, I usually opt for the buffet breakfast and sample most of the fruits, cereals, and yogurts, with just a dab of meat and eggs. For dinner, Mrs. Duke likes to go to places where you sit down and order from the menu. I usually go for soup and salad. I actually prefer to go to those low-priced buffets where they offer several kinds of meat dishes; marvelously varied salad, fruit, and vegetable bars; choices of two or three soups; and—regrettably for those who can't resist—dozens of dessert choices. This is good grazin' for me. I take very small portions of most of the salad items, even mixing the salad dressings, and very small, Jeffersonian portions of the meats, along with minimal servings of most of the veggies. This is my first tasting, and then I return for more of the more pleasantly flavored items if they still appeal to me. Often though, the samplings fill me up so I don't need to go back to the buffet. By grazing this way, I've probably consumed small portions of dozens of fruits and veggies.

Now think about this. Each of the 50 or 60 plants I've tasted may contain up to 5,000 identifiable "chemistries," all biologically active. And because my genes have co-evolved with many if not most of these chemistries, just as I selected what I wanted from the buffet, I maintain that our bodies select what they need from those thousands of chemistries. By grazing at the buffet, I offer my body thousands of gentle, natural compounds to choose from, many of which homeostatically get my body back to normal. That's what I sometimes call Duke's Diversity Diet.

So if you're forced by circumstance or seduced by opportunity to eat at restaurants, try to find places with great salad bars or buffets. They're great opportunities to eat for health!

CHAPTER 3

Duke's Dozen

My 12 Greatest Disease-Fighting Foods

WITH SO MANY GREAT HEALING FOODS out there, narrowing the list down to a top 12 (a top 10 list would have been just too short) certainly wasn't an easy task. But after careful consideration, my humble opinion is that these dozen foods offer the biggest nutritional bang for your buck.

Among the 12, you'll find a whole host of potential healers for common ailments—Alzheimer's, arthritis, cancer, colds and flu, gout, heart disease, menopause symptoms, motion sickness, and many others. And all 12 can be incorporated into your daily diet with relative ease.

Before we get into my Duke's Dozen, however, I want to offer just a quick note: You'll notice that for several of these, I've included the entire family of foods (for example, beans instead of just lima beans). This is because many foods in a given family share common nutritional traits, so it would be a disservice to leave several of them off the list in favor of just one, especially when the whole family provides a boatload of benefits.

But enough buildup—we have a lot of ground to cover! Without further ado, here's my list of the all-time top 12 healing foods.

Food #1: Beans

Few foods offer the unique combination of healthy nutrients and easy accessibility that beans do. Eating more can provide a multitude of benefits.

Nutrient Nuts and Bolts: Beans get a lot of good press for being low in fat and high in protein, which makes them a great alternative to animal-based protein sources like red meat. They're also brimming with soluble fiber. This means that they are adept at whisking cholesterol out of your system via the intestines, making them good for your heart.

A lesser-known benefit of beans, though, is their high levels of isoflavones, compounds that are similar in structure to the estrogen produced by your body (which is why they are also called phytoestrogens). These isoflavones may ease the symptoms of menopause, prevent some forms of cancer, reduce your risk of heart disease, and improve your bone and prostate health, among other benefits.

How to Get More: The nice thing about beans is how easily you can add them to any meal. Pour them into soups and salads or use them in spicy Mexican dishes. You also can't go wrong with hummus, a mix of chickpeas, lemon juice, and garlic often served with pita bread or crackers. Or try substituting tofu for meat in some of your dishes.

Making the Most of Them: Dried beans may give you a slight nutritional edge, but not that much, so if you don't have time to soak and prepare beans, don't worry. You can still gain a great benefit from canned beans. They're often high in sodium, though, so you may want to drain and rinse them before using.

Other Eating Tips: We all know the one drawback to eating a lot of beans; let's just say it's why they're called the musical fruit. But you can ease that problem by soaking dried beans overnight and discarding the soaking water before preparing them. Personally, I'm convinced that the Mexican herb epazote can lessen flatulence. Some studies also suggest that adding ginger or savory to a bean dish can reduce gassiness. Why not add all three?

Food #2: Bulbs

I usually don't play favorites, but when it comes to foods, garlic tops my list of healers. Though a recent high-profile study called its cholesterol-lowering ability into question, it still has enough heart-protective benefits to rank high on my list. It has other great qualities as well, including immunity-boosting and antiseptic properties. Onions share many of the properties and healthful benefits of garlic, so they also deserve a mention here. And in my Farmacy, I grow a nice batch of ramps, members of the garlic/onion family that you won't find in many supermarkets (unless it's ramp festival time in West Virginia and Ohio). All of these plants contain the very important compound alliin, which converts to the super-medicinal allicin.

Nutrient Nuts and Bolts: When it comes to the heart, you can thank garlic's many sulfur compounds, including diallyl disulfide, which prevent clotting and allow for smooth blood flow. Of course, garlic also contains over a dozen immunity-boosting compounds that can fight off colds and other infections, maybe even more effectively than popular herbs like echinacea. Recent research has also shown that several compounds in garlic can prevent cellular changes within the body that lead to cancer.

Onions offer many of the same sulfur compounds as garlic, but they bring even more to the table with their high amounts of flavonoids, specifically quercetin. This flavonoid has been shown in studies to reduce platelet clumping and even prevent some forms of cancer. So far, there is no better food source of quercetin than onion skins.

How to Get More: The other advantage of garlic and onions is just how easy they are to incorporate into your menus. I add both to virtually all my soups and stews. And when it comes to salads, just about the only dressing you'll see me use is vinegar and oil mixed with fresh garlic and fresh diced onion, often with hot sauce or diced hot pepper. That mixture alone has hundreds of healthful compounds. Sometimes I even roast garlic and put it on toast for breakfast.

Making the Most of Them: Now I know what you're thinking: "But Dr. Duke, what about the smell?" Well, as much as it pains me to say it, studies have shown time and again that the more garlic stinks, the better it works. That's why I often use it raw in salads or even eat whole cloves of the stuff if I don't have anything social going on that day.

This isn't to say that you can't get benefits from cooked garlic; you can. But you lose 40 percent of the original potency after garlic is cooked for 10 minutes, and you lose much more after 20—but you never lose it all. So if you're making a soup or stew, it might be a good idea to wait until near the end of the cooking time to add garlic. Green tea, parsley, and coriander all have a unique ability to partially quell the smell, so you may want to consider brewing green tea and garlic together or adding parsley to a garlicky salad. Or if you have a new potential client or lover or relative coming over, eat some parsley or coriander and drink some green tea quick!

Other Eating Tips: If you're going for full effect and eating whole cloves of garlic, it's important that you nick the surface of a clove first; that is, don't swallow it intact. I thought that was the way to go until my garlicologist, Larry Lawson, PhD, told me the skin should be broken before garlic enters the GI tract to get its benefits. This ensures that the medicinal compounds of the bulb are released and will begin working more quickly in the body.

Now back to onions for a minute. In one of those funny quirks of nature, most of the helpful flavonoids, such as quercetin, are found in the skin of the onion. That's why I always put the skins in a mesh bag and steep it in soups and stews when I'm making them. Just remove the bag before serving.

Food #3: The Caffeinators

A few years ago, recommending caffeine-laden foods that are popular in our diet—chocolate, coffee, and tea—would have been quite controversial. Even now, many people are hesitant to call coffee and chocolate health foods because of the risk of overconsumption. But the sheer number of helpful compounds, called polyphenols, found in these three foods makes them a shoo-in for this list. After all, there's a reason worldwide consumption of caffeine is 120,000 tons per year.

All three of these foods are such potent disease fighters that there's a battle in the nutritional community about which one is most important, and for which disease. I can't pretend to be able to answer that question, and neither can most other people. That's why I felt it was best to group all three together as "the caffeinators."

Nutrient Nuts and Bolts: The active compounds in chocolate, coffee, and tea are known as polyphenols. Some polyphenols, such as theobromine and theophylline, are common to all three foods. And some, like theanine in tea and anandamide and phenylethylamine in chocolate, are unique to individual plants. But all the polyphenols are in essence "super" antioxidants. In fact, when it comes to fighting free radicals, these three foods beat out all others, including the berries you always hear so much about. Based on their antioxidant status alone, you'd expect them to be superstars when it comes to heart disease and cancer protection, and studies have certainly supported that idea.

There may be even more benefits from these polyphenols, though: Some of them seem to boost mood and alertness. With coffee, this may be a result of the caffeine content alone, but chocolate has unique polyphenols that boost levels of dopamine, a brain chemical that improves mood and allows you to experience pleasure, in your body.

How to Get More: For many of the healing foods on this list, the more, the merrier. However, too much caffeine from coffee and tea can have adverse effects on the body. That's why most experts recommend limiting your intake to 2 cups a day or less. And since chocolate is so calorie dense that eating too much can lead to obesity, your intake shouldn't exceed 3 ounces a day.

Making the Most of Them: One other note about chocolate—not just any type will do. Milk chocolate and white chocolate have large amounts of sugar—and not enough polyphenols to really do you any good. That's why you need to stick to dark chocolate. Choose a brand with 60 percent or higher cocoa content to get the greatest benefit.

There's also a bit of a debate about which type of tea is best—black, green, oolong, or white. Since all of them are brewed from the leaves of the *Camellia sinensis* plant, it would stand to reason that the benefits would be roughly the same for each type of tea. However, because green and white teas are less processed, they seem to exhibit more antioxidant activity. On the flip side, black tea has cholesterol-reducing theaflavins, which form when the polyphenols in the tea ferment and turn orange-red.

Other Eating Tips: When it comes to our favorite hot beverages, black vs. green tea isn't the only question up for debate; another common one is caffeinated vs. decaffeinated. While some effects, such as enhanced mood and alertness, come

Staying in the Family

It wasn't easy narrowing this list down to just 12 foods—which is why I cheated and put food families in several of the spots. But I did this for another good reason as well: Variety is a critical factor in any healthy diet. And while related foods share many of the same healing compounds, they each have distinct nutrients that are helpful in their own unique ways.

Take garlic and onions, for example. If I had to pick just one of these, I'd go with garlic for its high amount of immunity-boosting and heart-helping sulfur compounds. But onions bring something substantial to the table that garlic doesn't—the flavonoid quercetin.

I could do the same thing with many families of foods. Pecans, for example, offer serotonin and omega-3's, but not in the same high quantities as walnuts, so walnuts made the cut. But I can't emphasize enough the importance of striving for variety in your daily diet. I grazed on both walnuts and pecans today.

from caffeine, studies on both coffee and tea have shown that the benefits of the polyphenols still exist in the decaffeinated forms. What's more, tea seems to offer roughly the same benefits whether it's prepared hot or cold, although home-brewed versions are more potent than commercially prepared teas.

One more note on the caffeinators: You may have heard about a recent study reporting that drinking as few as 2 cups of coffee a day can increase the risk of miscarriage. So if you are pregnant or thinking about becoming pregnant, you may want to consider cutting out coffee or tea, or at least discussing the risks with your doctor.

Food #4: Celery

I have to admit that I originally included celery on this list for personal reasons, as it has helped me prevent gout flare-ups. However, this super stalk is good for a lot more, including lowering cholesterol and blood pressure and even fighting off cancer. Here's how celery does it.

Nutrient Nuts and Bolts: Celery fights gout with an anti-inflammatory compound called apigenin, which the stalks contain in abundance—in addition to more than a dozen other anti-inflammatories. Researchers think that another celery compound, 3-n-butyl phthalide, may be the reason that celery lowers blood pressure so dramatically.

Celery is also a great source of soluble fiber, which may explain why it helps lower cholesterol. And the acetylenics, phenolic acids, and coumarins in celery make it a potential cancer fighter, as well.

How to Get More: Celery isn't the most flavorful vegetable, but that works to its advantage when it comes to incorporating it into soups, stews, and salads. You can be sure it isn't going to overpower the other flavors. And unlike a lot of other foods, celery doesn't lose many of its healthful compounds during cooking. I like my celery raw with a bit of peanut butter, but it's also good with pesto, guacamole, and salsa.

Making the Most of It: If you really want to derive health benefits from celery, you have to eat a lot of it. If I'm without gout preventive medicines, I try to eat four stalks a day, and research shows that it takes four to five stalks to show a positive benefit on your blood pressure reading. But don't overdo it; celery has a lot of sodium, which can have the opposite effect on your blood pressure if you eat too much.

Other Eating Tips: Most people chop the leaves off their celery and eat just the stalk, but I recommend eating it leaves and all. Those leaves contain even more calcium, potassium, and vitamin C.

Food #5: Cinnamon

For some, seeing cinnamon on this list is almost as surprising as seeing chocolate. And when you consider that almost every food product with cinnamon in its name—rolls, candy, etc.—is unhealthful, I can understand the skepticism. But strip the spice down to its purest form, and it's one of the most potent antioxidants on the planet. It also has a unique impact on blood sugar that can be comparable to that of the diabetes medication rosiglitazone (Avandia)—but without the prescription drug's heart-damaging side effects.

Nutrient Nuts and Bolts: What makes cinnamon work so well for controlling blood sugar may be a flavonoid compound known as methylhydroxy chalcone polymer, or MHCP. This antioxidant seems to activate the insulin receptors inside your cells, making it easier for them to take in blood sugar for energy. Other studies indicate that cinnamon may help lower cholesterol, too.

How to Get More: Many of us mix cinnamon with sugar when we sprinkle it on toast, which can negate its healthful properties. Instead, try it in oatmeal or coffee, and if you must use a sweetener, make it a nonnutritive sweetener, such as stevia. Cinnamon has its culinary drawbacks, but medicinally, it actually offers some antidiabetic properties. You can also suck on a cinnamon quill like a piece of candy. I know several people who tried to quit smoking by doing this instead of lighting a cigarette whenever they had the urge to smoke.

Making the Most of It: As with anything else, huge doses of cinnamon can be toxic, so it's a good idea to stick to a teaspoon or less daily. And naturally, not everything that says "cinnamon" on the label is healthy! You'll want to steer clear of sugary desserts and cereals.

Other Eating Tips: Cinnamon's strong effect on your blood sugar is remarkable, but it could be a problem if you have diabetes and are taking any medication to help control it. If that's the case, you may want to speak with your doctor about the risks involved.

Food #6: Citrus Fruits

When people think about citrus fruit, most of them think of vitamin C. But that's just the tip of the nutritional iceberg when it comes to these delectable foods. So far, I have identified close to 200 anti-carcinogenic compounds in citrus fruits—or at least compounds that may synergistically cooperate in helping to prevent the onset of cancer.

Nutrient Nuts and Bolts: The vitamin C found in citrus fruits is nothing to shake a stick at—it's a powerful antioxidant, and the latest research suggests that it works more quickly than other antioxidants such as vitamin E and the carotenoids. What's more, citrus fruits all contain a rather unique type of fiber called pectin. Like other types of soluble fiber, pectin gloms onto cholesterol and ushers it out of the body. Pectin may also serve as a cancer fighter, slowing the growth of cancer cells by soothing inflammation.

While tomatoes get all the press for being loaded with the potent carotenoid lycopene, pink (and only pink) grapefruit is also a rich source of this compound. And grapefruit of any color, along with its cousins lemons and limes, contains limonene and limonin. These compounds may increase the activity of a protein that eliminates estradiol, a hormone that's been tied to breast cancer. Along with these other compounds, oranges have hesperidin, which studies show can raise good cholesterol, lower bad cholesterol, and reduce inflammation.

How to Get More: Citrus fruits (and their juices) are great on their own, but they are so healthful that I'd recommend looking for other ways to work them into meals as well. Put fresh orange or grapefruit slices on salads or stir-fry dishes. Squeeze fresh lemon juice into your herbal teas for even more benefits. Even spreading orange marmalade on your morning toast has more benefit than you might imagine, especially if it's a low-sugar marmalade.

Making the Most of Them: The reason marmalade and citrus juices with extra pulp are so good for you is that they contain the whole fruit—including bits and pieces of the rind and the white pith in the middle. Although they aren't as appetizing as other parts of the fruits, these are where a lot of the pectin, limonoids, hesperidin, and other potent compounds lie. The fruit may be delicious, but it contains mostly water and fructose (fruit sugar). So opt for extra pulp in citrus juice when possible, and when you eat the whole fruit, don't be afraid to leave a little bit of the white stuff around it.

Other Eating Tips: I'd be remiss here if I didn't get in an extra word about grapefruit. This uniquely American fruit actually began as a mutation, which is why it has some properties that are different from those of other citrus fruits. For example, grapefruit contains substances called furanocoumarins and naringins, and the unique combination of these compounds can actually prevent certain pharmaceutical medicines from breaking down in the body, so it magnifies their effects—sometimes to dangerous levels. Keeping this in mind, you'll want to ask your doctor if any medications you're taking can react adversely with grapefruit or juice.

I'd like to reiterate that even with citrus, you should focus on consuming a variety of fruits with lots of different shapes and colors. Each type confers its own special benefits.

Food #7: Ginger

Ginger's roots (pun intended) go all the way back to Traditional Chinese Medicine, and for many, it's still the go-to treatment for preventing motion sickness or morning sickness. (For motion sickness, it has consistently outperformed the drug Dramamine in clinical studies.) But as with many other foods, ginger's power goes beyond its unique stomach-soothing properties.

Ch-Ch-Ch-Chia for Omega-3's?

Do you remember Chia Pets, those little clay sculptures that grew green, grassy "hair" and that people often received as gag gifts? If so, you'll get a kick out of this nutritional news.

It turns out that chia seeds, which are members of the mint family, actually have more omega-3 fatty acids in them than the oft-praised flaxseed—and they're available at health food stores for about the same price. So if you're tired of the same old seeds, you may want to make the switch to chia.

Better yet, go with both on alternating days. Variety, variety, variety! We're adding chia to the Green Farmacy Garden this year.

Nutrient Nuts and Bolts: Ginger is chock-full of COX-2 inhibitors, powerful anti-inflammatory compounds that inhibit a particular pain-causing enzyme in the body. This may make it helpful for preventing some of the symptoms of osteoarthritis. And the more we learn about inflammation's role in other illnesses (including Alzheimer's disease and cancer), the greater the role the anti-inflammatory COX-2 inhibitors in ginger may play in disease prevention.

How to Get More: It doesn't take much ginger to derive its healing benefits (about an ounce a day will do it), so adding it to a stir-fry dish or using it in a meat marinade will usually give you enough to help. For more immediate results to relieve motion sickness, try eating ¼ teaspoon of raw ginger. Candied ginger or ginger syrup is easier to take, but there's all that added sugar.

Making the Most of It: One thing you may notice about ginger is that the root is kind of stubborn and tends to hold onto its flavor when you try to make it into a tea. That's why I recommend grating it very finely before adding it to boiling water. I'd also recommend adding lemon or honey (or stevia if you're weight conscious) to give the tea a bit more flavor.

Other Eating Tips: I use a ginger elixir, which is ginger in liquid form, and add several drops to my herbal teas to gain even more benefits. Dried ginger powders and capsules that retain most of the benefits of fresh ginger are also available. And yes, ginger ale is another way to enjoy this health food—but check the ingredients. Many commercially produced ginger ales actually contain no ginger.

Food #8: Mints

To most people, "mint" means spearmint, peppermint, and fresh flavors that are associated with mouthwash or gum. Actually, there are hundreds of plants in the mint family—I have over 70 of them in my garden alone. Many of them are herbs that you'd recognize from your spice cabinet, such as basil, rosemary, thyme, oregano, lavender, sage, and lemon balm.

All these spices are known for the great flavor they impart to foods, but they can do much more for your health. Perhaps the most exciting breakthrough for the mint family is in the field of Alzheimer's research.

Nutrient Nuts and Bolts: Members of the mint family, with their pleasant taste and aroma, are traditional stomach soothers, often in tea form. Many of them also contain central nervous system stimulants, which work rather like caffeine, so they are nice alternatives to traditional coffee or tea. These are the "uppers," which include peppermint and spearmint. Some mints, such as lemon balm and lavender, are actually "downers," with sedative effects. They're also loaded with healthy-heart antioxidant compounds.

Perhaps the most exciting thing about the mint family is that most of its members contain at least a half dozen compounds that prevent the breakdown of acetylcholine. Acetylcholine is the neurotransmitter that carries messages from one synapse to another in your brain. When you're deficient in this substance, the messages have a harder time getting through. Keeping those connections strong may help us stay mentally sharp as we grow older, and adding more of the mint family to your diet just may be one of the keys to doing that.

How to Get More: The mind is certainly not something to trifle with, which is why I make mint tea part of my everyday routine. By including a variety of mints (I often use rosemary, peppermint, and thyme), you can create an infusion with more than a dozen acetylcholine-preserving compounds.

Making the Most of Them: People often ask me about my recipe for mint tea, and I have to admit that I don't really have one. I generally take a pinch of this and a pinch of that, pour boiling water over it, and let it steep for 10 to 20 minutes before drinking it. Over time, you'll find that you like some flavors more than others, in which case you can add more of the mints you enjoy and less of the ones you don't. I have been known to make mint teas (and liqueurs) with a mixture of all the dozens of good-tasting mints in my garden.

Other Eating Tips: Another option for getting the benefits of fresh mint is to chop the leaves and add them to salads. And, of course, many members of the mint family are ideal seasonings for a variety of healthful dishes. You can also put them into a muslin bag and steep them in your bath, since most of the acetylcholine-sparing compounds are transdermal, meaning they will go through the skin.

Food #9: Peppers

The pepper, or capsicum, genus includes a wide range of interesting fruits, from the spiciest hot peppers to the sweetest bells. And though these plants are related, they have very different healing properties. Chile peppers may help with weight loss, stomach protection, cold treatment, and arthritis pain prevention. Sweet peppers are antioxidant superstars, so they can help ward off heart disease and cancer. Both, however, are great for your health, and I recommend making them part of your daily diet.

Nutrient Nuts and Bolts: Many of the healing properties of hot chile peppers come from the compound capsaicin, which is what gives the peppers their heat. Capsaicin interferes with the transmission of pain, so it can be helpful in managing arthritis. And when you bite into a pepper, capsaicin increases your internal pain-killers (endorphins), improves your circulation, and even helps you lose weight. That spicy heat also makes chile peppers powerful decongestants that can help you

Make It a Baker's Dozen?

If your favorite health food didn't make my Duke's Dozen, don't despair. As you can imagine, narrowing any list of healthy foods down to just 12 was not an easy job, and I had to make difficult decisions based on the potency of the compounds in certain foods vs. others. In the end, the 12 listed here rose to the top.

However, a lot of other great foods were no less worthy. If my brother were to create a similar list, he would probably include cherries, as they have done wonders for his gout. (In my case, cherries did nothing, but celery did the trick—so celery made the cut.) You could make an equally compelling case for berries, flaxseed, cold-water fish, and a number of other foods. In the end, my contention remains the same: Duke's Dozen is a great place to start, but make sure your diet is built around a wide variety of healthful foods.

get fluids out during the course of a cold by making your eyes water, your nose run, and the mucus in your lungs loosen.

Bell peppers also have capsaicin but in much lower concentrations (although if you grow them close to the chiles in your garden, your bells may develop a bit of heat near the seeds). Their strength lies elsewhere—in their high levels of antioxidants. Green peppers provide a healthy dose of vitamin C, but for even more antioxidant potential, go with reds. A half cup of chopped red pepper provides 142 milligrams of vitamin C, which is 236 percent of the recommended daily intake. One pepper also has about half the daily value for beta-carotene, along with other healthy-heart antioxidants like beta-cryptoxanthin and lycopene.

How to Get More: Few of us eat enough peppers to enjoy the full effects of their healing properties, but they're easy to incorporate into all kinds of dishes. Hot peppers are a perfect complement to any spicy Asian or Mexican recipe, and bell peppers are great in soups, salads, stir-fries, fajitas, and pasta dishes. You can also roast peppers to release their sweet, smoky flavor. Stuffed bell peppers are good, but at times I prefer chiles rellenos, or stuffed hot peppers.

Making the Most of Them: Vitamin C is most potent in raw peppers, but their beta-carotene is better released when they're heated. What to do? A happy medium is to sauté peppers lightly so they still have a little crunch when you eat them. Beta-carotene and other carotenoids need a little fat to be absorbed, so serve them in a salad with olive or peanut oil or eat fresh peppers with a dash of avocado dip.

Other Eating Tips: Hot peppers may be good for your health, but they can be tough on your skin and eyes. If you're working with anything hotter than a jalapeño, wear plastic gloves when cutting it. Also, use soap afterward to make sure to get the juice off your hands. And if you're planning on grinding the peppers, goggles and a dust mask are not out of line.

If you do get burned by capsaicin, my good friend Art Tucker, PhD, senior author of *The Big Book of Herbs,* recommends chlorine bleach *or* ammonia (not both) for the skin, and vodka (capsaicin is alcohol soluble) or dairy products for mouth irritation. The casein in dairy products apparently breaks the bond of the capsaicin with the pain receptors in the mouth.

Also, when it comes to eating chiles, hotter is not necessarily better, so don't feel that you have to force down the hottest pepper. A jalapeño is pretty close to a habanero when it comes to beneficial healing properties.

Food #10: Pomegranates

Most people think the "forbidden fruit" in the Garden of Eden was an apple, but I have it on good authority that it was a pomegranate. The apple was not native to that part of the world, but the pomegranate was. And *pomegranate* literally means "many-seeded apple."

The pomegranate certainly is not forbidden when it comes to your health. It has an abundance of compounds that can help your body fight off cancer, heart disease, and menopause symptoms, among other conditions. Pomegranates have been used for centuries in the Middle East, Iran, and India as a folk remedy.

Nutrient Nuts and Bolts: Like many other fruits and vegetables, pomegranates are rich in antioxidants. But what sets this fruit apart is that it contains polyphenols, some of the same "super" class of antioxidants found in coffee, tea, and chocolate. Pomegranates have been shown to be cholesterol and heart disease fighters in many studies.

As powerful as it is, however, that antioxidant potential pales in comparison to the phytoestrogens in a pomegranate. Just half a fruit may contain the estrogenic equivalent of a daily dose of hormone replacement therapy (HRT), a common treatment for women struggling with menopause symptoms. As a matter of fact, the pomegranate contains several human-identical hormones, which have become the subject of much controversy these days. Wyeth Pharmaceuticals and the FDA are trying to slow the burgeoning interest in two of these hormones, called alpha and beta estradiol. But pomegranates have many other equally or less potent phytoestrogens. These compounds also make the fruit a potential cancer fighter.

What's more, it may also help with some of the conditions that together constitute metabolic syndrome, including diabetes and obesity. There's even a pomegranate diet that makes sense to me. My friends Robert Newman, PhD, and Ephraim

Lansky, MD, in their book *Pomegranate—The Most Medicinal Fruit,* attribute pomegranate's anti-obesity activity to punicic acid, another of the many compounds in the fruit. Of all the super-fruits out there, this one excels.

How to Get More: A lot of people have a hard time tearing open a fresh pomegranate without making a mess of themselves and the kitchen. If you want a more convenient option, choose pomegranate juice, available from a number of companies, including Pom Wonderful (www.pomwonderful.com). In fact, the juice may be even more healthful than the fruit, since manufacturers juice the entire fruit, including the seeds and part of the husk, which contains most of the polyphenols.

Making the Most of Them: Although pomegranates may be as potent as HRT, they're by no means a replacement for it. HRT is standardized, so you know exactly how much you are getting of specific hormones, but there's no such guarantee with pomegranates. If you're already taking HRT, you may want to ask your doctor if there's any problem with eating this fruit. (I suspect that you don't want to do both.) A single fruit or a glass of juice should be fine, but you don't want to overdo it, because these fruits are possibly the most powerful dietary sources of estrogenic compounds.

Other Eating Tips: You've probably noticed a growing number of pomegranate supplements, including capsules from more mainstream companies like Pom Wonderful. As with most supplements, these vary in quality and may deliver a powerful dose of estrogenic compounds. You may want to speak with your doctor before adding this supplement to your regimen.

Food #11: Turmeric

Turmeric is an essential ingredient in many of the different spice mixes that go under the generic name "curry." It's also what goes into commercial brands of mustard these days to make them yellow.

Turmeric's history as a healer is thousands of years old. It is one of the staples of Ayurvedic medicine, the traditional healing art of India. Today, I know a lot of people who swear by turmeric as the answer for their arthritis pain. Although the evidence is not yet definitive, it may also help prevent cancer and possibly even Alzheimer's disease.

Nutrient Nuts and Bolts: There's a reason turmeric has been used medicinally for so long and by so many people. Of all the plants I have studied, it ranks with garlic, ginger, and pomegranate as offering some of the strongest health benefits. I know a lot of people who find turmeric a better treatment for their osteoarthritis than the drug celecoxib (Celebrex). This is due to the high concentration of a COX-2 inhibitor called curcumin in the spice.

What's also interesting about turmeric is that, like the mint family, it has compounds that prevent the breakdown of acetylcholine. This makes a lot of curry fans say that they may be preventing mental decline, and this contention has certainly held true in epidemiological studies of the Indian population. And since COX-2 inhibitors are anti-inflammatory compounds, turmeric has also shown promise in colon cancer prevention.

How to Get More: Turmeric in the form of curry is a staple in Indian cooking, but if that's not your regular cuisine, you're probably not getting much of the spice in your diet. It has a pungent, somewhat bitter taste that takes some getting used to, but it's a unique flavor that many people grow to love.

A good way to start incorporating turmeric into dishes is to use it to spice up chicken, turkey, rice, vegetables, soups, or salad dressings. You can also buy curry paste and work it into your stir-fries. Or pick up an Indian cookbook; it will give you loads of turmeric dishes and open a new world of possibilities.

Making the Most of it: One way you'll definitely want to try using turmeric is to sprinkle it on cruciferous vegetables like cauliflower, broccoli, Brussels sprouts, or kale. In one study, scientists discovered that the combination of the phenethyl isothiocyanates in cruciferous vegetables and the curcumin in turmeric seems to prevent the growth of prostate cancer tumors in lab animals. Plus, the combination is delicious!

Other Eating Tips: Whatever dish you decide to make with turmeric, be sure you grind plenty of black pepper on top. For some reason, the pepper seems to enhance the absorption of the curcumin significantly.

Food #12: Walnuts

Since several of my Duke's Dozen are food families rather than individual foods, you might think I'd go with just nuts in this spot. Considering the fiber, healthy monounsaturated fats, and protein—especially arginine—found in most nuts, they wouldn't be a bad choice. Walnuts, however, have enough unique properties to let them stand above the rest of the pack, in my opinion. Butternuts, hickory nuts, and pecans belong to the same family.

Nutrient Nuts and Bolts: Have you ever noticed that a walnut half looks a lot like the human brain? I find this to be a strange coincidence since few foods are better for your brain than walnuts. They're a great source of serotonin, a neurotransmitter that the body also manufactures on its own. Serotonin has the secondary advantage of curbing appetite, which I'll get into in greater detail below. Additionally, few plant sources are higher in omega-3 fatty acids than walnuts.

By the way, although omega-3's get a lot of good press for preventing heart disease and reducing inflammation, they're also a known antidepressant. I suggest walnut oil with saffron to fight seasonal affective disorder.

How to Get More: I enjoy walnuts most as a snack. I keep them around my kitchen along with dried fruits and other nuts. (It sure beats crackers and cookies, if health is your objective!) Walnuts are also good mixed into a salad, as a topping for cereal, or sprinkled over pasta dishes or vegetables. And walnut halves go wonderfully well with that other health food, chocolate (as well as with my health nemeses, ice cream and maraschino cherries).

Making the Most of Them: Although this is anecdotal, I know some people who swear by walnuts as an appetite suppressant; it's probably because of the serotonin, which signals the brain that you're full. They claim that eating just three walnut halves before lunch makes them eat much less. Another way to enjoy the health benefits of walnuts is to use walnut oil for cooking or salad dressings.

Other Eating Tips: As healthful as they are, walnuts are still nuts, so they're extremely fat and calorie dense. That means you don't want to go overboard with them. Still, if you stick to just a handful at a time between meals, or just sprinkle a few chopped walnuts onto your dishes, you should be just fine.

CHAPTER 4

Making the Most of What You Eat

How to "Super-Size" the Nutrients in Your Diet

ONCE YOU'RE COMMITTED to adding more healthful foods to your diet, you'll want to get the maximum amount of nutrients possible from each food. That only makes good sense. But you may be surprised to learn that many of our basic assumptions about how to do that are false.

For example, many people assume that raw vegetables offer the most health benefits. After all, cooking only breaks down those helpful nutrients, right? While it's true that eating foods raw is optimal in many cases, especially if you're after enzymes, there are a number of foods that are actually better for you when cooked. What's more, some foods need to be combined with a little fat to give you better absorption.

Similarly, not all raw fruits and vegetables are created equal. In fact, I'll really go out on a limb here and say that in some instances, nonorganic foods may actually trump organic ones—at least medicinally. Ditto for dried, canned, or frozen vs. fresh. In each case, some phytonutrients are increased and others diminished.

Not All Foods Are Created Equal

Modern agriculture and transportation are amazing things. Never has such an abundance of fruits and vegetables been available right at our fingertips whenever we want them. But while this is undoubtedly a positive development, it does have its downside. The more that scientists and farmers engineer and breed our foods to be sweeter, juicier, bigger, and better looking, the less nutrient dense they often become.

Several researchers have looked into this trend, and the evidence seems pretty clear. One Canadian study found that potatoes have lost 100 percent of their vitamin A, 57 percent of their vitamin C and iron, and 28 percent of their calcium over the past 50 years. Several other fruits and vegetables, including oranges and broccoli, showed similar drops. In the United States, Donald Davis, PhD, a biochemist at the University of Texas, reported similar findings. He says that in the past 50 years, 6 of 13 major nutrients showed significant declines—calcium, iron, phosphorus, protein, riboflavin, and vitamin C. No wonder the government keeps increasing the recommended daily intake of fruits and veggies.

When you think about it, none of this should come as a surprise. Most of the good taste of produce often comes from more fructose (sugar) and more water. That's why fruits and vegetables that are smaller and not as tasty may sometimes be better for you. Another problem with modern foods is how far they often have to travel. Pick up any produce during the winter months (and sometimes even in summer), and there's a good chance that it came from some exotic, faraway destination such as Argentina, Australia, Chile, or China.

This is a problem, because many of the healing compounds in foods are volatile chemicals, which means they quickly lose their potency. So the fresher the food, the more volatile compounds it's going to retain. A freshly picked pomegranate, for example, has a lot more going for it than one that's been on a truck for several days. To test this theory, smell some freshly picked mint, then let it sit for a couple of days and smell it again. Not only will the aroma's strength have diminished, but it will have a different quality.

Think Globally, Eat Locally

Luckily, the dual problems of overbreeding and long journeys can be solved in the same way: by buying as much produce as you can locally. This is why the proliferation of farmers' markets in the past decade has been such a great thing for our health and well-being. We're also beginning to see local produce show up in a growing number of supermarkets.

The fruits and vegetables found in farmers' markets are often not as overbred as their mass-produced supermarket counterparts, so they're likely to retain more of their healthful nutrients. They also go on sale shortly after they're picked, which is the best way to ensure the highest nutrient dose. You also get a tomato that tastes the way a tomato is supposed to, not a mass-produced Frankenstein bred to travel better rather than taste better.

Of course, there's one way to get even fresher produce than you can purchase locally, and that's to grow it yourself. Granted, not everyone has a 6-acre farm like I do. But you'll be amazed by how many healthful fruits and vegetables you can grow in a modest yard or a few containers. Even growing a small herb garden indoors can contribute to getting significantly more nutrients in your diet!

The Organic Argument

Farmers' markets also feature a variety of organic foods, which most people perceive as being a more healthful choice. I can certainly agree that organics are worth buying and eating simply to avoid harmful pesticides, which may cause cancer in humans. But I have a somewhat unorthodox viewpoint on organic foods. At the risk of angering organic supporters, let me try to explain.

All plants are actually made up of two kinds of compounds—primary metabolites, which are normal nutrients, and secondary metabolites, which are often the ones we use as medicinal compounds. Organic plants as a whole receive more care when they're growing, so they produce more primary metabolites, making them a healthful choice—especially since they contain no synthetic and possibly carcinogenic pesticides! I emphasize that last point because there's little question in my mind that synthetic pesticides are causing cancers, and you should avoid them at all costs.

Pesticide-free, however, is a relative term. My farm has not been sprayed in 35 years, but I've seen the characteristic herbicide curl of my grape leaves when neighbors sprayed on a windy day. The leaves contort like gnarled arthritic hands.

However, as someone interested in the medicinal properties of plants, I think it's worth noting that a plant that is less "pampered" generally produces more secondary metabolites. I'll even generalize that almost any kind of stress in a plant increases levels of secondary phytochemicals (read *medicinals*) at the expense of primary metabolites (read *foods*). Fungal diseases are one type of stress on plants. If a soybean plant gets a fungus, its production of estrogenic isoflavones may go up a hundredfold. The same holds true for a fruit that gets bitten by a bug. Drought also increases the proportion of secondary metabolites, as does injuring a plant.

Now I'm not advocating that you eat fungus-infested soybeans or bruise your apples before you eat them—and I'm not trying to disparage organics. I just thought you might be interested in knowing that organic foods don't necessarily have more "medicine" in them than nonorganic ones. In fact, in many cases, the opposite is true.

Still, I believe the threats posed by pesticides are real, and for that reason, it's probably a good idea to choose organics in place of the most pesticide-heavy fruits and vegetables. For help with this, see the sidebar on page 34.

The Great Debate: Fresh, Frozen, or Canned?

The facts in another nutrition debate that may defy conventional wisdom have to do with fresh, frozen, and canned fruits and vegetables. Most people assume that fresher is better—and if you can get produce locally or pick it from your own garden, that is usually true.

If the "fresh" produce is off-season, though, and has taken several days or even weeks to get to your supermarket, then believe it or not, you're probably going to get a lot more nutrients from the frozen variety. Those products are usually frozen

The Most Pesticide-Heavy Foods

The biggest advantage of organic foods is the absence of potentially harmful pesticides. The biggest drawback? Most people say it's the price.

If you can't decide whether to go organic, an approach many experts advocate is to replace some of the most pesticide-heavy foods with organic options. In 2005, the Environmental Working Group compiled a guide to the amount of pesticides in foods to help you do just that. Here are some of their findings.

Most-Contaminated Fruits

Fruit	Samples That Tested Positive for Pesticides (%)
Nectarines	97.3
Peaches	96.6
Apples	93.6
Strawberries	92.3
Cherries	91.4

Most-Contaminated Vegetables

Vegetable	Samples That Tested Positive for Pesticides (%)
Celery	94.1
Cauliflower	84.6
Carrots	81.7
Bell peppers	81.5
Potatoes	81.0

Least-Contaminated Fruits

Fruit	Samples That Tested Positive for Pesticides (%)
Avocados	1.4
Mangos	7.1
Pineapple	7.7
Kiwifruit	15.3
Papayas	23.5

Least-Contaminated Vegetables

Vegetable	Samples That Tested Positive for Pesticides (%)
Onions	0.7
Frozen sweet corn	3.8
Asparagus	6.7
Frozen sweet peas	22.9
Broccoli	28.1

within a few hours of being picked, which means they retain a lot of nutrients and flavor. Studies have shown that frozen foods retain almost all their vitamin C but lose some vitamin B_6 and E.

Canned foods also fare a lot better than most people realize. Recent studies have shown that canned fruits and vegetables retain most of their vitamin C, B vitamins, potassium, and carotenoids.

As I'll discuss below, some nutrients from the carotenoid family, such as beta-carotene and lycopene, are better absorbed in the presence of fats. Others may actually need some heat to release them, which is why foods like carrots and peppers are often better cooked. The same applies to the canned versions of these foods. Canned pumpkin, for example, contains more carotenoids than fresh pumpkin, and canned tomato sauces, pastes, and juices, and even ketchup, have more lycopene than fresh tomatoes. Of course, this is also due to the fact that a lot of the water has been removed in the transition from fresh to canned or bottled, which makes the carotenoids more concentrated.

Creative Cooking

Whether they're fresh, frozen, or canned, in most cases we still cook our foods before we eat them, and cooking methods offer yet another way to maximize their nutritive value. Just as I recommend a great variety of fruits, veggies, nuts, and herbal teas, I also recommend variety in the way you prepare them—some raw, some stir-fried, some stewed or made into soups—but too late in my redneck life have I come to discourage deep frying and long, hard boiling.

Of course, the preparation technique that maximizes a food's nutrients varies greatly from food to food and nutrient to nutrient. To use one of my favorites as an example, garlic is most potent raw, but it needs to be cut up (or at least nicked or chewed) to release its medicine. As I've mentioned before, cooked garlic retains some medicinal potential, but it's significantly reduced: Cook it for 10 minutes, and it loses 40 percent of its medicinal properties; after 20 minutes, it loses much more.

The contradiction between vitamin C and vitamin A is another interesting case. Vitamin C is best fresh, and it begins to break down in the presence of heat. But the carotenoids that provide us with our vitamin A actually need a bit of heat to release them from the fibers of most foods. Since a lot of foods contain both vitamin C and carotenoids, you need to walk a fine line to derive the benefits of both. That's why you'll find me nibbling raw carrots and celery between meals but having them cooked at mealtime. I also eat raw greens in my salads and cooked greens in my soups.

Undercook it. Before we proceed, I have to admit a weakness here: I have an unfortunate tendency (inherited from my Southern ancestors) to boil the heck out of a lot of my dishes. And when it comes to getting the most nutrients out of foods, this is one of the worst things you can do. But here's the good news: Many of the nutrients leach into the "pot-liquor," as my mother called it, so you can consume that, too. If you discard the cooking liquid, however, even the water in which you boiled your asparagus or corn on the cob, you also discard many of the nutrients.

If anything, you're probably better off undercooking. Since many foods contain some nutrients that are better raw and others that are better cooked, this is a good way to make sure you get a little of both. In fact, many nutrients need only a little heat to set them free and make them ready for digestion. Too much heat destroys them.

Serve up some soup. While too much heat can wipe out a lot of healthful nutrients, cooking them in water can suck them up and out. Unless you keep and drink that water, there's no way to get the nutrients back.

That's why soups and stews are such good choices—they contain the vegetables *and* the broth! By eating both, you avoid losing much of anything in the cooking process.

Leave the peels on. It's funny how the parts of plants that we don't eat are often some of the most healthful parts. The peels of apples and onions are rich in the flavonoid quercetin. Eggplant skins have anthocyanins. Citrus peels are full of limonoids.

When Mrs. Duke makes a stew, she not only peels the potatoes, she also peels the carrots, but I've solved this dilemma when I prepare meals simply by leaving the skins on a lot of foods that others would peel. I always cook eggplants and potatoes this way. I also try to leave oranges and grapefruits a little "dirtier" (with more of the white pith on them) when I eat them. And let's face it—there's really no reason to ever peel an apple (especially if it's organic). The peel is delicious and contains proportionally many more of the fruit's medicinal phytochemicals.

Put the peels in the pot. If you're hesitant to eat the skins of certain foods—onions and carrots, for example—you can still derive benefits by adding the shavings to soups and stews. Carrot peels can go directly in, but put onion skins into a mesh bag so they don't end up floating around in the broth. They'll add both flavor and flavonoids.

Add some pepper. Turmeric, one of the super foods of India, has an interesting quirk. It turns out that adding freshly ground black pepper to it increases the absorption of its active ingredient, curcumin, several-fold. So the next time you're having curry, don't hold the pepper! Apparently, cooking turmeric in milk, as many Indians do, also enhances the bioavailability of the curcumin, so cream of curried celery soup comes to mind, using curry, black pepper, and milk (or cream if you're not worried about the fat content).

Use oil. As I mentioned earlier, carotenoids need help with absorption, and a little fat does the trick. As you might imagine, this is pretty easy to accomplish with most dishes. It can be as simple as adding some olive oil to a salad or stir-fry or even having fresh vegetables with dip. And of course, pizza parlors appropriately brag about their "oils" (read *grease*) enhancing the uptake of the lycopene in the tomato sauce.

PART II

Food Remedies That Work

Altitude Sickness

I ONCE BECAME ILL WITH *SOROCHE* during a trip to Peru. It sounds like an exotic disease, but it's actually the name the Andean people have for altitude sickness. After ascending to Machu Picchu, the famous high-altitude city ruins in Peru, I found myself short of breath, dizzy, and weak. When I returned a few months later, I was determined to avoid altitude sickness with the help of a remedy that's been used by Peruvian mountain hikers for thousands of years—the coca leaf. And it worked!

My companions and I munched on a few leaves before our excursion, and our bodies were then able to withstand the disabling effects of the high altitude. Not only that, we felt energized (one of my companions told me I tackled those climbs like a mountain goat). I celebrated my 65th birthday hugging the rock face of sister peak Huainu Picchu and singing "Rock of Ages."

The coca plant is commonly found in Peru and Bolivia, where the Andeans use it to brew tea. Often, though, you see Andean peasants whose jaws appear to be swollen. They've actually got a big chaw of coca—often mixed with plant ashes to facilitate the extraction of alkaloids—stuffed in there.

Coca is also the source of cocaine, so it's out of legal reach here in the States. This doesn't mean that the streets of Peru are a narcotic free-for-all. There's very little cocaine in coca tea—just enough to act as a stimulant, to about the same degree as coffee. Of course, I would never recommend trying to import the leaves to the United States, but if you're planning to visit a country where coca is legal, try sipping some coca leaf tea before any high-altitude adventure. Or take a chew. Or do both. If your climbing expeditions are more domestic, don't despair. Fortunately, other remedies are plentiful in the United States.

Into Thin Air

As we all know, gravitational forces bring even the mightiest to their knees. It's this force that keeps air molecules close to the Earth's surface. The farther you are from Earth, the less dense the air is, and the more likely you are to experience altitude sickness. At high elevations, your body struggles to adapt to decreased levels of oxygen. Fluid leaks into the tissues and begins to build up in the lungs and brain, and the body begins to dehydrate. Most people can climb to elevations of 8,000 feet above sea level without any ill effects. Higher elevations, however, can cause even the fittest bodies to experience something akin to a terrible hangover: headaches, dizziness, nausea, and vomiting.

The best thing you can do to prevent altitude sickness is ascend at a sensible rate to give your body a chance to adapt to the changing atmospheric pressure. According to experts at Apex, a team of high-altitude medical researchers, limiting your ascents to 300 feet a day should keep altitude sickness at bay.

Healing Foods for Altitude Sickness

There are other steps you can take to alleviate symptoms or even avoid falling ill at high altitudes. Here are my favorites.

★★★**Clove** Clove oil is extremely rich in eugenol, a compound that thins the blood to allow for more efficient distribution of nutrients in the body. For this reason, I've created a recipe appropriately called Altitude Adjustment Tea that includes clove oil as a key ingredient. I also mix in some of these other high-eugenol herbs that I usually have on hand: allspice, bayrum leaf, galangal, carrot seed, shrubby cinnamon, bay leaf, and marjoram. Here's my personal concoction: Steep cloves in very hot but not boiling water (boiling dissipates too much of the eugenol). Add allspice, bay leaf, cinnamon, and marjoram to taste. For an added boost of protection (and flavor), mix in these mints, as available, which contain thymol, another compound that thins the blood: balm, basil (also rich in eugenol), dittany, savory, and thyme.

★★★**Garlic** The scientific community has firmly established that garlic compounds afford the heart many protective benefits. A recent study at the University of Alabama at Birmingham found that garlic helps the blood produce hydrogen sulfide, which allows the blood vessels to relax. It also contains more than a dozen blood-thinning compounds. The ability to keep the vessels relaxed and the blood fluid is a valuable asset for bodies that are exposed to high altitudes. Finally, garlic clears the lungs and bronchial passages. Those are just some of the reasons that garlic is one of my preferred remedies for altitude sickness.

FOODS TO WATCH

I would recommend avoiding foods that contribute to inflammation. Some of the worst offenders are refined foods, which contain high amounts of added fat, sugar, salt, additives, and preservatives. Snack foods, in particular, are likely to contain large amounts of pro-inflammatory trans-fatty acids, omega-6 fatty acids, and high-fructose corn syrup, which also is a major player in our nation's obesity epidemic.

Other plants with blood-thinning properties include tomatoes, dill, fennel, onions, hot peppers, soybeans, celery, carrots, and parsley. All of these ingredients are ideal for what I call my Anti-Aggregant soup. Just cook as many of these as you have available in a big pot of water. One caution though: Be sure to cook the vegetables thoroughly, as raw veggies will challenge the intestinal fortitude of any mountain climber!

★★★**Thyme** When I was still with the government, they made me take a pharmaceutical diuretic, acetazolamide (Diamox), and they would have pronounced me insane if I'd said that I'd rather take oil of thyme, as Japanese mountain climbers do. Thyme can contain at least a dozen blood thinners and nine diuretics. I suspect many of the aromatic mints at Machu Picchu contain even more of these phytochemcials that are useful in treating *soroche,* but thyme works well.

★★★**Water** One of the most important defenses against altitude sickness is hydration. As your body takes in larger volumes of dry air, it loses fluids. The blood thickens and dehydration sets in, affecting the distribution of nutrients and oxygen. Replacing fluids may lessen the severity of altitude sickness or even prevent it altogether. Researchers from Spain, studying the effects of fluid intake on mountaineers staying at high altitudes, found that aggressive hydration had a protective effect against acute altitude sickness. So drink plenty of liquids before and during your climb, even if you don't feel thirsty. Aim for at least 3 to 4 quarts of water a day. You'll know you're properly hydrated when your urine is clear.

★★**High-carbohydrate foods** As triathletes, cross-country skiers, and other endurance athletes know, foods high in carbohydrates help to fuel the muscles. The body uses carbohydrates to create a reserve of glycogen, an acid your muscles need for energy. But carbohydrates have an added benefit at high altitudes: They process oxygen efficiently. Carbohydrates require less oxygen to metabolize than proteins and fats, an important distinction when oxygen is at a premium. Many mountaineers find that small meals of high-carb, low-fat foods prior to and during the first 3 or 4 days of an expedition work best to combat altitude sickness.

★★**Reishi** I rarely push mushrooms because I know so little about them, but this one I have seen growing on the wood steps in my Green Farmacy Garden in Maryland and in the ReNuPeRu Garden in Peru. It's fairly easy to recognize and not very likely to be confused with poisonous mushrooms. Almost all my Amazonian tours start out in the lowlands below Iquitos, Peru. The steps between the garden and the Canopy Walkway at the Explonapo Camp are constantly being "consumed" by the reishi. As my shaman puts it, singing his eerie *jicaro* (chant) of the mushroom, it is sucking the last power from the fallen tree of which these steps are constructed. He's right. The mushroom that he calls generically *cayampa* (or *cajampa*) is taking its nutrients from the dead tree. But apparently *cayampa mau* have the power to control *soroche*. Nowhere have I heard Andean Indians profess to have used reishi for *soroche,* but their Himalayan counterparts use reishi much as the Andeans use their coca, as an energizer, especially at high altitudes. I'd certainly give it a try if I couldn't get coca, or maybe even with coca.

From the Herbal Medicine Chest

Some studies show that ginkgo increases blood flow through the body, particularly the brain. This may be why mountain climbers have found that it helps stave off the effects of altitude sickness. In one study, researchers transported participants from sea level in northern Chile to an elevation of over 12,000 feet. A third of them received 80 milligrams of ginkgo, another third were given an altitude sickness medication, and the rest took a placebo 24 hours before their ascent and during their 3-day stay. The group that received ginkgo had significantly fewer incidents of severe altitude sickness than did the other two groups. When trying this herb, limit yourself to 60 to 240 milligrams of standardized extract a day. Any more than that could result in diarrhea, irritability, and restlessness.

Angina

ANGINA, TECHNICALLY CALLED ANGINA PECTORIS, is a symptom of heart disease that causes moderate to severe chest pain. It's really a warning sign that blood is having a hard time getting to your heart, probably because of a buildup of plaque in the arteries that feed it. There are two main forms: stable angina, in which the pain strikes during some type of physical exertion, whether you're jogging or simply weeding your garden, and unstable angina, when the pain occurs even while you're resting. Angina is serious; you need to be under a doctor's care. You should also consider it a warning sign that a heart attack may be skulking right around the corner. Your angina may require medication, including nitroglycerin to open blood vessels during the painful attacks and cholesterol- and blood pressure–reducing drugs. But you can also find some benefit from certain foods, including the following.

Healing Foods for Angina

★★★**Fish** Fish, especially cold–water marine fish, have so many heart-healthy benefits that I consider them part of my farmacopia. For angina, I recommend at least two fishy meals a week because they're a great source of coenzyme Q10 (CoQ10). This chemical is an important ingredient in the recipe that cells need to make energy. The majority of CoQ10 in your body lies in your heart, where it's a powerful antioxidant and energy enhancer. The typical American diet, however, which is high in polyunsaturated fats, can lead to low CoQ10 levels. Studies find that supplementing with this enzyme can decrease blood clots and the thickness, or viscosity, of blood, which helps reduce angina attacks. In one study of 73 people with serious heart disease, those who took 120 milligrams a day had only 9 angina attacks compared with 28 in those who took a placebo. I think it's best to get your nutrients from food, however—hence the fish recommendation.

I also suggest that you make one of your fish meals codfish. Cheap and readily available, it's also the best source, after beef steak and ground beef (neither of which I can bring myself to recommend on a regular basis for heart health), of the amino acid L-carnitine. Like CoQ10, carnitine is important for helping cells—particularly heart cells—produce energy. Studies evaluating its use in people with angina find it increases their ability to exercise without an angina attack (a sign of improved blood flow to the heart) and improves other indications of heart function.

★★**Avocados** Not only are avocados high in heart-healthy monounsaturated fats, they're also high in the amino acid L-arginine. This compound enhances the action of nitric oxide, a molecule that enables blood vessels to dilate. When researchers asked 36 patients with angina to eat either of two energy bars high in arginine a day or two placebo bars, they found that those who ate the arginine bars were able to exercise on a treadmill 20 percent longer without an angina attack than those who ate the placebo bars. Other studies found that people improved their physical function by a third after supplementing with arginine. These improvements, researchers report, are even better than those found in studies of patients taking angina medications such as ranolazine (Ranexa) and diltiazem (Tiazac).

FOODS TO WATCH

The caffeine in coffee stimulates your heart and increases your heart rate, leading to more blood pumping through your body. That, in turn, can overwhelm partially clogged arteries, leading to an angina attack. Studies find that more than five cups a day is the danger point, increasing your risk of unstable angina or even a heart attack.

Love Your Heart—Go Vegetarian

You may not be ready to give up meat altogether, but studies by cardiologist Dean Ornish, MD, who directs the Preventive Medicine Research Institute in Sausalito, California, find that following a diet that includes no animal foods except fat-free milk, egg whites, and low-fat yogurt relieves angina pain within just a few weeks. If you're tired of being chained to medication, I'd suggest trying this diet for a month. You have nothing to lose but some pain!

As a side note, many nuts and seeds are great sources of arginine, including sunflower seeds, carob, butternuts, watermelon seeds, peanuts, sesame seeds, almonds, and Brazil nuts.

★★**Bilberries, blackberries, blueberries, and cherries** These fruits are high in compounds called anthocyanins, which help dilate blood vessels. Anything that helps blood vessels dilate reduces the risk of an angina attack because wider blood vessels make it easier for blood to get through. Anthocyanins can also help prevent blood clots. A 1993 evaluation of anthocyanins in fruits found the highest amount in bilberries and then, in descending order, blackberries, black currants, blueberries, cherries, cranberries, and red raspberries.

★★**Carrots and parsnips** These vegetables, along with fennel, parsley, celery, and a Chinese herb you may not have heard of—angelica—belong to the carrot family, a class of veggies packed with compounds that mimic the actions of prescription drugs called calcium channel blockers. These drugs, which include amlodipine (Norvasc), diltiazem (Cardizem, Dilacor XR), and nifedipine (Adalat, Procardia), work by keeping calcium out of cells in the heart or blood vessel walls, which, in turn, prevents those muscles from contracting. All of this reduces blood pressure, increases blood flow, and limits the likelihood of an angina attack. In one study involving angelica, also called dong quai, 72 people with angina received either a concoction of various herbs, including angelica, chrysanthemum, safflower, licorice, and dried leech, twice a day for 4 weeks or the angina drug isosorbide dinitrate (Isordil, Sorbitrate) three times a day for 4 weeks. Ninety-four percent of those who got the herbal mixture saw their angina disappear entirely compared with 86.1 percent of those who received the medication. Other studies in animals find that a compound isolated from angelica, called n-butylidenephthalide, also relaxes blood vessels. Since you probably can't find angelica in your local supermarket, make a juice or soup with carrots, parsley, fennel, and celery and drink it daily.

★**Cantaloupe** I'll single out the biblical melon that we call cantaloupe, but many fruits, like many veggies, can help prevent heart problems (and cancer). You can buy and enjoy whole melons as we do, or you may want to make juice with a blender or juicer (I prefer a blender because juicers tend to eject fiber from the juice). Cantaloupe contains the compound adenosine, which is used in heart patients to thin the blood and prevent angina attacks. Aim for two 8-ounce glasses a day.

★**Pineapple** This tropical fruit is a vast reservoir of bromelain, which has anti-inflammatory, anti-clotting, and diuretic properties. More than 400 scientific articles, primarily from Germany, attest to the medical uses of bromelain, ranging from treating sinusitis, face and head trauma, and post-traumatic inflammation and swelling to helping reduce swelling and pain from having teeth pulled! One study from the early 1970s found that a daily dose of bromelain eradicated angina symptoms in participants within 4 to 90 days. Only after they stopped taking the supplement did their pain return.

Asthma

FOR 20 MILLION AMERICANS, the simple act of breathing is not something to take for granted. They have asthma. They live with a chronic cough, shortness of breath, wheezing, chest tightness, and the constant fear of having a full-on attack.

Asthma causes inflammation in the bronchial tubes, the passageways in your lungs, making it harder to breathe in and out. The inflammation, in turn, causes thick mucus to line the tubes, which makes breathing even harder.

The inflammation also makes the airways more sensitive to irritants and allergens such as animal dander, dust mites, pollen, mold, cigarette smoke, indoor and outdoor air pollution, industrial chemicals, and even strong scents—any of which can trigger an attack. So can hay fever allergies, because a type of protein called histamine, which causes allergy symptoms, also plays a role in asthma. Other triggers include exercise, respiratory infections, aspirin, sulfites in food, and stress.

During an attack, your airways constrict, and less air reaches your lungs. If the attack is severe, your organs can stop getting the oxygen they need, which could lead to death. Asthma causes about 5,000 deaths a year.

More and more children are coping with asthma, too. In the United States, nine million kids under age 18 have it, a number that has risen sharply since 1980. Doctors don't know why it's more common today, but I believe it has something to do with an increase in airborne chemical pollution and a tendency to eat fewer and fewer natural foods.

It's important to take the medications your doctor prescribes, but looking at the foods you're eating and making some changes in your diet can also help. Nature has enriched our foods with healing compounds. Some, such as minerals, come out of the ground; others are manufactured by our green friends. Given the choice, I prefer these green, nature-made chemicals, what I call green farmaceuticals, over the man-made products that come out of a box, often with black-label warnings (though often black enough, in my opinion).

Here's how you can take control of your asthma by choosing carefully among the healing foods that nature provides.

Healing Foods for Asthma

First, a caution: Asthma can be life-threatening, so if your doctor recommends particular treatments, use them. Many doctors prescribe inhalers containing drugs called bronchodilators that open the bronchial tubes. Some also prescribe powerful hormone-like drugs called corticosteroids to reduce inflammation. You would be wise, however, to find a broadminded general physician who is also knowledgeable about green alternatives.

There is one prescription medication to avoid if you can: salmeterol (Serevent, Advair), a drug taken with an inhaler. Shelly R. Salpeter, MD, and her colleagues performed a meta-analysis of 19 randomized, placebo-controlled trials that included more than 33,000 people with asthma and found that although salmeterol can help improve asthma in some people, it can actually make symptoms worse and even life-threatening in others. Some researchers believe the drug may be responsible for about 4,000 of the 5,000 annual deaths from asthma in the United States. (Hmm. . . makes me want to write a new rhyme: "Salpeter et al on salmeterol; possibly kills more than no drug at all!")

Although other medications may not carry such high risks, they aren't risk free. Checking out safer, natural approaches to controlling your asthma remains a good bet. In fact, you'll find that some foods work remarkably well at reducing inflammation and opening the bronchial tubes, making it easier to take a deep breath of fresh air. Here are some to try.

★★★**Citrus fruits, strawberries, broccoli, and other foods high in vitamin C**
Vitamin C stops the release of histamine, the chemical in your body that causes wheezing, watery eyes, and a runny nose. That's what makes this nutrient great for people with asthma.

Studies have found that vitamin C intake (along with vitamin A and carotenoids) has an effect on how severe asthma symptoms can be. In 2004, researchers studied more than 4,000 children and found that those with lower levels of vitamin C in their bodies were more likely to be diagnosed with asthma.

Another study, done on adolescents in 2007, found that those who had the lowest intake of antioxidants such as vitamin C had a greater chance of developing respiratory problems such as asthma.

Foods high in vitamin C also contain flavonoids, which work to block the release of histamine. For that reason, I recommend eating bell peppers (especially red ones), broccoli, Brussels sprouts, butternut squash, cantaloupe, grapefruit, kiwifruit, oranges, papayas, strawberries, sweet potatoes, and tomatoes. Camu-camu, an Amazonian fruit, contains more vitamin C than any other food. It's not widely available here, but that may change.

★★★**Coffee, tea, and other sources of caffeine** People with asthma have been turning to strong coffee and tea to relieve their symptoms since as far back as the 1830s. More recently, doctors have compared the effects of caffeine and theophylline (a bronchodilator used in inhalers that occurs naturally in the same plants as caffeine) and found that caffeine works as well as or even better than the drug at reducing asthma symptoms.

When researchers looked at the results of the Second National Health and Nutrition Examination Survey, they found that adults over age 30 who drank coffee regularly had 29 percent fewer asthma symptoms than those who didn't drink it. In fact, coffee, tea, caffeinated soda, cocoa, and dark chocolate all contain theophylline and theobromine, another anti-asthmatic compound.

Some experts say that if you don't have your inhaler and you feel an asthma attack coming on, drink two or three cups of coffee. Coffee has the highest amount of caffeine (about 100 milligrams per cup), while 12 ounces of soda, a cup of tea, or a cup of cocoa has about 50 milligrams. Chocolate has even less: 1½ ounces of chocolate contains a little less than a can of soda. It's always important to keep in mind, though, that caffeine can cause insomnia and make you jittery, so you don't want to overuse it.

As I've said, asthma is life-threatening, so I recommend following your doctor's advice about using pharmaceutical drugs to treat your asthma and use caffeine as a supplement to that treatment.

★★★**Onions, garlic, and leeks** Dr. Walter Dorsch, of Johannes Gutenberg University in Mainz, Germany, has identified compounds in onions and onion juice that help reduce inflammation. He found that compounds in onions called thiosulfinates and cepaenes (for *cepa* in the scientific name *Allium cepa*) have

FOODS TO WATCH

Just as there are foods that help you breathe more easily, the foods listed below will make your asthma symptoms worse.

Salt. Americans get several times their share of salt. According to the Center for Science in the Public Interest, Americans get 4,000 milligrams of sodium a day, but experts advise getting half that amount: 1,500 to 2,400 milligrams. Limiting your sodium is worth your while if you have asthma. Research has found that following a low-sodium diet for 2 to 5 weeks improves lung function and reduces asthma symptoms. Even following a low-sodium plan for just a couple of weeks lessened constriction of bronchial tubes, the data shows.

The key to cutting sodium intake is to avoid processed foods. Only 11 percent of the sodium Americans eat is added at the table or while cooking; a whopping 77 percent comes from processed foods such as snacks, canned vegetables and soups, lunchmeats, frozen foods, and even bread. You can stay within the guidelines above by eating natural foods such as fresh fruits and vegetables, using fresh herbs and spices instead of salty condiments, and sticking with low-sodium breads and soup broths. And don't forget about restaurant fare: It's loaded with sodium. A good reason to eat in.

Milk, eggs, peanuts, tree nuts, soy, wheat, fish, and shellfish. Some people have allergic reactions to these foods, and that could trigger an asthma attack, according to the American Academy of Allergy, Asthma, and Immunology in Milwaukee. If you notice that your symptoms worsen after you eat these, it's a good idea to take note and try to avoid those foods in the future.

Sunflower, corn, or safflower oil. These oils contain omega-6 fatty acids, which promote inflammation that leads to constriction of the airways. It's a good idea to avoid them and use olive or canola oil instead.

Foods that trigger acid reflux. Many people who have asthma also have gastroesophageal reflux disease, or GERD. Frequent heartburn can damage your lungs and make asthma worse, so try to avoid foods that trigger GERD symptoms, such as acidic foods, fried foods, and heavy sauces.

anti-inflammatory and anti-asthmatic properties. Onions are also very rich in quercetin, another anti-inflammatory compound. Onion skins are perhaps our richest—and least expensive—source.

In fact, people have used onion and garlic for asthma for centuries. Rabbi Jacob Zahalon wrote in his book *Otzar Hachayim* (*The Treasury of Life*) in 1683 that garlic and onion had beneficial effects for asthma and for neutralizing poisons.

Add onions and garlic to salads, soups, tomato sauce, chili, or stews, or simply rub a garlic clove over a slice of toasted bread.

★★★**Wasabi and other spicy foods** Spicy foods can help you breathe better when you have asthma, says Richard N. Firshein, DO, medical director of the Firshein Center for Comprehensive Medicine in New York City and author of *Reversing Asthma*. That includes hot peppers, horseradish, and spicy dishes like chili.

If you're a fan of extremely hot foods, try wasabi, the Japanese equivalent of horseradish. Some research has shown that it can relieve allergies such as hay fever, which probably means it's helpful for asthma as well. You'll find it in the international foods section of your supermarket; eat it with crackers or dip or with sushi.

★★**Citrus peels** Citrus fruits have more to offer than their vitamin-packed flesh. Their peels contain limonene, a chemical that helps reduce asthma attacks, especially those triggered by air pollution. Limonene may work by saturating the cells in your lungs to protect them against ozone. Researcher Ehud Keinan, PhD, of the Israel Institute of Technology experimented on rats and found that those that inhaled limonene had significant protection from bronchial obstruction.

You can squeeze citrus peels by folding a piece between your fingers. When folded, some immediately emit a small cloud of aromatic compounds that contain limonene. Carefully inhale the aroma to see if you notice any benefit. Eating citrus peel will also help, but be sure to wash it thoroughly to remove pesticides.

Another option: Grate lemon, orange, and grapefruit peel into stir-fries, bread and cake batter, salad dressings, and rice. And use marmalade as a spread. In addition to helping your asthma, limonene may help prevent breast, colon, and prostate cancers.

Since limonene is also absorbed through the skin, you can add crushed citrus peels to your bathwater.

Although there haven't been any human clinical trials testing citrus inhalation (and there probably won't be), I would bet that citrus peels would score well alongside pharmaceuticals, and they would be cheaper and probably safer.

★★**Low-fat foods** Eating healthful foods that are low in fat, such as fresh fruit and vegetables, can help control your asthma symptoms because they help control your weight. Scientists surveyed more than 3,000 people with asthma and found that those who were obese were more likely to have severe, persistent symptoms; use more pharmaceutical drugs to control those symptoms; and miss work more often than people who had asthma but maintained a healthy weight.

★★**Salmon and other fatty fish.** If your asthma symptoms flare up after exercise, you may find relief with the omega-3 fatty acids in oily cold-water fish. These fatty acids help reduce inflammation in the lungs and decrease tissue damage after an asthma attack.

In one study of 20 elite athletes (half of whom usually experienced asthma symptoms after exercise and half of whom didn't), researchers randomly assigned the participants to a diet supplemented with either fish-oil capsules or placebos containing olive oil. The athletes maintained the diets for 3 weeks, took a week off, and then returned to using the supplements for another 3 weeks. Results showed that those who usually experienced asthma after working out and took the fish-oil supplements saw an 80 percent improvement in their symptoms.

The athletes' omega-3 supplements contained eicosapentaenoic acid (EPA) and docosahexaenoic acid (DHA), two kinds of fatty acids abundant in salmon, mackerel, herring, tuna, and sardines.

★**Brazil nuts** Doctors believe that not getting enough selenium can lead to chronic asthma. This trace mineral makes antioxidant enzymes, which means it helps keep free radicals from forming, damaging the body, and possibly leading to asthma symptoms. In a review of trials that looked at supplementing with selenium to treat asthma symptoms, researchers found that it does seem to help. You can get it from Brazil nuts—an average-size nut contains 70 micrograms of selenium—as well as fish such as tuna and cod and lean beef.

★**Cereal, bananas, potatoes, and other sources of vitamin B$_6$** A vitamin B$_6$ deficiency is associated with higher levels of inflammation, and some asthma drugs can deplete your stores. The Daily Value for this vitamin is only 2 milligrams, so to make sure you're getting vitamin B_6–rich foods in your diet, simply enjoy some fortified cereal or oatmeal in the morning; have a banana as a snack; sprinkle chickpeas or sunflower seeds over your salad; or have a baked potato with chicken breast, pork loin, or roast beef. All of these foods contain B_6. Because too much B_6 can damage your nerves, I don't recommend taking a supplement unless directed by your doctor.

★**Halibut, soybeans, spinach, and other magnesium-rich foods** People who have asthma often have low levels of magnesium, and studies suggest that getting more of this mineral may improve lung function. Halibut, soybeans, spinach, oatmeal, cereal, potatoes, nuts, and peanut butter all contain magnesium. If nuts cause your asthma symptoms to act up, however, be sure to steer clear of them.

★**Honey** Some say adding honey to tea, milk, and other foods—or even inhaling its aroma—can help asthma symptoms. Honey is one of the most popular forms of complementary and alternative medicine used by parents of children with asthma in Turkey, according to a study published in the *Annals of Allergy, Asthma, and Immunology*. Garlic can be added to the honey as a treatment, and I might even experiment by also adding some grated lemon peel.

★**Mediterranean foods** Children living on the Greek island of Crete rarely experience allergic reactions such as asthma, so researchers set out to see if their Mediterranean diet might be the reason. They looked at 690 kids ages 7 to 18. A survey revealed that 80 percent of the children ate fresh fruit and 68 percent ate fresh vegetables at least twice a day. Further study showed a close relationship between the amount of fresh, locally grown grapes, oranges, apples, nuts, and tomatoes the children ate and how free they were of symptoms of asthma and nasal allergies.

Another study suggests that expectant mothers who follow a Mediterranean diet during pregnancy may give their children the gift of long-term good health. Researchers tracked the health of 460 children on an island in Spain from birth to 6½ years. Those whose mothers had eaten a high-quality Mediterranean diet during pregnancy proved less likely to experience wheezing and allergy symptoms.

★**Parsley** People in Peru have been known to juice parsley, heat it, and add it to milk and honey to relieve asthma and other conditions. You can try adding parsley to omelets, salads, salsa, tabbouleh, spaghetti sauce, and soups.

★★**Vitamin E–rich leafy greens** Several studies have found a connection between vitamin E intake and asthma. Vitamin E helps the body release chemicals that relax the muscles in the lungs and opens the airways. Doctors also believe that it targets free radicals caused by air pollution.

In a study conducted by the Harvard School of Public Health of more than 77,000 women, those who consumed the most vitamin E from their diets had the lowest risk of asthma. However, there is one important point to mention: The researchers didn't count the vitamin E present in nuts, which can cause an allergic reaction in many people with asthma. In another study, researchers asked more than 68,000 French women about their diets and found that those who had the highest intake of leafy vegetables, along with carrots and tomatoes, had the lowest prevalence of asthma.

The fact that the vitamin E in all of these studies came from food rather than supplements is key when it comes to asthma and allergies. In another experiment done on rats, researchers showed that gamma-tocopherol, the form of the vitamin you get from food, was more effective for asthma and allergy relief than alpha-tocopherol, the form found in supplements.

Leafy greens such as spinach are loaded with vitamin E. So is wheat germ. Try sprinkling it on oatmeal, salads, yogurt, or ice cream or using it as a coating on fish or chicken. Wheat germ can also be used in place of ½ cup of flour when you bake muffins, bread, or pancakes.

From the Herbal Medicine Chest

The leaves of the ginkgo plant *(Ginkgo biloba)* have been used for thousands of years in Asia to treat asthma, allergies, bronchitis, and coughs, and today researchers are finding that this Eastern healing tradition may be on the right track. In a recent study by Chinese researchers, 75 people with asthma were given either a steroid alone or a steroid plus ginkgo extract. Those who received the extract had a significantly greater decrease in inflammation than did those who took only the steroid.

I recommend taking this herb as a 50:1 extract (meaning 50 pounds of leaves yields 1 pound of extract) according to the package directions. Don't take more than 60 to 240 milligrams of standardized extract a day because large amounts can cause diarrhea, irritability, and restlessness.

Athlete's Foot

LIKE MY SON, I used to have clammy, highly aromatic feet, especially when I stayed in my work shoes for any length of time. But unlike my son, I like to go barefoot, and I haven't had a serious foot problem in a long time. I've even walked barefoot in the jungles of Amazonian Peru, picking up God knows what, and I've still eluded the fungal skin infection known as athlete's foot.

Athlete's foot, or tinea pedis, is caused by common superficial fungi that attack the feet. However, they can migrate north to other parts of the body, like the groin and underarms. And because the organisms can persist over long periods of time, they can spread through clothing and bed sheets that haven't been washed.

The fungi thrive in warm, dark, humid places like swimming pools, showers, and sweaty feet trapped in socks and shoes. To prevent and treat athlete's foot, doctors often recommend keeping your feet clean and dry and to wear flip-flops in areas that are likely to harbor foot fungi. That comes close to my recommendation to go barefoot for reasonable exposure to antiseptic sunlight.

Athlete's foot is very common. Reportedly, 70 percent of all adults will be infected at one time or another. My personal first line of defense would be a barefoot weekend at a saltwater beach. The germ-killing combination of sun exposure and salt is usually enough to destroy foot fungus. But if going barefoot stops working and I start feeling the telltale signs of burning, itching, and skin cracking between my toes, I reach for these foods.

Healing Foods for Athlete's Foot

★★★**Garlic** Garlic is my first choice of treatment for athlete's foot. It's one of the most widely recommended fungal antiseptics—and for good reason. Fresh garlic contains allicin, a compound that has antibacterial, antiviral, and antifungal properties. Many scientifically rigorous studies show that it's effective for treating athlete's foot and other fungal infections. In one study of 47 soldiers with athlete's foot, those treated with garlic were fungus free after 60 days.

Garlic kills fungi on contact, so a garlic footbath is the best way to treat itchy, burning toes. Simply put crushed, diced garlic in a basin with warm water and a little rubbing alcohol, then soak your feet for up to 30 minutes.

If steeping your feet in a tub of malodorous cloves isn't appealing, you might try a traditional Chinese remedy: Crush several cloves of garlic and steep them in olive oil for 1 to 3 days. When you're ready to use it, strain out the plant material and apply the oil to the affected areas with a clean cloth or cotton ball once or twice a day. You can also put crushed garlic in a pair of clean, dry socks and wear them while you're sleeping.

Garlic can cause skin irritation and blistering in some people, so if you use it topically and find that it burns your skin, stop using it.

Eating garlic could be a second line of defense. If you're in a serious battle with fungi, why not engage the enemy on all fronts? You've certainly noticed that if you consume a lot of garlic, you can smell it in your sweat, so you know that it can attack fungi from the inside out. It also boosts the immune system, which can help fight athlete's foot. Garlic is the most common herb in my Green Farmacy Garden because it is so far, on an evidentiary basis, the most versatile. And I can't emphasize enough that it's important to consume garlic as a whole food, not just a supplement of garlic extract. The whole food contains a whole shotgun shell of antifungals, while the supplement contains only one.

★★★**Licorice** With more antifungal compounds than any other herb and an ability to reduce inflammation, licorice is up to the task of eradicating athlete's foot. You can buy licorice cream, but a cup of my Tinea Tea is a more pleasant (and cheaper) experience. The primary ingredient is licorice, but I like to add ginger and cinnamon, two spices that are antifungal powerhouses. Just steep them in hot water, strain, and enjoy—but don't throw away that potent sediment. Apply the dregs right to the affected areas of your feet.

★★**Baking soda** Sweaty feet are a fun place for fungi. When you remove the moisture, you're effectively evicting them, which is why keeping your feet dry is key in preventing and treating athlete's foot. Sprinkling your feet with baking soda after your shower will absorb moisture and kill offending fungi. You can also make a paste with warm water and baking soda and rub it on the affected areas. Leave the paste on for 15 minutes, rinse it off, and dry your feet thoroughly, especially between the toes where fungi like to hide.

To give baking soda an antiseptic boost, use it as a base to make your own foot talc by mixing in a few herbs and spices with germ-killing properties. The more potent choices are clove, oregano, rosemary, and thyme. If you don't have those on hand, however, almost any dried herb or spice that isn't outdated will do. They all have varying degrees of antiseptic compounds.

★★**Tomato sauce** I don't imagine you'll ever see tomato sauce marketed as a fungus treatment, but it certainly contains plenty of fungicides. Many of the traditional ingredients that make pasta sauce so *delicioso* also happen to contain antifungal compounds. You can cook up your own special sauce by going heavy on ingredients that are rich in fungicides, mainly basil, celery, carrots, dill, fennel, garlic, sage, and thyme. Just add what you have on hand, heat it up, and pour it over your favorite pasta dish. If you're feeling adventurous, you can even spread the sauce between your toes and leave it there for a few hours.

★★**Vinegar** Some studies indicate that vinegar inhibits the growth of certain microorganisms, including bacteria and fungi. Many doctors recommend soaking your feet in a mixture of 1 part white vinegar and 2 parts warm water for 15 to 20 minutes. Be sure to thoroughly rinse the solution off and dry your feet well. To really amp up the antifungal effects of vinegar, add a dash of garlic powder or fresh diced garlic (which is usually deemed more effective right after dicing). Researchers at the University of Iowa discovered that white vinegar effectively reduced the growth of fungus, but there was an even greater reduction when garlic powder was added to the vinegar.

★★**Walnut** The meat of the walnut has great nutritional value, but the best fungicidal activity is in the hull, which is discarded before it reaches the market. Around the Green Farmacy Garden, walnuts roll around all over the place in fall, sometimes making walking a little hazardous. But my old Green Pharmacy recommendations still hold: After you take out the meat of those walnuts, throw the garbage into a bucket of water to steep for about 24 hours. Remove the hulls, and you're left with a strong mix of topical fungicides to which you can add some garlic. Soak your feet for 15 to 30 minutes.

From the Herbal Medicine Chest

Tea tree oil is a terrific antiseptic that many experts recommend for athlete's foot.

Australian researchers gave 158 people with athlete's foot a 50 percent tea tree oil solution, a 25 percent tea tree oil solution, or a placebo. The patients applied their solutions to the affected areas twice a day for 4 weeks. At the end of the study, 64 percent of the group using the 50 percent solution were cured, and 55 percent of those using the 25 percent solution were cured. Only 31 percent of the patients using the placebo were cured.

To make your own tea tree oil solution, dilute the oil with an equal amount of water or vegetable oil and apply it directly to the affected areas with a clean cloth or cotton ball three times a day. Tea tree oil can cause an allergic reaction in some people, so if your skin becomes irritated, discontinue use. And never ingest the oil; even small amounts can be fatal if it's swallowed.

Backache

As A PERSON WHO HAS LONG HAD BACK PROBLEMS, I'm astounded by the number of Americans who share my affliction. The most recent estimates, published in a 2008 issue of the journal *Arthritis and Rheumatism*, show that a whopping 59 million Americans have had lower-back pain within the past 3 months! Another 30 million have had neck pain within that time period. That means that at any given moment, nearly one in three Americans are coping with distress that can dramatically affect their quality of life and at worst be totally incapacitating.

According to researchers at Stanford University School of Medicine, who conducted a nationwide survey of 1,200 adults in 2005, 25 percent of respondents cited the back as their most common source of pain. They said it had adverse effects on their work and other duties, mood, day-to-day activities, sleep, and overall enjoyment of life.

Unfortunately, good pain relief is hard to come by. Although respondents relied most on prescription drugs and prayer, only 50 percent of them said these methods were effective. About 1 in 10 took daily over-the-counter painkillers, while 2 in 10 relied on daily prescription painkillers. That means a sizable number of Americans are gobbling mounds of drugs each day but more often than not are getting little benefit.

Not so long ago, doctors treated back pain with rest, long-term medication, and surgery. Fortunately, surgery is no longer as commonly recommended, yet Americans are still about 20 times more likely than Canadians and Europeans to "go under the knife" for back pain.

If your doctor recommends surgery, I strongly suggest getting several other medical opinions. I regret not having done that when I underwent cervical fusion at the behest of my HMO. That operation was a waste of blood, sutures, and recovery time. It didn't make me feel any better. Only later did I learn that 80 percent of patients with the same diagnosis—those who had the wisdom to forgo surgery—gradually rid themselves of pain in just 4 months.

That said, I don't have the same negative opinion about the short-term use of medications—prescription and nonprescription—to treat a nasty flare-up of back pain. Aspirin and other nonsteroidal anti-inflammatory drugs—and, in severe cases, codeine or slow-release morphine (both of which come from an herbal source: the opium poppy)—can provide temporary relief.

Healing Foods for Backache

To help prevent backache—or manage lingering or lessening pain—a number of food remedies can prove useful.

A Triple Whammy for Back Pain

I would give this one only two stars because I haven't yet tried it. But if I had a killer backache and needed to attack it with my entire arsenal, I'd start by eating some stinging nettle greens, an excellent painkilling food that unfortunately must be either grown or foraged; I've yet to find it in any supermarket (when you cook the leaves, they lose their sting). Then I'd mix up a salve made of mashed chile pepper, ground mustard seed, and vinegar, possibly with a little wintergreen oil (which contains painkilling methylsalicylate), clove oil (which contains painkilling eugenol), and one of the mint oils listed on page 60. After rubbing this pungent concoction on my sore back, I'd take a bite of red pepper (which, in addition to capsaicin, contains painkilling salicylates) or a spoonful of horseradish or mustard (both of which contain painkilling isothiocyanate). I think this whammy of a remedy has great potential for treating out-of-whack backs.

★★★**Chile peppers** Hot peppers contain a resinous, pungent substance known as capsaicin, which is number one among my painkillers. When applied topically, capsaicin temporarily depletes substance P, a chemical in nerves that transmits pain sensations. Without substance P, pain signals can no longer be sent. Dozens of studies show that capsaicin can temporarily relieve many painful conditions, including back pain.

You can buy a commercial topical cream containing 0.025 to 0.075 percent capsaicin and apply it to your aching back three or four times a day. Or you can do what people outside the United States often do: buy a chile pepper, mash it, and apply it directly. You can also mix mashed chile with a skin cream such as cold cream. Either way, you'll save money. A fresh hot pepper costs a few pennies, whereas a commercial capsaicin product such as Zostrix can cost up to $16.

No matter which route you choose, you may experience a burning sensation the first few times you use capsaicin, but it usually subsides with repeated use. Just be sure to thoroughly wash your hands after using it. If you get any in your eyes, nose, or mouth, it may be almost as painful as your aching back.

Although capsaicin is best used topically, it may be helpful to add more peppers, pepper-derived hot sauce, and cayenne powder to your diet. Another option is taking a cayenne tincture (0.3 to 1 milliliter) three times a day. You can also make an infusion by stirring ½ to 1 teaspoon (2.5 to 5 grams) of cayenne powder into 1 cup of boiling water, letting it stand for 10 minutes, and taking 1 teaspoon mixed with water three or four times daily.

Besides being potent COX-2 inhibitors, peppers are a pretty good source of natural analgesic salicylates (aspirin-like compounds). You can bet I add some to my curried celery dietary analgesic. (See my Curried Celery COX-2 Inhibitor recipe on page 286 and my COX-2–Inhibiting Chile Drink recipe on page 323.)

★★★**Ginger** Ginger contains high amounts of a powerful anti-inflammatory substance called zingibain. According to some experts, it's even more potent than the bromelain in pineapple or the papain in papaya. Ginger reportedly contains 180 times more proteolytic enzymes than the papaya plant and may be even more effective at relieving inflammation-related conditions, including backache. It also contains at least four natural COX-2 inhibitors, and, unlike prescription COX-2 inhibitors such as celecoxib (Celebrex), it's not associated with any serious side effects.

It's easy to get enough ginger in your diet to help reduce pain. You can take it as an herb in tea by steeping three or four slices of fresh ginger in a cup of boiling water, or, if you prefer, you can get medicinal doses in tinctures or capsules. I, however, prefer ginger as a liberal and tasty addition to my daily diet. Sprinkling ½ teaspoon of powdered ginger into your foods or eating about an ounce (2 tablespoons) of fresh ginger provides a medicinal dose every day. Even ginger ale helps and is easy it to take—but be sure it's the real thing, made with ginger.

Recently, I've been enjoying New Chapter's commercial ginger salve in honey. It reminds me of an exotic pain remedy I encountered during my travels down the Amazon River. I dubbed it Soccorro's Secret, after Soccorro Guerrero, who brewed it in her kitchen. Her salve is made of ginger, honey, rum, and other ingredients, including the herb dragon's blood. Of course, you could always try drinking a tea made with a tablespoon of dried ginger and sweetened to taste with honey or—if you're feeling adventurous—just a splash of rum.

FOODS TO WATCH

Although no specific foods will increase your risk of backache, eating too much food on a regular basis can. Being overweight or obese places a lot of strain on your lower back. So does a lack of exercise. Although it sounds counterintuitive, one of the worst things you can do for an aching back is to stop exercising. The YMCA has an excellent program for people with back pain, which combines stretching, strength training, and relaxation.

★★★**Mint** Peppermint, spearmint, Chinese mint, and other mint oils contain high amounts of menthol, which when applied topically can help relieve the pain and muscle tightness associated with backache. Although you can buy commercial products containing menthol, it may be a better (and cheaper) bet to apply mint oils directly to your back—but beware that such oils are toxic when consumed internally. Another option is to drink peppermint tea two or three times a day. Although many commercial mint teas are available, I'd recommend making your own by pouring 1 cup of boiling water over 1 heaping teaspoon (5 grams) of dried peppermint leaves and steeping for 5 to 10 minutes; drink three to four cups daily. For extra benefits, consider stirring a delicious peppermint/chamomile tea with a licorice stick, which will give you a host of analgesic and anti-inflammatory compounds. Another option is taking 3 to 6 grams of peppermint leaf tablets or capsules a day. In the Green Farmacy Garden and the Amazon medicinal plant gardens I visit, we have many weedy mints, and I often just pick a handful of leaves, mash them with my hands, and apply locally to achy areas.

★★**Cherries** If you have a really bad backache, I doubt that eating cherries will make you feel much better. But if you're prone to backaches, regular consumption of cherries may help prevent some of the muscle damage to your quadratus lumborum, the muscle most commonly involved in lower-back pain. In a 2006 study published in the *British Journal of Sports Medicine,* researchers studied 14 healthy male college students who drank either a bottle of tart cherry juice (which contained the equivalent of 50 to 60 tart cherries) or a placebo drink before engaging in a muscle-damaging exercise. They found that muscle soreness and pain scores were considerably lower among the students who drank the cherry juice. (See page 195 for more information about cherries.)

★★**Pineapple** This exotic fruit is rich in a number of substances that can help people with conditions such as back pain. Foremost among them is bromelain, a proteolytic enzyme that helps reduce the swelling and inflammation of many painful "-itis" (inflammatory) conditions. Its anti-inflammatory effects are so profound that the German government has approved its use for healing after injuries and surgical procedures. Pineapple also contains high amounts of manganese, which is essential for the formation of collagen, the tough, fibrous protein that builds connective tissues such as bone, skin, and cartilage. You can get 100 percent of the Daily Value for manganese (2 milligrams) from just a cup of fresh pineapple chunks or pineapple juice. Pineapple is also a rich source of vitamin C, also necessary for collagen formation: A cup of fresh chunks contains 24 milligrams, or 40 percent of the daily value. To get the maximum antioxidant punch, try "Gold" pineapple, which is imported from Costa Rica and contains four times as much vitamin C as other pineapples.

Unfortunately, recent research suggests that the levels of both bromelain in fresh pineapple and papain, a related enzyme in fresh papaya, may be too low to relieve a bad episode of back pain. While I would encourage enjoying these fruits—either whole or as juice—you'll probably need to go the supplement route to get seriously effective levels. Or spice things up with ginger, with its proteolytic enzyme zingibain. Naturopaths suggest taking anywhere between 250 and 750 milligrams of bromelain three times a day. In human studies, a daily dose of up to 2,000 milligrams has not been shown to be harmful.

★★**Turmeric** This yellow curry spice is a rich source of curcumin, a strong antioxidant that protects against free radical damage. Curcumin is also a natural pain-relieving COX-2-inhibitor, which makes it an attractive, side effect–free alternative to prescription COX-2 inhibitors such as Celebrex. It also reduces inflammation by lowering histamine levels and possibly stimulating the adrenal glands to produce more cortisone, the body's natural painkiller. Lately, I've had two students who switched from Celebrex to either curcumin or curried celery and thought it was a good tradeoff. (See my Curried Celery COX-2 Inhibitor recipe on page 286 and my COX-2–Inhibiting Chile Drink recipe on page 323.)

Human studies of curcumin have found that it can reduce the pain and stiffness associated with rheumatoid arthritis as well as help relieve postsurgical inflammation. I prefer a whole-foods approach whenever possible because I believe you get more healing power from whole foods than from individual components, so I often use liberal amounts of curry in rice and other dishes and would consider adding it to other anti-inflammatory foods such as pineapple and papaya. You also can make tea with turmeric.

Unfortunately, it's difficult to get medicinal doses of curcumin from diet alone. According to naturopaths, that dose is 250 to 500 milligrams of pure curcumin a day between meals, which translates into 5 to 25 teaspoons of dried turmeric daily. That's a good deal more than even a curry fan like me would want to add to my food. I would recommend adding as much turmeric as possible to your diet to help prevent pain and taking turmeric supplements—standardized to contain 90 to 95 percent curcumin—to help relieve acute pain. And always take it with freshly ground black pepper, which increases its absorption significantly.

From the Herbal Medicine Chest

The results of many studies suggest that devil's claw may be an effective alternative to conventional drugs for back pain. One study found that a dose of 600 to 1,200 milligrams a day reduced lower-back pain. Another study, which involved 316 patients, found that devil's claw relieved back pain as well as did a standard dose of rofecoxib (Vioxx), the COX-2 inhibitor that was pulled from the market because it increased the risk of heart attacks. When you feel those twinges coming on, try taking 1,200 milligrams of devil's claw a day. Just be sure it's a water-soluble extract product containing 50 milligrams of the compound harpagoside. Because the herb could be dangerous for people with low blood pressure and those taking blood thinners, it's best to consult your doctor before trying this remedy.

Bad Breath

BAD BREATH, HALITOSIS, ORAL MALODOR—all of these terms are used to describe a skunky or otherwise unpleasant aroma emanating from the mouth. No one is immune to bad breath, not even those who are persnickety about dental care (and that includes dentists). That unpleasant aroma can be caused by any number of things, not the least of which is bacteria on the teeth, gums, and tongue that produce sulfur compounds. Even the most advanced toothbrushes can't reach into all the nooks and crannies where foodborne bacteria hide. Fortunately, our bodies produce about 3 pints of saliva a day to wash away particles that toothbrushes and floss miss. Saliva even contains minerals to help repair microscopic tooth decay. Conversely, when your mouth is dry, bacteria multiply and create a stench that can cause even your dearest friend to recoil in horror. (A drink of water should put you back on speaking terms.)

Certain foods are notorious for causing bad breath. The biggest offenders are members of the allium family: garlic and onions. As your body metabolizes these foods, it produces gases that are carried to your lungs and released in your breath.

There are other, less obvious reasons for bad breath that can indicate health problems. Respiratory and sinus infections, diabetes, and liver and kidney diseases are some conditions that can cause halitosis. If you have persistent bad breath, be sure to see your dentist or primary care doctor to get to the bottom of things.

Healing Foods for Bad Breath

Stores are bulging with products that claim to freshen your breath, but deciding which one works best is no easy task. Before you begin sifting through them, consider taking a more natural approach.

★★★**Yogurt** There are times when you need to fight fire with fire, or in this case, fight bacteria with bacteria. Our bodies are teeming with all sorts of flora to keep harmful microorganisms from proliferating out of control. Bacteria that thrive at the back of the throat produce hydrogen sulfide, a common cause of malodorous mouths. Fortunately, bacteria found in yogurt may keep the "bad bugs" in check. When Japanese researchers gave study participants 3 ounces of unsweetened yogurt twice a day for 6 weeks, hydrogen sulfide levels decreased in over half of those with confirmed halitosis. As an added benefit, plaque and gingivitis were significantly reduced. The scientists aren't exactly sure how yogurt bacteria reduce hydrogen sulfide, according to lead researcher Kenichi Hojo. It's possible that the beneficial organisms in yogurt, *Streptococcus thermophilus* and *Lactobacillus bulgaricus*, simply crowd out the foul bacteria or create a hostile environment for them. Eating unsweetened plain yogurt with active cultures will work best, but artificially sweetened varieties should be effective, too, says Hojo.

There were times when we had excess goat's milk, and I ended up trying to make some yogurts and cheeses from it. I wasn't fond of them and would rather use store-bought. I think adding small bits of anti-halitosis mint leaves may help, but too much herb may damage the beneficial bacteria a bit.

★★**Cinnamon gum** When we suspect our mouths of smelling foul, we may reach for a stick of sweet-scented chewing gum. Some of these gums simply mask odors, and once the flavor fades, bad breath comes back with a vengeance. But gums that contain the essential oil cinnamaldehyde can actually eliminate odors and even prevent the

FOODS TO WATCH

When it comes to bad breath, garlic and onions would seem to be the most logical foods to avoid. However, these alliums contain so many nutritional benefits that to suggest banning them would be irresponsible, not to mention unethical. If you have persistent bad breath and have eliminated any health condition as the culprit, it may be wise to cut back on your intake of protein.

One of the most common complaints by dieters who follow a high-protein diet is halitosis. Sure, they may lose weight, but that bad breath can lead to lost friendships. Bacteria love to feast on protein-dense foods like milk, cheese, eggs, and poultry. If you're eating a lot of high-protein foods, try to replace some of them with healthy carbohydrates, and be sure to brush or rinse your teeth after every meal.

growth of new stinky bacteria. In a University of Chicago study, researchers asked volunteers to chew one of three different types of gum: Big Red, a popular gum with cinnamaldehyde; the same brand of gum without cinnamaldehyde; or a gum base without any essential oils or flavorings. After 20 minutes of chewing, the gum with cinnamaldehyde reduced mouth bacteria by 50 percent. The population of bacteria at the back of the tongue was decreased by an impressive 43 percent.

★★**Cranberries** These berries are like traffic cops. They keep bacteria from loitering around smooth tissue surfaces and wreaking havoc. That's why they're touted as a strong preventive against bladder infections. Cranberries employ these same "move along" directives to prevent bacteria from sticking to the teeth. When a solution of 25 percent cranberry juice was applied to plaque-covered surfaces, the adherence of bacteria was reduced by 40 to 85 percent. Since bad breath is often the result of bacterial buildup in the mouth, these results should be encouraging news to anyone battling halitosis. However, before you drink a glass of cranberry juice, take heed. The researchers caution that most juices are made with sugar to make the natural mouth-puckering tartness of the berries more palatable. Also, the cranberries' acidity can have corrosive effects on teeth.

★★**Oregano** Many aromatic mints, like aromatic cinnamon, score well for battling halitosis. In my Multiple Activity Menus, oregano scored highest for antioxidant activity—even better than rosemary and sage, which also score well.

★★**Parsley** Sometimes it takes just one sprig of parsley to neutralize breath odor. Why? Parsley contains chlorophyll, a plant pigment that happens to be a powerful deodorizer. All green leafy vegetables contain varying amounts of chlorophyll, but parsley is among the richest sources. Munch on it after having a meal, drinking a cup of coffee, or eating anything that causes malodorous breath. You can always keep a fresh supply on hand in the refrigerator. When choosing parsley at the store, pick the greenest you can find.

★**Celery** Generally, any food that's good for your body is good for your breath, but celery seems custom made for fighting halitosis. Most experts believe that the most common cause of bad breath is poor dental hygiene. In the absence of proper brushing and flossing, food particles on the teeth and the back of the tongue breed pungent bacteria. Munching on a stalk is helpful in two ways; its roughness helps scrub bacteria from the back of the tongue, and its natural fibers assist in cleaning the teeth. It's like using an edible toothbrush. In fact, if you ever find yourself without a toothbrush, chomping on a celery stick after a meal or first thing in the morning will do in a pinch.

★**Coriander** Whenever I leave Panama, I smell like coriander because it's indispensable in their national chicken soup/stew called *sancocho*. Coriander has not only two anti-halitosis compounds, cineole and thymol, but also dozens of antibacterial and antiseptic compounds.

★**Lemon** I happened to be talking to Martha Libster, RN, author of *Delmar's Integrative Herb Guide for Nurses*, when she suggested that a well-known deodorant—a.k.a. lemon—might help with bad breath. What with its two anti-halitosis and two dozen antibacterial phytochemicals, it sounds to me like a good bet. You might try fresh lemon juice flavored with one or more of the aforementioned herbs (cinnamon, oregano, or parsley).

★**Mushrooms** As you know, feasting on lasagna and pasta sauces with loads of garlic can leave you *solo mio* for a few days. Why not do yourself and your *paisans* a favor by adding some white button mushrooms to those dishes? Research conducted at the University of California, Davis, revealed that an extract made from white mushrooms appeared to deodorize the breath of participants who rinsed their mouths with a garlic solution.

★**Raisins** On the surface, raisins may seem like dental disaster waiting to happen. They're sweet and sticky—ideal conditions for odoriferous bacteria to get a foothold. However, a phytochemical in raisins called oleanolic acid actually fights those bacteria, according to researchers at the Chicago College of Dentistry at the University of Illinois. In a laboratory analysis, oleanolic acid inhibited the growth of two strains of oral bacteria: *Streptococcus mutans,* which causes cavities and bad breath, and *Porphyromonas gingivalis,* which causes gum disease. The lead researcher, Christine Wu, notes that added sugar, or sucrose, is what promotes cavities. Natural foods like raisins contain mainly fructose and glucose. Other culinary delights that contain breath-freshening oleanolic acid include clove, rosemary, thyme, lavender, oregano, basil, and sage.

★**Sage** So far, there's only a phytochemical rationale for using sage against halitosis. I've never tried it myself, but it's well endowed with three different anti-halitosis phytochemicals: 1,8-cineole, menthol, and thymol. Some people used to use sage for all of their oral care by rubbing its rough leaves on their teeth and gums.

From the Herbal Medicine Chest

No one's breath is minty-fresh first thing in the morning. Salivation slows down during the night, and oral pH levels shift from acidic to alkaline, encouraging odor-producing bacteria and "morning breath." An herbal mouthwash can alleviate morning breath just as well as many of the store-bought mouthwashes.

Since alcohol and eucalyptol (cineole), key ingredients in many mouth-washes, are effective against halitosis-inducing bacteria, you can mix up your own unique "Halitos-ade" by steeping cineole-rich herbs in cheap vodka. I prefer to use eucalyptus, rosemary, and spearmint, but there are plenty of other herbs to consider, including basil, bee balm, cardamom, cinnamon, fennel, ginger, hyssop, lavender, lemon leaf, lemon verbena, nutmeg, peppermint, sweet Annie, tansy, tarragon, turmeric, and yarrow.

Put several ounces of herbs and a pint of vodka in a wide-mouth jar with a screw-on lid, and let it steep indefinitely. If you don't like the look of all those herbs swimming around, just strain them out after a few days.

The Chinese have long known about the power of magnolia bark. References to the health-giving qualities of this woody plant date back to 1083. Magnolia bark is used primarily as a remedy for lung and intestinal disorders, but now scientists are finding that it brings a breath of fresh air to oral malodor research. When volunteers were given mints containing magnolia bark extract after lunch, their saliva showed 61 percent fewer oral bacteria after 30 minutes. Participants given magnolia bark gum had a 43 percent reduction in the offensive bacteria after 40 minutes.

Bladder Infections

ONE IN EVERY FIVE WOMEN will have at least one bladder infection during their lives, and about 11 percent of those will get them annually. Men can develop bladder infections, too, especially if they have prostate enlargement, but this problem strikes mostly women.

Bladder infections, also called urinary tract infections (UTIs), result in nearly 8.3 million doctor visits and 1.6 million hospitalizations annually, according to the National Kidney Foundation. Two-thirds of office visits are by women of childbearing age. Some 80 percent of bladder infections are caused by bacteria from the anal area, notably *Escherichia coli,* a microorganism that lives in the digestive tract. Since women have much shorter urethras (the tube through which urine exits the body) than men do, *E. coli* can travel more easily into their bladders. Luckily, most infections aren't serious and can be easily treated with antibiotic medications.

The first sign of a bladder infection may be a strong urge to urinate or a painful burning sensation during urination. Even though you may feel that you have to go

CysTea

Two chemicals from foods, cineole (eucalyptol) and thymol, are urinary antiseptics. I think that herbs with cineole make a more pleasantly flavored tea, but thymol is perhaps the more potent of the two. You can wander into the herb section of your supermarket or natural foods store and find the ingredients to concoct your own CysTea—what I call an herb tea that fights cystitis—to taste. Some culinary plants with high amounts of cineole include cardamom, basil, cinnamon, spearmint, rosemary, ginger, nutmeg, peppermint, fennel, tarragon, and turmeric. If you want the power of thymol antisepsis, you might use basil, oregano (which also reportedly contains arbutin), savory, or thyme. I'd also add some teaberry, for both its arbutin and its delightful aroma. I'd go with a few cardamom berries, a handful of spearmint and rosemary, some cranberry and/or blueberry, and a dash of ginger and turmeric. That would provide a flavorful mix of dozens of antiseptic phytochemicals.

frequently, you may produce little urine each time. You may also have soreness in your lower abdomen, back, or sides. Your urine may look cloudy or have a reddish tinge from blood, and it may smell foul or strong. You may also feel tired, shaky, and washed out. If the infection spreads to the kidneys, you may have fever, chills, nausea, vomiting, and back pain in addition to the frequent urge to urinate and painful urination. If you develop these symptoms, don't wait to see your doctor for treatment, or you may end up with more complicated health problems.

Healing Foods for Bladder Infections

★★★**Celery** With loads of analgesic, anti-inflammatory, and diuretic compounds, as well as some calcium blockers, celery seed extracts seem appropriate for treating bladder infections. Celery seed is said to improve the quantity and quality of urine and is a useful diuretic for UTIs. Along with parsley and carrots, celery stalks should be consumed liberally, as all three promote urine flow and generally support the urinary tract.

★★★**Cranberries** For ages, grandmothers and other folks, as well as a few wise doctors, have recommended cranberry juice to clear up bladder infections. Scientists were a little later coming on board, but they now agree. Research suggests

> Drinking more fluids, such as cranberry juice and water, encourages frequent urination, which helps flush bacteria from the bladder, but some fluids can be irritating. When you feel a bladder infection coming on, avoid drinking alcohol and coffee, tea, and colas that contain caffeine.

cranberry may be effective against UTIs because it prevents *E. coli* from attaching to the walls of the bladder.

Along with helping to prevent and treat garden-variety UTIs, it turns out that cranberries may also help prevent more serious bladder infections. In a very small study at the University of Washington in Seattle, researchers gave three women cranberry juice cocktail after collecting urine samples. The scientists took more samples 4 to 6 hours afterward, combined both sets of samples with human bladder cells, and incubated them with *E. coli*. They found that the number of bacteria able to stick to the bladder cells (which is the first thing bacteria have to do to cause an infection) was significantly reduced in the women's urine after they drank the cranberry juice. The most protective dose was 8 ounces.

Although this was a very small study, several larger ones show similar results. A team of Cochrane Collaboration researchers recently identified 10 studies that included a total of 1,049 participants. Their review of the studies concluded that cranberry juice decreases the number of UTIs over a 12-month period, particularly for women with recurrent infections. The effectiveness for other groups wasn't as clear. But the scientists also identified a problem with the cranberry juice studies: Lots of participants dropped out. People just may not want to drink that much cranberry juice over long periods of time.

Thus, the problem with the cranberry juice prescription is that you have to drink a lot of it; naturopaths suggest drinking 17 ounces a day to treat UTIs. The juice is naturally tart, so you'll want to sweeten it, meaning that this prescription is rather high in calories unless you sweeten with stevia, and some folks find that distasteful.

★★★**Yogurt** For an infection-fighting breakfast, you might try tossing a handful of blueberries into a bowl of yogurt and chasing it with a glass of cranberry juice. Yogurt is a good natural healer. Studies show that the probiotics (active bacterial cultures) in yogurt help prevent both bladder and yeast infections.

Another way yogurt may help is by stimulating the production of several cytokines (molecules that help regulate immune function), according to recent research from the department of nutritional sciences at the University of Vienna, Austria. Although both conventional and probiotic yogurt enhanced immune function in the study, I'd look for yogurt that lists live cultures on the label.

On his Web site, Andrew Weil, MD, professor at the University of Arizona College of Medicine in Tucson, warns us not to be fooled by the words "made with active cultures." All yogurts are made with live cultures, but some manufacturers heat-treat yogurt after fermenting it, which kills the cultures. The FDA requires them to label these products "heat-treated after culturing." Avoid these products and look for yogurt labels that say "active yogurt cultures," "living yogurt cultures," or "contains active cultures."

You might improve the action of probiotics by pairing them with herbs rich in inulin, such as Jerusalem artichoke, dandelion, and chicory.

★★**Blueberries** As with cranberries, folk practitioners have claimed for a long time that blueberries help UTIs. Blueberries contain constituents similar to those in cranberries and may also prevent bacteria from attaching to the lining of the bladder. However, there isn't much research on the effectiveness of blueberries in preventing bladder infections.

Banish Bladder Infections

All of the foods mentioned here, along with your doctor's prescription, can help treat bladder infections, but I'd be remiss if I didn't include the following standard self-care guidelines for preventing this condition.

All women, whether or not they're prone to bladder infections, should:

- Drink eight glasses of water a day
- Urinate whenever they feel the urge (a full bladder is more prone to infection)
- Avoid douching
- Wipe from front to back after using the bathroom, to prevent anal bacteria from being introduced into the urethra

Women with recurrent bladder infections should:

- Take showers instead of baths
- Drink a glass of water before and after sexual intercourse
- Urinate within 15 minutes after intercourse

An early study published in the *Journal of the American Medical Association* showed that certain compounds in cranberry and blueberry juice may prevent bacteria from clinging to the bladder walls so they can't cause infection there. Both blueberries and cranberries, as well as many other herbs and fruits in the heather family, contain arbutin, an antibiotic and diuretic compound that helps relieve water retention. In another study of seven juices, cranberry and blueberry both lowered *E. coli* adhesion, while grapefruit, guava, mango, orange, and pineapple did not.

★★**Teaberry (wintergreen)** You probably won't find this at the supermarket except in chewing gums and herbal teas, but if you can find it, I think this one really belongs in every spice chest. In midwinter, I steep the leaves and berries in vodka for my homemade liqueur called Teaberry Trip. In summer, I like to add wild ginger and bee balm. Old-timers steeped the leaves in brandy as a tonic liqueur. In Maine, we also use it to make wintergreen tea. Northern Indians revered the leaves almost as much as the Incas revered the leaves of coca. There are at least four painkilling compounds in them: methyl salicylate, caffeic acid, ferulic acid, and gentisic acid. For bladder complaints, it contains the important urinary antiseptic arbutin plus a lot of other bladder-friendly phytochemicals.

★**Papaya and other produce** After cranberry and blueberry, UTI-fighting juices include carrot, celery, cucumber, papaya, and parsley. Papaya, in particular, has a long history of use for bladder problems, and no wonder. Good research shows that it's a diuretic that helps empty the bladder.

From the Herbal Medicine Chest

Bearberries, close relatives of cranberries and blueberries, contain a good amount of arbutin, a natural diuretic and antibiotic. The herb was highly recommended by my late friend Varro Tyler, PhD, dean and professor emeritus of pharmacognosy (natural product pharmacy) at Purdue University in West Lafayette, Indiana. In his excellent book *Herbs of Choice*, Dr. Tyler relied on the recommendations of Germany's Commission E, a government agency that evaluates the safety and efficacy of medicinal herbs. Calling bearberry the "most effective antibacterial herb for urinary tract infections," Dr. Tyler offered the Commission E prescription: Take 10 grams a day (about ½ ounce) to treat bladder infections. This much bearberry contains anywhere from 400 to 700 milligrams of arbutin. Maximum antibacterial activity occurs 3 to 4 hours after taking this herb.

Body Odor

SCIENCE IS PROVING what I've suspected all along: Male body odor can be a turn-on. Researchers at the University of California, Berkeley, discovered that male sweat has a physiological effect on women. In two trials, 48 heterosexual female students at the university took 20 whiffs of androstadienone, a derivative of testosterone found in male perspiration. They reported greater sexual arousal and better moods than participants who sniffed a control odor. The women also had increased blood pressure, heart rate, and breathing. Androstadienone is an additive in some perfumes and colognes. Kind of makes you think twice about the typical male's mating habits—he washes all of those naturally seductive scents down the drain and then splashes on cologne that's spiked with the same components.

Despite what the folks at Berkeley say, however, my 79 years have taught me that many women are distinctly turned *off* by male body odor. Scientists at Rockefeller University in New York City and Duke University in North Carolina presented 400 people with a variety of odors, including male sweat, and asked them to rate the pleasantness of each. Some described the sweat odor as sweet and vanilla-like, while others found it foul. How can something smell "lovely" to one person and "locker room" to another? The answer is genetics. The way you perceive androstadienone is genetically determined. And for the hundredth time, I repeat, none of us is average. Average is theoretical, even though conventional medicine often treats us as though we were average.

The effect of body odors on others is rather complex. Fortunately, the reason body odor occurs is much simpler. We're all equipped with glands that produce sweat in response to body temperature, emotions, diet, and medications. As for the scent, perspiration doesn't actually have an aroma until it comes in contact with bacteria on the skin. That's why bathing remains the best way to control odor. However, since bacteria tend to colonize every 6 hours, most people need reinforcements between baths in the form of deodorants. Before buying commercial roll-ons and sprays, though, try using these foods to keep your body odor from becoming someone else's problem.

Healing Foods for Body Odor

★**Chamomile tea** A sip of this tea just may do the trick. Chamomile is an herb of many talents. It's antimicrobial and sedative, so while it's helping your underarms resist bacteria, it's also coaxing your mind to relax and let go of the stresses that make you sweat in the first place. If you prefer a more direct approach to body odor,

FOODS TO WATCH

The human digestive system is meant to function like a well-oiled machine. It breaks down food and propels it through into the intestines, where blood cells absorb and taxi its nutrients throughout the body. Since not much is known about how the ingestion of specific foods may influence our aromas, curious researchers from the Czech Republic decided to compare the body odor of vegetarians to the body odor of red meat eaters. Seventeen men maintained either a "meat" or "nonmeat" diet for 2 weeks. The men on the meat diet were fed beef for lunch and dinner during the final 4 days. Then 30 brave women sniffed underarm pads worn by the men during the last 24 hours of the diets and rated the samples according to their pleasantness. The scent of the pads worn by the nonmeat eaters was rated as considerably more pleasing and less intense than that of those worn by the meat eaters.

If your diet is largely carnivorous and your natural scent is something akin to a goat's, do yourself a favor and opt instead for heart-friendly vegetables or white meat. Both your heart and your friends will thank you.

put chamomile in a cloth bag and add it to your bath or apply spent tea bags directly to your armpits. They've come in handy whenever I've needed a quick underarm wipe.

Chamomile is near the top of the list when it comes to antibacterial effectiveness and safety, but there are other herbs with deodorant properties that you can either brew or bathe with: thyme, myrrh, licorice, oregano, rosemary, ginger, nutmeg, cinnamon, lemon balm, peppermint, spearmint, and bay.

★**Parsley** Ever wonder why your dog vomits after eating grass? It could be because grass contains chlorophyll, a compound that binds to toxins and escorts them from the body via vomit and sweat. It's that bonding action that makes chlorophyll one of the most powerful internal deodorants you can buy (or grow). In the mid-1950s, doctors administered chlorophyll to patients with colostomies and foul-smelling wounds to control the odor. Today, some people swear by chlorophyll supplements to freshen everyday body odor. Before buying supplements, though, try munching on sprigs of parsley or adding this savory herb to omelets, salads, and soups. If you're not a fan of its slightly peppery taste, there are plenty of other greens to choose from. Anything green and leafy, including spinach, kale, endive, and alfalfa, is chock-full of chlorophyll. Broccoli and green beans are good sources as well.

★**Spinach** Inside those dark green leaves is a powerhouse of zinc, an essential mineral that the body needs for overall immune system support. It's been reported that a zinc deficiency can aggravate body odor. Breastfeeding, dieting, bouts of diarrhea, and heavy sweating can deplete zinc stores. A diet that includes spinach will help replenish this life-giving nutrient and may just make your armpits less pungent. To really give your zinc stores a boost, accent your spinach dishes with two more zinc-rich vegetables, cucumbers and cowpeas. If you favor a different flavor, choose other foods high in zinc, such as parsley, collards, Brussels sprouts, spring beans, endive, prunes, and asparagus. (If you suspect you have a zinc deficiency, be sure to see your doctor.)

★**Vinegar** Vinegar could be the world's oldest medicine. It's been said that Hippocrates used it as an antibiotic and a general health elixir in 400 BC. Sweat-munching bacteria thrive in alkaline environments, and acids such as vinegar neutralize the alkalinity, making your skin inhospitable to bacteria. Simply pour white distilled vinegar on a soft cloth and give your underarms a good wipe. To avoid stinging, don't apply it to freshly shaved or irritated skin.

From the Herbal Medicine Chest

Sage is one of several special herbs in the mint family that are known to dry up bodily secretions, most notably sweat. You can make your own soothing underarm massage lotion that will reduce perspiration and deodorize with just a few ingredients. Dilute sage essential oil in vegetable oil (try a drop or two of essential oil per tablespoon of vegetable oil) and rub the mixture into your armpits.

Bronchitis

IF YOU HAVE A COLD OR THE FLU and develop a cough that produces phlegm (what doctors call a purulent cough), you may have bronchitis. It causes wheezing, difficulty breathing, chest pain, a sore throat, and fatigue. You may also have a fever, chills, muscle aches, and nasal congestion.

More than 12 million people get bronchitis every year. It can happen at any age, but children are hit the hardest. It's diagnosed more than two times as often in kids under age 5 than in other age groups.

In adults, smoking and exposure to toxic gas, dust, or pollution put you at risk for chronic bronchitis, which is defined as having a cough almost every day for at least 3 months of the year for 2 years in a row. Smoking and pollution cause inflammation and thickening of the bronchial tubes.

There's a misconception, though, about the pathogen that causes bronchitis. It's often blamed on bacteria, but more and more, I think that other pathogens, such as fungi and viruses, are involved in any "-itis," or inflammation. Until you're positive of the pathogens, you can't know which antibiotics, if any, are best.

In fact, research has been unable to demonstrate that they help acute bronchitis at all, and the Centers for Disease Control and Prevention has advised against their use in most cases. Doctors, however, continue to prescribe them for up to 80 percent of bronchitis patients, both adults and children.

I advise against using an antibiotic unless your doctor says it's right for the particular pathogen that's causing your bronchitis. If your condition is viral, an antibiotic won't help. I also recommend loading your food and herbal shotgun with a broad spectrum of phytochemicals that can nip away at the enemies causing your bronchitis and possibly boost your immune system.

Most of the foods and culinary herbs you'll read about in this chapter are what I call broad-spectrum antiseptics that contain antibacterial, antifungal, and antiviral compounds, which can help subdue most of the pathogens that could be caus-

FOODS TO WATCH

Bronchitis hits when your immune system is already weak from a cold or the flu, so keeping yourself as healthy as possible, even when you're sick, will help you avoid the problem. That means avoiding or limiting your consumption of certain foods such as those listed below.

High-fat and high-sugar foods. When you're eating french fries instead of a salad and drinking soda instead of vitamin C–packed orange juice, you're missing out on the nutrients and phytochemicals you need from immunity-boosting foods. Save lower-nutrient foods for an occasional splurge on a healthier day, and stick with those that offer only the best protection from bronchitis.

Dairy products. Milk and other dairy foods can increase the amount of mucus in the airways, so you may want to avoid them when you have bronchitis.

ing the bronchitis. When it comes to an upper respiratory infection caused by a virus, plant medicines are the best medicine.

Healing Foods for Bronchitis

★★★**Elderberries** Wine, juice, or jam made from these berries provides antiviral, immunity-boosting agents for anyone who has a cough or cold, the flu, allergies, or a fever.

Studies have found an elderberry extract called Sambucol effective for stimulating the immune system because of its flavonoids and anthocyanins, which have anti-inflammatory activity. New research even hints that Sambucol may work as well as the prescription drug zanamivir (Relenza).

I'm sure that all genuine elderberry wines contain many of the same ingredients as Sambucol. Although it is the only formulation that's been effective in clinical trials, elderberry jam, juice, and wine haven't been studied yet. I trust the food first and the extract second because our bodies have evolved to respond to what we find in nature.

Of course, if you're taking a cold medicine, you shouldn't drink wine, but I'd rather go the other way and drop the pharmaceutical in favor of elderberry wine while getting other immunity boosters from my food.

★★★**Garlic and onions** For bronchitis, garlic is my supreme immunity-boosting broad-spectrum antiseptic of choice. The pungent garlic bulb contains antiviral and antibacterial chemicals along with a menu of compounds with anti-bronchitic activity. And the Jews of Yemen used onion to treat respiratory ailments by crushing it, mixing it with sour goat's milk and crystallized sugar, and drinking it.

We still need well-designed human studies on garlic's effect on respiratory diseases, but preliminary research suggests that it helps make upper respiratory infections less severe. In one study done on mice, researchers found that garlic extract inhibited an antibiotic-resistant microorganism, called *Pseudomonas aeruginosa*, that causes chronic lung infections in people with cystic fibrosis. I suspect that many other pathogens that are resistant to monochemical antibiotics will respond favorably to polychemical garlic, especially in humans with generally healthy immune systems.

Once you've eaten garlic, it actually releases chemicals that travel to the lungs and protect them from inflammation. That's why you get garlic breath when you eat hummus or anything else with a strong garlic taste. (You can take care of that problem by chewing on a few sprigs of parsley, by the way.) When I have a deep-seated bronchial problem, I begin to expectorate shortly after ingesting raw garlic or even garlic capsules.

★★★**Guava** This sweet fruit from the Caribbean is packed with vitamin C, which means it can go a long way toward helping you get over a bout of bronchitis. Vitamin C from a supplement has been shown in studies to help with allergies, asthma, respiratory infections, nasal congestion, and watery eyes.

In one study, researchers gave 57 elderly patients, who were in the hospital because of bronchitis and bronchial pneumonia, either 200 milligrams of vitamin C or a placebo each day in supplement form. After 4 weeks, the patients who received vitamin C showed significant improvement in their respiratory function.

Eating a medium guava gives you 165 milligrams of vitamin C. Of course, reaching for citrus fruits such as oranges, grapefruits, and tangerines also boosts the vitamin C in your diet. Even adding ½ cup of chopped red bell pepper or a medium papaya adds 95 milligrams to your daily total.

Making fresh fruits and vegetables part of your meals throughout the day should always be your goal, but it wouldn't hurt to take 500 to 1,000 milligrams of supplemental vitamin C, says Richard N. Firshein, DO, medical director of the Firshein Center for Comprehensive Medicine in New York City and author of *Reversing Asthma*.

★★★**Thyme** Germany's Commission E—a government agency that evaluates the safety and efficacy of medicinal herbs—has approved thyme for bronchitis and other upper respiratory conditions. This culinary herb stimulates the immune system, works as an antiseptic, and helps clear mucus from the respiratory tract. My friend Martha Libster, RN, author of *Delmar's Integrative Herb Guide for Nurses*, points out that early patent medicines for respiratory problems like bronchitis, laryngitis, sore throat, and whooping cough contained thyme.

I recommend making a thyme decoction to use as a gargle for bronchitis and sore throat. A tea decoction involves putting the herb in water and boiling or sim-

Cough Crucifix Soup

Anyone with bronchitis, a cough, a cold, the flu, or sinusitis should try what I call Cough Crucifix Soup, which contains vegetables that fall under the label crucifers. Crucifers include all members of the cabbage or mustard family, including broccoli, cabbage, collard greens, cresses such as watercress, kale, turnip, and kohlrabi (a cabbage with a turnip shape). The hot compounds in cabbage and mustard greens have antiseptic properties and tend to open the sinuses. Add those vegetables, along with horseradish, wasabi, or garlic, to help with a cough. The hotter, the better.

mering it for 10 or 20 minutes, allowing the medicinal phytochemicals to be released. You can also add cardamom, cinnamon, peppermint, or a licorice stick to the tea, but the thyme itself contains more than a dozen different antiseptic compounds, making it another broad-spectrum antiseptic.

★★**Bran cereal** Oat bran and bran cereal help heal bronchitis because they contain a good amount of magnesium. If your magnesium levels are low, you're at higher risk for respiratory diseases such as bronchitis. In a study from the 1990s, researchers asked 2,633 adults in the United Kingdom about their dietary habits to measure how much magnesium they got in their diets. Those with higher magnesium intakes had better lung function and had experienced less wheezing during the previous year. Some naturopaths recommend taking 300 to 600 milligrams of magnesium a day to prevent respiratory problems.

A ½ cup of 100 percent bran cereal has 93 milligrams of magnesium, and the same amount of dry oat bran packs 96 milligrams. Another option is brown rice, with 1 cup of cooked rice providing 86 milligrams of magnesium. It would be a good idea to eat the whole grains along with other sources of magnesium, such as almonds, hazelnuts, peanuts, spinach, and okra, throughout the day.

Other good sources include purslane, green beans, poppy seeds, cowpeas, licorice (the root, not the black or red candy twists), lettuce, and nettle. Or you could turn to soybeans, nuts, fish, dairy products, and lean meats. Even better, make a vegetable "MagneSoup" with some or all of these ingredients to get a good amount of magnesium.

★★**Camu-camu** It may be difficult to find, but this grape-size fruit from the Amazon has even more vitamin C than guava. Eating just a few of these delicious fruits will give you 500 milligrams of vitamin C, and ½ cup contains some 2,000 milligrams. I just returned from the Amazon, where I introduced 40 North American ecotourists, including several nurses, pharmacists, and physicians, to the marvelous camu-camu.

★★**Cayenne, chile peppers, ginger, horseradish, and mustard** Irwin Ziment, MD, of the UCLA School of Medicine, routinely recommends hot spices such as red and black pepper, ginger, horseradish, and mustard for asthma, bronchitis, and other chronic respiratory problems.

Using spicy foods was probably part of an old Mayan tradition, and some Mayans even added hot pepper to their hot chocolate. Peppers dilate blood vessels and help relieve chronic congestion, while other hot foods irritate the mucous membranes in the nose and throat and cause them to weep a watery secretion, which helps release mucus when you cough or blow your nose.

Mustard Blaster Salad Dressing

For bronchitis, pneumonia, and other respiratory conditions, I like to make a salad dressing called the Mustard Blaster. Using a mortar or pestle, juice blender, or coffee grinder, grind 1 ounce of mustard seed (pure, mixed white, black, or garlic mustard), then add enough vinegar to keep it nearly liquid. Add a dash of ground horseradish and/or wasabi, followed by 5 to 10 drops of lemon juice. For texture and taste, add enough cornmeal to thicken the mixture. If you'd like to increase the medicinal qualities of the dressing (but possibly lose the taste), add a dash of thyme and/or some finely chopped fresh garlic. (Be aware that these ingredients can pack a wallop, causing a burning sensation in your mouth; you can turn down the heat by adding more cornmeal.) After you finish your salad, chew on a licorice stick (not anise candy) to add another superfood to your arsenal against bronchitis.

Dr. Ziment recommends eating a chile pepper a day with meals. In addition to easing bronchitis, it can be helpful for colds, coughs, and hay fever. Chicken soup with hot pepper added may also be a pleasant decongestant.

As with garlic, hot peppers seem to induce expectoration; sometimes capsaicin, the substance that gives them their heat, is used experimentally to induce cough-like responses in animal models and humans. Capsaicin hasn't been declared an expectorant, to my surprise, but peppers do contain at least five other expectorant phytochemicals.

★★**Assorted spices** When I searched my database for foods that would help with bronchitis, I came up with a list that reads like a who's who of spices, with some herbs and foods thrown in. Anise and chamomile made the list, as well as apricot, caraway, cardamom, cinnamon, colt's foot, corn mint, couchgrass, dandelion, dill, elder, eucalyptus, fennel, galangal, garlic, horseradish, nasturtium, onion, radish, ribwort, and star anise. To fight bronchitis, it's a good idea to plan your meals around as many of these foods as possible.

★★**Mint** More than a millennium ago, water mint (a close kin to peppermint) was recommended for lung problems that produced phlegm. More recently, German scientists began recommending menthol or mint oil for allergies, pharyngitis, croup, laryngitis, sinusitis, and bronchitis. They found that using camphor, eucalyptus oil, and menthol as a nasal ointment helped improve nasal congestion. They also said that anise, chamomile, or peppermint simmered in a pot and inhaled as steam can help, as can putting a few drops of peppermint oil on a hankie or pillow and breathing it in several times.

You can also get benefits from drinking peppermint tea; eating peppermint candy, jelly, and sauces; and chewing peppermint gum.

★★**Watercress** This vegetable is part of the crucifer or mustard family and was approved by the German Commission E for respiratory infections. Add the leaves to your green salad, pasta salad, or stir-fry; layer them in a sandwich; or use them in soups.

From the Herbal Medicine Chest

Many of the herbs well known for fighting bronchitis contain compounds that act as antiseptics, relieve coughing, open the airways, and help clear phlegm from the respiratory tract.

In fact, pharmaceutical drugs work in the same way that these herbs do to relieve bronchitis. According to Linda B. White, MD, adjunct professor at Metropolitan State College in Denver and senior coauthor of *The Herbal Drugstore,* drugs that treat bronchitis rely on the same three activities as do the herbs. They suppress cough (antitussive), clear phlegm from the respiratory tract (expectorant), and open the airways in the lungs (bronchodilator).

Here are some herbs to consider.

Aniseed (Pimpinella anisum) If you have bronchitis and sinusitis, hot herbs such as anise can help open your sinuses. I enjoy aniseed and leaves in teas, soups (added sparingly), and liqueurs. Each imparts different proportions of many biologically active anti-bronchitic constituents.

Borage seed oil (Borago officinalis) In a study of patients with acute respiratory distress syndrome who were receiving treatment in a critical care unit at the Mayo Clinic, 150 people who were given borage seed oil, fish oil, protein, carbohydrates, and antioxidants via a tube inserted through the nose had a 35 percent increase in survival odds. The researchers think it was the gamma-linolenic acid in the oil that caused the beneficial effects. The oil has the highest concentration of gamma-linolenic acid found naturally (although it's also found in evening primrose oil and black currant seed oil).

Chamomile (Matricaria recutita) Inside a cup of chamomile tea lies an arsenal of compounds that can help with bronchitis. Chamomile is a good source of apigenin, an herbal COX-2-inhibitor (a pain reliever). Beneficial substances are especially abundant in chamomiles that come from Rome and Hungary, according to French scientists who compared those chamomiles with others in the US Department of Agriculture database. Just a quart of the tea has significant anti-inflammatory activity.

You may also benefit from inhaling the aroma of the chamomile flowers as you boil the water and when you pour it over the flowers. Be careful not to get too close to avoid being scalded.

Elecampane _(Inula helenium)_ Elecampane is well endowed with antiviral and antibacterial as well as expectorant compounds. Gazmend Skenderi, author of _Herbal Vade Mecum_, recommends using the root in teas for asthma, bronchitis, colds, and cough. However, certified lactation consultant Sheila Humphrey, RN, author of _The Nursing Mother's Herbal_, gives it a low score for safety with nursing mothers, as it's frequently reported to be allergenic.

Licorice _(Glycyrrhiza glabra)_ Licorice scored highest in my database search for anti-bronchitic foods. It has a long folk history, and laboratory evidence has confirmed its effectiveness. Theophrastus, the so-called father of botany who lived from 373 to 287 BC, suggested using licorice for asthma, bronchitis, and cough. I rank licorice (along with garlic) as tops for bronchitis and other pulmonary afflictions.

You can buy licorice as a standardized herb and add it as a sweetener to the aromatic teas mentioned in this chapter. But licorice also has its downside. Long-term use can lead to headaches, lethargy, sodium and water retention, loss of potassium, and high blood pressure. You shouldn't use it regularly for longer than 6 weeks, and don't take it if you're pregnant or nursing or if you have severe liver, kidney, or heart disease or high blood pressure. If you're taking a diuretic, you should also avoid licorice.

Bruises

WHEN I FIRST STARTED WORKING ON THIS CHAPTER, ironically, I had a bruise just above the elbow on my left arm. At first, I didn't know where it came from, but then I realized I probably had gotten it while shoveling snow earlier in the day. I had hit a block of ice frozen to the pavement, which made me lose my grip on the shovel and the shovel to strike my arm.

Most bruises are caused by similar mishaps: Some part of your body hits something hard like a desk or coffee table, or something hard hits you. The black-and-blue marks that result are caused by blood leaking out of the capillaries that lie just beneath the skin. Black eyes are more common in men, and bruises on the legs are more common in women. In my case, since there was no pain with my bruise—just the unsightly discoloration—I chose not to treat it.

As a matter of fact, I don't remember *ever* treating a bruise, on myself or anyone else. I could see myself trying to mask a black eye if I were about to lecture a bunch of Pacific herbalists, but I think I'd do that with nonfood "pancake" makeup. But I do believe that some natural foods can help prevent and treat bruises and the swelling, discoloration, and soreness that accompany them.

Healing Foods for Bruises

★★★**Pineapple** Because it contains the healing compound bromelain, pineapple seems to be an effective treatment for a black eye. In a 1960 study, 74 boxers with numerous bruises received bromelain supplements four times a day, and 72 bruised boxers received placebos. After 4 days, 78 percent of the boxers treated with bromelain had no signs of bruising compared with only 14 percent of those taking placebos (it took 7 to 14 days for their bruises to heal).

★★★**Pomegranate and guava** These show great promise for preventing bruising. You might try mixing the juice of both fruits, along with bilberry/blueberry juice and basil, oregano, and turmeric to taste.

★★**Blueberries** I truly believe that foods rich in vitamin C and bioflavonoids can strengthen weakened capillaries and help prevent the blood leakage that results in the black and blue of a bruise. Janet Maccaro, ND, PhD, a naturopath and holistic nutritionist in Ormond Beach, Florida, and author of *Natural Health Remedies A–Z*, points out that vitamin C– and bioflavonoid-rich foods also help build collagen. The quicker collagen is formed and the thicker it becomes, the shorter the healing time for bruises.

For a nice vitamin C–flavonoid combo, try eating some blueberries, which are a good source of both. They contain a type of flavonoid called proanthocyanidins, which are known to strengthen the walls of capillaries weakened by bruising. Blueberries also have the capillary-preserving compound rutin and two others (eascin and hyperoside) with similar qualities. Try adding them to some buckwheat pancakes in the morning. Buckwheat is also a significant source of rutin.

★★**Citrus fruits** These fruits are another excellent source of vitamin C and bioflavonoids, and I believe increasing your intake can help bruises heal faster.

In nature, vitamin C is usually accompanied by bioflavonoids, and there are proven synergies between the two. If you want to boost your intake of bioflavonoids, try açai juice, which comes from an Amazonian palm fruit. Another Amazonian gem is camu-camu, by far the richest known source of vitamin C. Both are

Following the Folklore

In addition to the remedies listed for bruise treatment and/or prevention, my ethnobotany database lists several other food species esteemed in folklore for treating bruises, including the following: among the nuts, coconut and pistachio; among the fruit-bearing species, cantaloupe, elderberries, grapes, passionfruit, peaches, and plums; and among herbs and vegetables, amaranth, carrots, celery, dandelion, dill, marigolds, plantain, poppies, radishes, thyme, and turmeric.

available online. Other, more familiar foods high in vitamin C and bioflavonoids include blueberries, citrus juices, citrus peel marmalades, guava, tomatoes, and peppers.

★★**Green leafy vegetables** Another vitamin that may help ward off bruising is vitamin K. For reasons that aren't exactly clear, people deficient in this vitamin seem to be more prone to bruising. To get more in your diet, eat leafy greens such as spinach and kale, as well as broccoli and Brussels sprouts.

★★**Pansies** These flowers are an outstanding source of the bioflavonoid rutin, which is more a preventive than a curative for bruises. I may be the only person I know who eats a fresh pansy every day when they're available. One flower could give you a significant dose of rutin—about 20 milligrams—and I think this little boost may lessen my susceptibility not only to bruises but also to glaucoma, hemorrhoids, and varicose veins. Not too keen on eating flowers? You can apply wild pansy directly to a bruise to treat it topically.

★**Chamomile** To soothe your nerves and the discomfort of a bruise, you might try some chamomile tea. Chamomile contains analgesics and anti-inflammatories, including a half dozen COX-2 inhibitors. While enjoying my chamomile tea, I might also apply the chamomile tea bag, or a regular green or black tea bag, to the bruise.

★**Parsley** As a topical remedy, Jim LaValle, ND, a pharmacist, naturopathic physician, and founder of the LaValle Metabolic Institute in Cincinnati, suggests using parsley. Chop some up, place it on the bruise, and wrap the area with an elastic bandage for about an hour. The parsley will decrease inflammation, reduce the pain, and help the bruise fade more quickly. It contains the preventive compound rutin, but more important, it contains nearly two dozen anti-inflammatories, more than a half dozen analgesics, and some compounds that deter swelling.

★**Potatoes** This topical remedy has withstood the test of time: Old-timers claim that placing a raw potato on a bruise is more effective than using a beefsteak, and I agree, even though I'm not a vegetarian. I'm cheap, though, so I would cook and eat the potato (and the steak) after I placed it on my black eye. I'm not sure I'd recycle my parsley, though.

From the Herbal Medicine Chest

Just as effective as bruise-healing remedies that take the form of foods are some treatments that fall more into the herbal category. Here are some herbs that may help prevent and/or speed the healing of a bruise.

Cayenne (Capsicum frutescens) Because of its anti-inflammatory, antiseptic, and capillary-strengthening properties, cayenne appears to be a potentially effective remedy for preventing and treating bruises. An ointment made from 1 part cayenne pepper and 5 parts petroleum jelly has been used successfully in China and Taiwan to treat bruises when applied every 1 to 2 days.

St. John's wort (Hypericum perforatum) This herb helps prevent and treat bruises because it acts as an antioxidant. Although I would have said St. John's wort is not a food, Francois Couplan, PhD, in his *Encyclopedia of Edible Plants of North America,* says "the leaves are edible in small quantities" and notes that they can be added to salads or made into teas. One study done at the University of Georgia College of Pharmacy looked at the antioxidant properties of St. John's wort in human vascular tissue and found that it inhibits free radical production, thus making it useful for treating bruises.

St. John's wort may also be used topically in the form of oil. The oil is rich in tannins, astringents that help control capillary bleeding and shrink tissue. For maximum effect, start applying it as soon as you spot a bruise and reapply it three times a day.

Burns

BURNS HAPPEN IN AN INSTANT. It takes only a slight touch on a hot stove, a flame, or an iron to cause one. But the pain, unfortunately, can linger for hours, days, or weeks, depending on the depth of the burn.

Burns come in three degrees of severity. First-degree burns, such as sunburns, injure only the outermost layer of skin. Although they hurt, they aren't nearly as painful as second-degree burns, which penetrate deeper into the skin and cause blisters. Oddly, the worst kind of burns, third-degree burns, often cause no pain at all because the injury has destroyed the nerves that transmit pain signals to the brain. Both second- and third-degree burns covering an area larger than a quarter need immediate medical attention—no food will suffice to treat them.

For first-degree and mild second-degree burns, however, there are some natural food remedies that appear to help. Take the potato, for example, touted by a fan of *The Green Pharmacy* in a letter to the editor.

You have a wonderful book. I just bought it. In looking at what you have about the potato, I see you have failed to mention how great it is when used for burns, either grated or thinly sliced. We have used this for years in our family. It stops all pain and helps the healing process, although I have never figured out why. I recently had a 3x4-inch hot oil burn on my arm, and I used grated potato on it for two days. I just washed it with soap and water and kept putting the potato on. Four days later, I still felt no discomfort. My doctor looked at it five days after the injury occurred and said it was a second-degree burn, and he couldn't believe it didn't hurt. The potato stops all pain and cools the burn immediately.

Well, I looked into his claim and did several of my Multiple Activity Menu (MAM) queries at www.ars-grin.gov/duke/dev/all.html, and lo and behold, potato had the highest synergy score for burns of any foods that I checked. This doesn't prove that potato can magically cure burns, but it does suggest that this vegetable has a lot of phytochemicals that may help soothe minor ones.

Healing Foods for Burns

Potato is certainly worth a try for mild burns or smaller second-degree burns (my reader's 3x4-inch hot oil burn is larger than recommended for self-treatment, but luckily, he came out okay). Below are some other food remedies that you may want to try.

★★★**Chamomile** Chamomile tea is an excellent brew and gets the seal of approval from my friend Adriane Fugh-Berman, MD, associate professor in the department of physiology and biophysics at Georgetown University School of Medicine and author of *The 5-Minute Herb and Dietary Supplement Consult*. She says that most teas made from chamomile are benign (do no harm) when applied topically, and they may help calm the pain of a burn. Chamomile reportedly can cause allergic reactions, but they are rare.

Why does it work? When I started my usual search for a chemical rationale, I saw that chamomile contains the chemical alpha-bisabolol, a powerful anti-inflammatory. In fact, it's the best source of the chemical that I've found.

★★★**Onions** These flavorful bulbs seem to aid in healing burns. From Africa and Italy to America, chopped onions, chives, and leeks have been applied—with or without reason—to burns. Perhaps antisepsis is the rationale. Or maybe, as new research suggests, the onion reduces burn-related scarring. A study published in the journal *Trauma* showed that the anti-inflammatory phytochemical quercetin, which is found in onions, was effective for preventing, and to a lesser extent, curing, raised red scars. Martha Libster, RN, author of *Delmar's Integrative Herb Guide for Nurses,* says mashed onions can be used as poultices on burns, and the skins, rich in quercetin, can be boiled gently and applied to burned skin. It just may help reduce scarring. To improve the poultice even more, I might add onion skins along with corn (with the silk intact) to boiling water. Then the water would contain both anti-scarring allantoin and quercetin. Or if I were more intent on making medicine than cooking a meal, I'd boil up a mixture of corn silk, onion skins, and ginger.

★★★**Water** It may sound simple, but one of the best remedies for burns is good old-fashioned H_2O. First, rinsing burned skin under cool water (not cold, which can do more harm than good) right after the injury occurs will immediately soothe the pain. And since burns can leave you dehydrated, sipping eight 8-ounce glasses of water per day can keep your skin moisturized and help healing at the same time.

★★**Garlic** As a great believer in garlic, I looked for new studies on garlic for treating burns. Unfortunately, the ones I found were more concerned with garlic causing burns. To be honest, some of my garlic-laden dishes, with raw garlic, do sometimes burn my mouth, although the sensation is generally more pleasant than uncomfortable. But some people are truly allergic to garlic, and other sensitive individuals can suffer mild chemical burns from it when it's freshly cut and raw. In one case cited in a medical journal, a nursing mother burned her breast with garlic while trying to treat herself for an undiagnosed skin condition, and the authors suggest that the lactating breast may be especially susceptible to garlic burns.

However, despite these exceptions, garlic generally aids healing. In their book *Garlic: Science and Therapeutic Application of* Allium sativum L. *and Related Species*, Heinrich Koch and Larry Lawson relate that garlic has long quickened the healing of burns, sores, and wounds. Its phytochemicals increase the regeneration of skin, preventing secondary infections. I recommend mashing garlic and applying the paste to a burn as a poultice.

★★**Oats** Both old-style oatmeal porridge and newer instant oatmeal seem to alleviate various skin irritations, including burns, when applied topically. Australians—who may be even more conservative about herbal alternatives than Americans—studied a product containing liquid paraffin and 5 percent colloidal oatmeal to reduce the itch experienced by burn patients. After acute burn patients used either the product with oatmeal or an oil containing just liquid paraffin for 10 months, the group using the oatmeal product reported significantly less itching than the group using the liquid paraffin alone.

★★**Tea** Kampo (Japanese alternative medicine) practitioners apply green tea to help heal burns. Western healers sometimes use spent tea bags, which are rich in tannins and polyphenols, on minor burns. Historically, tannins were once sprayed on serious burns, creating a protective membrane known as an eschar.

★**Apples** Rich in pectin, apples may act as yet another effective topical treatment for burns. A Russian study looked at the results of treating burn wounds with a 1 to 2 percent solution of apple or beet pectin. The best results occurred when the pectin was applied from the day the burn injury occurred. I would try rubbing a piece of raw apple on a burn for the first few days after the injury to see if it improves.

★**Cucumber** Not only does cucumber offer a refreshing taste, but its flesh is also cooling, making it a good remedy for burns. Carolyn Dean, MD, ND, and her Chinese medicine guru, Jeffrey Yuen, suggest you make a cucumber paste and apply it to a burn like a poultice to draw out the heat.

★**Elderberry** Early American eclectic healers used elderberry—more often the edible flowers than the fruits—for burns. I wouldn't hesitate to use the fruit of the elderberry to rub on sunburned skin. John Heinerman, PhD, an anthropologist and author of many books on herbal healing, recommends cold elderberry juice for burns and inflammation in his book *Heinerman's Encyclopedia of Healing Juices*. You may feel less pain if you drink fermented elderberry juice.

★**Flaxseed** You may want to try the biblical herb flaxseed on a burn. Over a thousand years ago, German abbess and author Hildegarde von Bingen wrote, "Whoever has been burned anywhere on his body should boil flaxseed [a.k.a. linseed] in water, dip a linen in it [remember, linen is derived from flax, too!], and place the cloth over the area of the burn." Today, trying this may help a bit, as long as you use a clean cloth to maintain sterility. Linseed oil mixed with an equal quantity of lime water, known as Carron oil, has been described as an excellent application for burns and scalds.

★**Ginger** The juice of the ginger root is useful for burns caused by heat (as opposed to chemical burns). In China, cotton balls soaked in ginger juice are used to treat first- and second-degree burns. The juice reportedly helps reduce pain, inflammation, and blisters. To soothe your own burn, try doing the same.

★**Honey** Ancient Egyptians used honey to treat burns, and it seems they were smart to do so. A study done in New Zealand, Nigeria, and the United Arab Emirates found that honey indeed helps burns. To help a burn heal faster, Janet Maccaro, ND, PhD, a holistic nutritionist in Ormond Beach, Florida, and author of *Natural Health Remedies A–Z*, suggests applying cold water for a few minutes, applying a coat of raw honey, then covering the burn with a gauze bandage.

★**Papaya** As healing takes place, perhaps a day or two after the burn, Dr. Maccaro suggests applying some papaya to the affected area since the enzymes in the fruit help remove dead cells from the wound. A Russian study substantiates her claim—it showed that the antioxidant activity of a papaya preparation decreased the severity of burn wounds in rats, specifically by reducing the risk of oxidative damage to burned tissue.

★**Sugar** For years, people have applied sugar to burns in hospitals. It sounds strange, but there is evidence that raw white sugar does a great job of protecting the wound and speeding healing. Jim LaValle, ND, a pharmacist, naturopathic physician, and founder of the LaValle Metabolic Institute in Cincinnati, suggests you run some water over the burned area and then apply sugar until it creates a glossy, glass-like barrier. Do this twice a day until the burn is healed.

★**Tofu** Admitting a long, perhaps hereditary bias, I care little for tofu. I'd much rather apply it to a burn than eat it, and my friend Martha Libster notes that tofu can be used to cool burns. You can make a paste with water, tofu, and ginger, then spread it evenly over gauze to apply to a burn. It helps reduce heat, inflammation, and swelling. Tofu may also be used internally to treat burns. Highly technical French studies suggest that when patients with severe burns are fed a soy formula, it seems to enhance their recovery.

From the Herbal Medicine Chest

Several herbs can help reduce the pain of a burn and speed healing. You may want to try one of the following.

Calendula (Calendula officinalis) Calendula is an age-old folk remedy for treating burns. Its flowers are best known for use in skin care. Extracts promote healing by stimulating the reproduction of epithelial cells (cells that are closely packed together and form the outer layer of your skin). For this reason, it has been used not only for minor abrasions but also for radiation burns, scalds, mild skin burns, razor burns, mild sunburns, and windburns. Calendula compresses applied promptly to injured skin inhibit bacterial, viral, and fungal microorganisms. The herb also contains three phytochemicals—caffeic acid, chlorogenic acid, and rutin—that help protect collagen in the skin from the ravages of sunburn.

Lavender (Lavandula angustifolia) Loaded with analgesics, antibacterials and anti-inflammatories, lavender is easy to take internally. The leaves, petals, and flowering tips of English lavender make a great addition to dressings, jams, jellies, salads, soft drinks, soups, stews, vinegars, and wines. Jim LaValle, ND, a pharmacist, naturopathic physician, and founder of the LaValle Metabolic Institute in Cincinnati, suggests you also apply some essential oil of lavender topically to minor burns.

Plantain (Plantago major) A barely edible plant (more likely to be found in Metamucil than in the produce aisle at the supermarket) that helps ease burns is the plantain, not to be confused with the banana relative also called plantain. Simply take juice from the fresh leaves of the plant and apply it directly to the burn. I have used this remedy many times and found it very soothing.

Bursitis

BETWEEN OUR BONES and the muscles or tendons near joints are fluid-filled sacs, which help cushion the joints. These are called bursae, and if they become inflamed, the result is bursitis, a painful condition that affects about 8.7 million Americans.

Bursitis is most often caused by overuse of particular joints, often the wrists and shoulders. I know that from personal experience, having been stricken with bouts of bursitis due to physical activities such as hunching over a computer, driving long distances, mowing the aisles in my Green Farmacy Garden, and playing guitar and bass fiddle in a bluegrass group.

If you get a diagnosis of bursitis, your doctor is likely to recommend over-the-counter nonsteroidal anti-inflammatory drugs such as aspirin and ibuprofen or a prescription COX-2 inhibitor such as celecoxib (Celebrex). However, all of these medications can cause side effects, some of them very serious. Instead of taking that chance, you may want to try some foods from nature's pharmacy instead. Below are some that I recommend.

Healing Foods for Bursitis

★★★**Turmeric** This yellow curry spice is a rich source of curcumin, a strong antioxidant that protects against free radical damage. Curcumin contains natural painrelieving COX-2-inhibitors, which makes it an attractive and safe alternative to prescription COX-2 inhibitors. It also reduces inflammation by lowering histamine levels and possibly by stimulating the adrenal glands to produce more cortisone, the body's natural painkiller. Lately, I've had two students who switched from Celebrex to either curcumin or curried celery and thought it was a good tradeoff. (See my Curried Celery COX-2 Inhibitor recipe on page 286.)

Human studies of curcumin have found that it can reduce the pain and stiffness associated with rheumatoid arthritis as well as help relieve postsurgical inflammation. I prefer a whole-foods approach whenever possible because as I've said elsewhere, I believe you get more healing power from whole foods than from individual components. I often add liberal amounts of curry to rice and other dishes and would consider adding other anti-inflammatory foods such as pineapple and papaya.

Unfortunately, it's difficult to get a medicinal dose of curcumin from your diet alone. According to many naturopaths, that dose is 250 to 500 milligrams of pure curcumin a day, which translates into 5 to 25 teaspoons of dried turmeric daily. That's a good deal more than even a curry fan like me would want to add to my food, so I would recommend adding as much turmeric as possible to your diet to help prevent pain and, to help relieve it, take turmeric supplements standardized to 90 to 95 percent curcumin.

One note: Curcumin isn't very efficiently absorbed, but you can increase absorption significantly by taking your dietary turmeric or supplemental curcumin with freshly ground black pepper.

★★**Celery** It wasn't long after Celebrex, rofecoxib (Vioxx), and other prescription COX-2 inhibitors were promoted as the new "miracle aspirin" that herbalists said, "Wait a minute. Many foods and edible spices contain natural COX-2 inhibitors, and they're unlikely to cause any adverse side effects." Two of the best sources of natural COX-2 inhibitors are celery and celery seed, which contain high amounts of painkilling apigenin. When I was diagnosed with gout and looking for an alternative to the prescription drug allopurinol (Zyloprim) as a way to reduce my uric acid levels, I found that either eating four celery stalks or taking two to four tablets of celery seed extract daily all but eliminated my gout attacks. If I were again stricken with a bout of bursitis, I know that celery would be a gentler medicine than the cortisone shot my doctor would want to give me. If you have bursitis, I'd recommend either trying the regimen I use for gout or sampling my Curried Celery COX-2 Inhibitor recipe. Alternatively, you might try preparing a tea by pouring boiling water over 1 teaspoon of freshly crushed celery seeds and letting it steep for 10 to 20 minutes before drinking.

★★**Chamomile** Although best known as a calming herb, chamomile also contains potent anti-inflammatory compounds such as apigenin, luteolin, and quercetin. If you sample my Curried Celery COX-2 Inhibitor, you might try chasing it with a cup of chamomile tea. Naturopaths recommend drinking three or four cups a day to treat painful conditions such as bursitis. You might also try taking 2 to 3 grams of the herb in tablet or capsule form or 4 to 6 milliliters of tincture three times a day between meals. You can also apply a topical chamomile cream or ointment to the affected area three or four times daily.

★★**Chile peppers** Hot peppers contain a resinous and pungent substance known as capsaicin, which is number one among my painkillers. In fact, you'll probably be surprised to learn that capsaicin is a potent COX-2–inhibiting anti-inflammatory. When applied topically, capsaicin temporarily depletes substance P, a chemical in nerves that transmits pain sensations. Without substance P, pain signals can no longer be sent. Dozens of studies show that capsaicin can temporarily relieve many painful conditions, including bursitis.

You can buy a commercial topical cream containing 0.025 to 0.075 percent capsaicin and apply it to your sore spots three or four times a day. Or you can do what people outside the United States often do: buy a chile pepper, mash it, and apply it directly. You can also mix mashed hot pepper with a skin cream such as cold cream. Either way, you'll save money. A fresh pepper costs a few pennies, whereas a commercial capsaicin product such as Zostrix can cost up to $16.

No matter which route you choose, you may experience a burning sensation the first few times you use capsaicin, but it usually subsides with repeated use. Just be

FOODS TO WATCH

I would recommend avoiding foods that contribute to inflammation. Some of the worst offenders are refined foods that contain lots of added fat, sugar, salt, additives, and preservatives. Snack foods in particular are likely to contain large amounts of pro-inflammatory trans fatty acids, omega-6 fatty acids, and high-fructose corn syrup, which is also a major player in our nation's obesity epidemic.

Food Remedies That Work

sure to thoroughly wash your hands after using it. If you get any in your eyes, nose, or mouth, it may be almost as painful as your bursitis.

Although capsaicin is best used topically, it may be helpful to add more peppers and pepper-derived hot sauces to your diet. Ingesting hot peppers increases your internal painkillers, called endorphins, and provides a bit of nature's aspirin, salicylic acid.

Another option is taking a cayenne tincture (0.3 to 1 milliliter) three times a day. You can also make an infusion by stirring ½ to 1 teaspoon (2.5 to 5 grams) of cayenne powder into a cup of boiling water, letting it stand for 10 minutes, and taking 1 teaspoon mixed with water three or four times daily.

★★**Ginger** Ginger contains high amounts of zingibain, a powerful anti-inflammatory enzyme that according to some experts is as powerful as the bromelain in pineapple or the papain in papaya. But ginger contains 180 times more anti-inflammatory enzymes than the papaya plant and may be even more effective at relieving the symptoms of bursitis. It's easy to get enough ginger in your diet to help reduce pain. You can take it as an herb in tea by steeping three or four slices of fresh ginger in a cup of boiling water, or, if you prefer, you can get medicinal doses in tinctures or capsules. I, however, prefer ginger as a liberal and tasty addition to my daily diet. You can get medicinal doses by sprinkling ½ teaspoon of powdered ginger into your foods or by eating about an ounce (6 teaspoons) of fresh ginger every day.

In Asia, ginger has an extensive history as a treatment for bursitis. To get an added anti-inflammatory effect, try using it in combination with pineapple and licorice. In moderate amounts—up to three cups of tea a day—licorice is usually safe. But in larger amounts, long-term use can cause some serious side effects (see From the Herbal Medicine Chest on page 93).

★★**Leafy greens** Because many alternative practitioners suggest that magnesium-rich leafy vegetables may be effective for bursitis, I've created my own Magnesium Medley, which includes purslane (which contains nearly 2 percent magnesium by dry weight), green beans, poppy seed, cowpeas, spinach, snake gourd, licorice, lettuce, and nettle. For even more benefits, you might try drinking apple cider vinegar and honey after rising in the morning or taking 1 tablespoon of cod-liver oil an hour or two before meals. I confess, when I'm on the road, I take a supplemental magnesium pill if I have nighttime leg cramps, which annoy me more often than bursitis. In this case, one capsule does the trick, but a second capsule can give me a touch of diarrhea.

★★**Mint** Peppermint, spearmint, Chinese mint, and other mint oils contain high amounts of menthol, which when applied topically can help relieve the pain associated with bursitis. Although you can buy commercial products containing menthol, it may be a better (and cheaper) bet to apply mint oils directly to your sore spots (but be aware that such oils are toxic when consumed internally in large quantities). Another option is to drink peppermint tea two or three times a day. Although many commercial mint teas are available, I'd recommend making your own by pouring 1 cup of boiling water over 1 heaping teaspoon (5 grams) of dried peppermint leaves and steeping for 5 to 10 minutes; drink three to four cups daily. For extra benefits, consider stirring a delicious peppermint/chamomile tea with a licorice stick, which will give you a host of analgesic and anti-inflammatory compounds. Another option is taking 3 to 6 grams of peppermint leaf tablets or capsules a day.

★★**Oregano** This is a welcome weed in the Green Farmacy Garden. For almost any inflammatory condition, it's a treasure house of active compounds—eight natural COX-2 inhibitors, more than a dozen analgesics and anesthetics, and more than two dozen anti-inflammatory compounds. Nowhere—not on PubMed or in any of my herbal reading—have I seen oregano prescribed or recommended for bursitis, but the chemistry tells me it is worth recommending. It's a key ingredient in some anti-inflammatory medicines, and I now add it to my celery curries. Even in mid-winter, I can go out and strip old dry florets off my oregano, pour boiling water over them, add lemon and stevia, and have an Organic Oregano Anti-inflammaTea. Many of the herb's useful phytochemicals are easily absorbed by the skin and can also be inhaled, so breathe in the wafting aromatics between draughts. You can make a poultice of the dregs and apply it topically near the sore bursa to get even more relief. By the way, everything I've said today about oregano can also be said about rosemary. You can stir Anti-inflammaTea with a licorice stick, thus adding some of the magic anti-inflammatories of licorice.

★**Flaxseed** Studies show that increasing your dietary ratio of anti-inflammatory omega-3 fatty acids to pro-inflammatory omega-6 fatty acids can benefit more than 50 common ailments, including inflammatory conditions such as bursitis. When I see such a long list for any nutrient or herb, I'm somewhat skeptical, but scientists I respect seem to think that omega-3's can make an enormous difference in your health. Although the richest sources are cold-water fish and fish oil, many plant species also contain high amounts of omega-3's. These include flaxseed oil, canola oil, chia oil, walnut oil, soybean oil, and wheat germ oil. So far, I haven't been bold enough to concoct a fish-oil salad dressing (which might make sense if you like anchovies in your salad). In most cases, walnut oil may be more pleasing to the palate.

★**Pineapple** This exotic fruit is rich in a number of substances that can help people with conditions such as bursitis. Foremost among them is bromelain, a proteolytic enzyme that helps reduce the swelling and inflammation of many painful "-itis" (inflammatory) conditions. Its anti-inflammatory effects are so profound that the German government has approved its use for healing after injuries and surgical procedures. Pineapple also contains high amounts of manganese, which is essential for the formation of collagen, the tough, fibrous protein that builds connective tissues such as bone, skin, and cartilage. You can get 100 percent of the daily value for manganese (2 milligrams) from just a cup of fresh pineapple chunks or pineapple juice. Pineapple is also a rich source of vitamin C, also necessary for collagen formation, offering more of this important vitamin than apples, cranberries, or tomato juice. A cup of fresh pineapple chunks contains 24 milligrams of C, or 40 percent of the Daily Value. To get the maximum antioxidant punch, try "Gold" pineapple, which is imported from Costa Rica and contains four times more vitamin C than other pineapples.

Unfortunately, recent research suggests that levels of both bromelain in fresh pineapple and papain, a related enzyme in fresh papaya, may be too low to relieve a bad bout of bursitis. While I would encourage enjoying these fruits—either whole or as juice—you'll probably need to take supplements to get effective levels. Naturopaths suggest taking anywhere between 250 and 500 milligrams of bromelain three times a day. In human studies, a daily dose of up to 2,000 milligrams has not proven harmful.

From the Herbal Medicine Chest

I consider licorice to be the poor man's herbal alternative to corticosteroids, mostly because it doesn't cause nearly as many adverse side effects. It contains at least 24 anti-inflammatory compounds, 5 of which are natural COX-2 inhibitors. It's also a potent antioxidant that's rich in flavonoids and magnesium, a mineral that has proven benefits in treating bursitis. You might try taking 5 to 6 grams of licorice-root capsules a day or 500 milligrams of licorice extract three times a day. You also can make a tea by boiling ½ ounce (14 grams) of licorice root in 1 pint of water for 15 minutes and drinking two or three cups a day. But don't use licorice for more than 6 weeks, since long-term use can cause high blood pressure. Avoid it entirely if you have high blood pressure; are taking diuretics; are pregnant; or have cardiomyopathy, diabetes, liver disease, or thyroid problems. I like to use a licorice stick to stir my chamomile tea, which adds bit more COX-2–inhibiting activity, but it's probably not enough to cause worrisome side effects.

Canker Sores

CANKER SORES MAY BE TINY, but the pain they inflict can be big. Unfortunately, we don't know what causes them, even though experts have been trying to figure that out for as long as people have been getting them. Researchers have noticed, however, that certain conditions can make some people more susceptible than others.

People frequently confuse canker sores with cold sores. Cold sores are blistering lesions that almost always occur on the outside of your lips and are caused by a type of herpesvirus. They can be quite contagious. Canker sores, on the other hand, are ulcers that appear on the inside of your mouth, usually at the base of your gums or on the inside surface of your cheeks or lips. They often appear as shallow, whitish, round depressions inside red rings. They aren't caused by herpesvirus, they aren't contagious, and they require their own special course of treatment.

Canker sores are quite common (up to 50 percent of people have had them), especially between the ages of 10 and 40. They also tend to run in families. Some doctors report that they're more common during winter and spring.

In a tiny minority of cases, recurring or persistent canker sores can be a symptom of certain intestinal diseases or HIV/AIDS, but this happens so rarely that you shouldn't worry about it. More common triggers include stress, mouth injuries, nutritional deficiencies, and food allergies.

Even though the underlying cause of these painful lesions has eluded scientists, there are precautions you can take to lower your chances of developing them. To begin with, avoid nuts, spicy foods, and acidic foods such as oranges and pineapple. Even though these are great foods, chock-full of phytochemicals that can help with other conditions, if cankers are your main concern, you should make other choices.

Also, canker sores can crop up after minor mouth traumas such as abrasions from ill-fitting dental appliances or accidental bites to the cheek or tongue. Talk with your dentist if an appliance is irritating your mouth. Accidental bites often result from chewing and speaking at the same time—so please, take your mother's advice and don't talk with your mouth full.

Finally, consider changing your toothpaste if it contains sodium laurel sulfate (SLS), a foaming agent that creates lots of froth when you brush. SLS is a powerful detergent that removes the protective mucous layer on the inside of the lips and cheeks, says David Kennedy, DDS, past president of the International Academy of Oral Medicine and Toxicology in San Diego. You can find toothpaste without SLS in many health food stores, he says.

The good news about canker sores is that they usually heal by themselves after 7 to 10 days. If they hang around for longer than that, prevent you from eating or talking, recur, or start getting bigger, make an appointment to see your doctor.

Healing Foods for Canker Sores

There are plenty of over-the-counter remedies that may take the sting out, but a simple (and inexpensive) saltwater rinse or a few ice cubes may work just as well. Your kitchen also holds an assortment of quick and easy remedies to quell the pain, so give these a try.

★★**Raspberries** Certain cultures, such as the Micmac population of Canada, have used raspberries to treat various kinds of sores. It's the astringent leaves or root bark, rather than the fruits, that appear to contain various analgesic, antiviral, anti-inflammatory, and antiseptic compounds. These properties make the raspberry plant a prime candidate for treating oral sores, including canker sores.

★★**Sage** Well known for drying out secretions, sage is admirably equipped to help heal oral sores. It has a long folk history as a remedy; in fact, certain cultures like to fashion the sage plant into toothbrushes. I'm not sure I'd want to rub a canker sore with sage, but I might try a sage tea as a mouth rinse.

★**Black tea** Several over-the-counter products contain tannins, astringent polyphenols that bind liquids, absorb toxins, and soothe inflamed tissues inside the mouth. Fortunately, you may have those same tannins right in your kitchen. Witch hazel, periwinkle, eucalyptus, and goldenseal are just a few of the many herbs that are rich in these astringents. If you don't have any of these on hand, however, any tea will do. Just place a spent tea bag right on the sore to relieve the pain.

★**German chamomile** Chamomile scores even better than black or green tea as a treatment for canker sores. I'd drink the tea, and maybe even suck on the spent tea bags. Like my other top scorers for canker sores, it is loaded with painkillers and sore- and ulcer-healing properties.

★**Yogurt** The kindest thing you can do for a mouth that's been "cankered" is to eat foods like yogurt that are soft and easy to swallow. And yogurt may help for another reason. Researchers agree that bacteria in the mouth aggravate cankers, so foods that make your mouth's pH less hospitable to bacteria, including yogurt, may relieve the pain and even prevent ulcers from coming back. If you're struggling with an eruption right now, try eating at least 4 tablespoons of yogurt with active cultures (check the label) every day.

From the Herbal Medicine Chest

For relief of canker sores, you may want to try one of these herbal remedies.

Licorice (*Glycyrrhiza glabra*) The sweet root of the licorice plant has soothing and coating abilities that people with canker sores are sure to appreciate. Researchers from the University of Washington and the American Academy of Oral Medicine in Seattle studied 46 adults with recurrent canker sores. Half of them applied a patch with licorice extract to their ulcers for 16 hours a day, while the other half agreed not to treat their sores with any medication. After 8 days, the group using the herbal patches had significantly smaller sores and less pain than did the group without the patches.

You can purchase oral patches with licorice extract, or you can easily brew your own treatment. Boil ½ ounce (14 grams) of licorice root in 1 pint of water for 15 minutes. Keep the pain at bay by drinking one to two cups a day when your canker sores are especially tender. Don't drink this tea for longer than 10 days, however, because licorice can cause high blood pressure and water retention. Instead, wash the area, swishing the liquid back and forth over the sore.

Myrrh (*Commiphora* spp.) Myrrh contains a veritable treasure chest of constituents that make it ideal for soothing and healing canker sores. It has impressive anti-inflammatory, antioxidant, and antimicrobial actions. In fact, Germany's Commission E, a government agency that evaluates the safety and efficacy of medicinal herbs, has given myrrh its stamp of approval for the treatment of mild mouth and throat inflammations. The commission recommends dabbing undiluted tincture right on the sore.

Carpal Tunnel Syndrome

INSIDE EACH OF YOUR WRISTS is a "tunnel" that allows blood vessels, ligaments, and a nerve called the median to pass through to the fingers. If tissues inside the tunnel become inflamed and swollen, they can compress the median nerve and cause carpal tunnel syndrome (CTS), a collection of symptoms that include pain, weakness, finger stiffness, and a pins-and-needles sensation that may be especially noticeable during sleep. CTS affects five times as many women as men and usually develops in people between the ages of 30 and 60.

Until recently, researchers believed that CTS results from repetitive stress on the hands and wrists during work or recreational activities. However, recent evidence suggests that genetics may play at least as important a role. According to a 2007 study of 4,488 twins published in the *British Medical Journal*, heredity is even more important than environmental stress on the wrists in predicting who will—and won't—develop CTS. New research presented at the 2007 annual meeting of the American Academy of Orthopaedic Surgeons showed that people who continuously use their hands at work—such as construction workers and court reporters—don't develop CTS more frequently than other people.

Although I spend up to 15 hours a day on my computer on cold winter days, I haven't yet developed CTS. That may be partly due to my genetics or my gender. Women are more likely to develop this disorder, due to the hormone fluctuations of menstruation, pregnancy, and menopause. I also make a habit of taking frequent breaks from my computer work, during I which roll Chinese balls in my hands for relaxation. Since the balls contain little bells, this is not only a physically soothing sensation but a psychically soothing one as well.

The most recent estimates, published in a 2008 issue of the journal *Arthritis and Rheumatism,* show that a whopping 4 to 10 million Americans have CTS. That means that as many as 1 in 30 Americans—at any given moment—are coping with distress that at best can dramatically affect their quality of life and at worst can be totally incapacitating.

The financial toll of CTS and similar conditions—which include osteoarthritis, rheumatoid arthritis, fibromylagia, gout, and back pain—adds up to an astounding $128 billion a year in lost wages and medical expenses. By the year 2030, it's estimated that 40 percent of American adults will be affected by some form of arthritic disease.

Unfortunately, good pain relief is hard to come by. CTS is often treated with over-the-counter and prescription nonsteroidal anti-inflammatory drugs. But 50 percent of respondents to a 2005 national survey conducted by the Stanford University School of Medicine reported that such medications were ineffective for pain.

If your doctor advises surgery for CTS, think twice. Although surgery can be effective, it's invasive and creates scar tissue that can make the condition worse. If you're overweight, losing a few pounds—which reduces pressure on the median nerve—may be as effective as surgery.

If I had CTS, I'd much prefer to wear wrist splints at night than undergo surgery. In a 2005 study published in the *Archives of Physical Medicine and Rehabilitation,* researchers from the University of Michigan randomly assigned 112 autoworkers either to wear splints at night or watch an instructional video. After 3 months, about 50 percent of the splint group reported significantly decreased hand, wrist, elbow, and forearm pain, and one patient even obtained complete relief.

Another conventional treatment—local steroid injections—may also be preferable to surgery. In a 2005 study published in *Arthritis and Rheumatism,* Spanish researchers compared outcomes in 101 patients—including 93 women—who either received injections or underwent operations. After three months, 94 percent of the injection group had significantly reduced nocturnal symptoms compared to 75 percent of the surgery group. After a year, outcomes were the same in both groups, suggesting yet another reason why you should avoid the scalpel if possible.

Healing Foods for Carpal Tunnel Syndrome

To help prevent CTS—or manage lingering or lessening pain—a number of food remedies can prove useful. Here are some to try.

★★★**Basil** The unholy basil in my Green Farmacy Garden contains at least eight natural COX-2 inhibitors and tastes good, too. I would use it in pesto and add oregano and rosemary, along with the hot pepper mentioned on page 99. I've made a carpal pesto that includes avocado, which would get some all-important vitamin B_6 into the system. For a double whammy, have a cup of chamomile or green tea with your pesto.

★★★**Turmeric** This yellow curry spice is a rich source of curcumin, a strong antioxidant that protects against free radical damage. Curcumin contains natural pain-relieving COX-2-inhibitors, which makes it an attractive, side effect–free alternative to prescription COX-2 inhibitors such as celecoxib (Celebrex). It also reduces inflammation by lowering histamine levels and possibly by stimulating the adrenal glands to produce more cortisone, the body's natural painkiller. Lately, I've had two students who switched from Celebrex to either curcumin or curried celery and thought it was a good tradeoff. (See my Curried Celery COX-2 Inhibitor recipe on page 286.)

Human studies have found that curcumin can reduce the pain and stiffness associated with rheumatoid arthritis as well as help relieve postsurgical inflammation.

I prefer a whole-foods approach whenever possible because I believe you get more healing power from whole foods than from individual components. I often add liberal amounts of curry to rice and other dishes and would consider adding other anti-inflammatory foods such as pineapple and papaya. You can also make tea with turmeric.

Unfortunately, it's difficult to get medicinal doses of curcumin from your diet alone. According to naturopaths, that dose is 250 to 500 milligrams of pure curcumin per day between meals, which translates into 5 to 25 teaspoons of dried turmeric daily. I would recommend adding as much turmeric as possible to your diet

FOODS TO WATCH

If you have carpal tunnel syndrome, don't use the artificial sweetener aspartame. One study found that people who consumed the most aspartame were most likely to develop CTS. It also found that symptoms subsided within 2 weeks in people with CTS who stopped using the sweetener.

to help prevent CTS and taking turmeric supplements—standardized to 90 to 95 percent curcumin—to help relieve acute symptoms.

An herbal supplement called Zyflamend contains turmeric and several other edible herbs, all of which have several phytochemcials that may help alleviate CTS. Available in health food stores, Zyflamend is a blend of turmeric, ginger, green tea, holy basil, oregano, rosemary, and other herbs with anti-inflammatory properties.

★★**Avocado** Avocados are high in vitamin B_6. Many studies suggest that a B_6 deficiency can either increase your susceptibility to CTS or make the symptoms worse. Many experts believe that the typical Western diet contains too little B_6. Avocado dip can be pleasant way to get your daily quota and possibly alleviate CTS. You can jazz up the dip with COX-2–inhibiting spices, such as hot pepper, basil, ginger, oregano, rosemary, and turmeric.

To ensure that you get enough B_6 each day, eat more avocados, bananas, barley, brown rice, cauliflower, chickpeas, mangoes, okra, prunes, salmon, sesame, spinach, sunflower seeds, sweet potatoes, and watercress. Many of these foods also contain antioxidants and other compounds that may help reduce the inflammation associated with CTS.

Some research suggests that much higher amounts of B_6 are needed to treat severe cases of CTS, and naturopaths often recommend getting 40 to 80 milligrams twice a day. Because you would be hard-pressed to obtain that dose from food, supplements may be an option. Andrew Weil, MD, professor at the University of Arizona College of Medicine in Tucson, suggests taking 100 milligrams of B_6 twice a day. Just be sure to get your doctor's permission beforehand. In daily doses over 200 milligrams, this vitamin can cause nerve damage, which may actually worsen your CTS.

★★**Chamomile** Although best known as a calming herb, chamomile also contains potent anti-inflammatory compounds such as apigenin, luteolin, and quercetin. If you sample my Curried Celery COX-2 Inhibitor, you might try chasing it with a cup of chamomile tea. Naturopaths recommend drinking three or four cups per day to treat painful conditions such as CTS. You might also try taking 2 to 3 grams of the herb in tablet or capsule form or 4 to 6 milliliters of tincture three times per day between meals. You can also apply a topical chamomile cream or ointment to your wrists three to four times daily.

★★**Chile peppers** Hot peppers contain a resinous and pungent substance known as capsaicin, which is number one among my painkillers. When applied topically, capsaicin temporarily depletes substance P, a chemical in nerves that transmits pain sensations. Without substance P, pain signals can no longer be sent. Capsaicin is a potent COX-2 inhibitor; dozens of studies show that it can temporarily relieve many painful conditions, including CTS.

You can buy a commercial topical cream containing 0.025 to 0.075 percent capsaicin and apply it to your aching wrists three or four times a day. Or you can do what people outside the United States often do: buy a chile pepper, mash it and apply it directly. You can also mix mashed hot pepper with a skin cream such as cold cream. Either way, you'll save money. A fresh pepper costs a few pennies, whereas a commercial capsaicin product such as Zostrix can cost up to $16.

No matter which route you choose, you may experience a burning sensation the first few times you use capsaicin, but it usually subsides with repeated use. Just be sure to thoroughly wash your hands after applying it. If you get any in your eyes, nose, or mouth, it may prove almost as painful as your tingling wrists.

Although capsaicin is best used topically, it may be helpful to add more peppers and pepper-derived hot sauces to your diet. Another option would be to take a cayenne tincture (0.3 to 1 milliliter) three times per day. You can also make an infusion by stirring ½ to 1 teaspoon (2.5 to 5 grams) of cayenne powder into 1 cup of boiling water, letting it stand for 10 minutes, and taking 1 teaspoon mixed with water three or four times daily.

★★**Flaxseed** Flaxseed is a rich source of omega-3 fatty acids—especially alpha-linolenic acid, which helps reduce levels of pro-inflammatory chemicals called prostaglandins. It also contains lignans, which help neutralize free radicals, the unstable oxygen molecules that contribute to inflammation. Based on the evidence I've seen, I'd try a daily regimen of 25 to 30 grams (about 3 tablespoons) of ground flaxseed or 1 to 3 tablespoons of flaxseed oil to combat the symptoms of CTS. Remember that store-bought flaxseed is often whole, but it can't be digested unless it's ground. If you eat whole flaxseed, you may reap a royal stomachache instead of any anti-inflammatory benefits. Try adding ground flaxseed to hot cereals or baking flour. Be sure to promptly refrigerate any unused ground flaxseed to prevent spoilage.

★★**Pineapple** This exotic fruit is rich in a number of substances that can help people with conditions such as CTS. Foremost among them is bromelain, a proteolytic enzyme that helps reduce the swelling and inflammation of many painful "-itis" (inflammatory) conditions. Its anti-inflammatory effects are so profound that the German government has approved its use for healing after injuries and surgical procedures. Pineapple also contains high amounts of manganese, which is essential for the formation of collagen, the tough, fibrous protein that builds connective tissues such as bone, skin, and cartilage. You can get 100 percent of the daily value of manganese (2 milligrams) from just a cup of fresh pineapple chunks or pineapple juice. Pineapple is also a rich source of vitamin C, also necessary for collagen formation; it contains more of this important vitamin than do apples, cranberries, or tomato juice. A cup of fresh pineapple chunks contains 24 milligrams, or 40 percent of the daily value for C. To get the maximum antioxidant punch, try "Gold" pineapple, which is imported from Costa Rica and contains four times as much vitamin C as other pineapples.

Unfortunately, recent research suggests that levels of both bromelain in fresh pineapple and papain, a related enzyme in fresh papaya, may be too low to relieve a bad case of CTS. While I would encourage enjoying these fruits—either whole or as juice—you'll probably need to go the supplement route to get seriously effective levels. Naturopaths suggest taking anywhere between 250 and 500 milligrams of bromelain three times a day. In human studies, a daily dose of up to 2,000 milligrams has not been shown to be harmful.

From the Herbal Medicine Chest

Willow bark—the original source of aspirin—is rich in salicylates, which reduce pain as well as inflammation. To make a tea, steep 1 to 2 teaspoons of dried, powdered bark or 5 teaspoons of fresh bark in hot water for about 10 minutes, then strain. You may wish to flavor it with something sweet like honey in order to blunt the bitter taste. If I had carpal tunnel syndrome, I'd drink two or three cups of this tea daily. If you're allergic to aspirin or can't tolerate its side effects, however, avoid willow bark.

Cataracts

THE WORD CATARACT HAS TWO MEANINGS, and neither one of them is pleasant to experience. The first meaning is a huge waterfall or deluge of water, and the second meaning—the one that concerns us now—refers to a medical condition in which the lens of an eye becomes cloudy or opaque. I have the dubious distinction of having experienced both.

While I can only imagine plunging over a waterfall to be immersed in the white water below, I did canoe into the cloudy whiteness of some class 2 cataracts (my son seeks out even more adventurous ones). And I have "slid" down some of those slippery-sloped stones in the mountains of North Carolina. The other type of cataract affects the lens that sits behind the eye's pupil, and it slowly causes your vision to become blurred—as if you're looking at life through a waterfall. If left untreated, a cataract can lead to blindness.

More than half of all Americans either have cataracts or have had cataract surgery by the age of 80, according to the National Institutes of Health, and I fell into that group myself at age 77. On February 15, 2007, Cupid's arrows were put aside in favor of a surgeon's knife, a process that took only 6 hours from the start of surgery until my return home. I can say, after my cataractomy, that if you have cataracts and can afford to remove them, it's worth the cost and effort.

Even better, of course, would be to improve your diet in order to lessen the chances of needing such surgery in the first place. While foods and herbs can't cure cataracts, I won't hesitate to say that they can delay the formation or progression of cataracts.

What causes cataracts in the first place? Most cataracts are related to aging, and they occur when the protein in the lens starts to clump together and cloud the vision. Over time, more clumping occurs and your vision progressively becomes more blurred. Why the protein clumps isn't clear, but possible causes include exposure to ultraviolet rays or radiation, smoking, and diabetes. As a chain-smoking heliophile, I had my share of UV and smoke. These factors lead to free radicals—highly reactive oxygen molecules that cause lots of damage inside the body.

To combat oxidative damage, you naturally want to pull out the antioxidants, specifically by turning to the following foods.

Healing Foods for Cataracts

★★**Almonds** While wheat germ oil may have the highest concentration of vitamin E, you're unlikely to eat it on its own. Almonds, on the other hand, have 40 percent of the Daily Value of vitamin E in a 1-ounce serving, and you can eat dry roasted almonds plain or mix them into salads or other meals.

★★**Broccoli and spinach** A study in the *American Journal of Clinical Nutrition* looked at a specific group of antioxidants—carotenoids, which are natural pigments that color vegetables yellow, orange, and red—and concluded that among the list of foods high in carotenoids, broccoli and spinach were most associated with a lower risk of cataracts.

Why did those two catch the researchers' eyes? Both of them are packed with lutein and zeaxanthin, the only two carotenoids that accumulate in the retina and other ocular tissues. The men in the study who were in the highest fifth in terms of lutein and zeaxanthin intake had a 19 percent lower risk of cataracts than those in the bottom fifth. The FDA hasn't set Daily Values for lutein and zeaxanthin, but from the results of this study you can see that more is better. (The only possible risk of overdose from lutein is carotenoderma, in which the skin takes on a slight yellow-orange discoloration. If you cut down on the foods that contain lutein, this unnatural coloring will vanish over time.)

★★**Carrots** As you might guess from the name, carrots are a decent source of beta-carotene, with one large carrot providing 6 milligrams. Carrots fit well into soups, sandwiches, salads, and other dishes, so you can mix them into a variety of meals.

★★**Kale, collard greens, and turnip greens** A few vegetables that top even broccoli and spinach in the amount of lutein and zeaxanthin they contain are kale, collard greens, and turnip greens—yet they didn't show up in the previous study. Why? Very few participants included them in their diet! It's hard to get any benefit from vegetables if they're not on your plate (and, needless to say, not going into your mouth). Ounce for ounce, kale far surpasses all other vegetables in the amount of lutein and zeaxanthin it contains. Mrs. Duke, a Northerner, and I, a Southerner, speculate that Yankees prefer spinach, beet greens, lambsquarters, and chard (in the bland lambsquarter family), and Southerners prefer the more pungent cabbage family (collards, kale, and turnip greens). I like the latter. She doesn't. Two years my junior, she hasn't experienced the cataract surgeon's knife.

Note that turnip roots themselves contain no lutein and zeaxanthin; all of that goodness is kept in the leaves.

★★**Sunflower seed kernels and hazelnuts** Other sources of vitamin E include these crunchy goodies. Dry roasted sunflower seed kernels boast 30 percent of the Daily Value in 1 ounce, and hazelnuts have 20 percent in 1 ounce.

★★**Sweet potatoes** One of the big risk factors for cataracts is smoking, but a 12-year-long study that was published in the *Archives of Ophthalmology* in 2003 found that men who smoked and took 50 milligrams of beta-carotene on alternate days had a 26 percent reduced risk of cataracts compared with smokers who didn't take beta-carotene.

The best long-term action that you could take to improve your health would be to stop smoking, but I realize that not everyone is willing to take this step. If you fall into this group, maybe you can balance your smoking with a snack of sweet potatoes. A cup of sweet potatoes has 11 milligrams of beta-carotene, enough to get you started toward that goal of 50 milligrams every other day.

★★**Wheat germ oil** In addition to lutein and zeaxanthin, a 2008 report in the *Archives of Ophthalmology* found that participants who consumed the most vitamin E also had a lower risk of cataracts. While the Daily Value of vitamin E is 30 International Units (IU), most nutritional labels list the amount of vitamin E in milligrams; vitamin E exists in multiple forms, and 1 milligram of one type isn't the same as 1 milligram of another type.

Those details aside, you can turn to wheat germ oil for all the vitamin E that you need in a day. One tablespoon of wheat germ oil includes 20 milligrams of the alpha-tocopherol form of vitamin E, which equals 100 percent of the Daily Value. You can use wheat germ oil in salad dressings or mix it with freshly cooked pasta.

★**Capers, onions, and peppers** Believe it or not, rats develop cataracts just as humans do, but research has shown that ingestion of quercetin slows down oxidative damage to the lens in rats and may play a role in preventing the formation of cataracts. Quercetin is a flavonol, which is a specific type of flavonoid, and flavonoids have antioxidant properties.

There's no recommended level for quercetin in rats, much less in humans, but the foods that contain the most quercetin are capers, peppers (but only the hot varieties, especially hot yellow wax peppers), and onions.

★**Cranberries, elderberries, and bee pollen** You don't have to stick with strong savory flavors to have quercetin in your diet. These sweet treats feature the flavonol as well, as do less common berries such as the crowberry, chokeberry, and bog whortleberry.

★**Dried tea leaves** By far the food item that boasts the most quercetin is dried tea leaves, both black and green. But the US Department of Agriculture database for brewed tea shows almost no quercetin. This means that the only way to get the quercetin from the leaves into your body would be to ingest the leaves, so brew up a batch of tea from the leaves and drain the cup dry without using a filter.

Colds and Flu

SOME ESTIMATES SAY that Americans get a billion colds a year, and there are more than 200 viruses that can cause them. Millions of people get the influenza virus each year. About 200,000 develop complications from the flu and have to be hospitalized, and nearly 36,000 die from it.

Both of these viral diseases can spread easily. All it takes is close contact, whether you inhale a virus or pick it up from a surface an infected person has touched.

Cold symptoms tend to last 1 to 2 weeks, with the first signs being sneezing, a scratchy throat, and a runny nose; later, you can have nasal congestion, cough, muscle aches, and a headache. Colds can lead to bronchitis, pneumonia, ear infections, sinusitis, and an increase in asthma symptoms.

The flu, on the other hand, hits suddenly and can give you a high fever, headaches, a dry cough, a sore throat, a runny or stuffy nose, muscle aches, and an upset stomach that last from 2 days to 2 weeks. It may also make you feel extremely fatigued and may lead to pneumonia in some people.

At the first sign of a cold or the flu, I feed my aching body garlic soup with onions. Unfortunately, too few Americans look to their pantry for relief. Instead, they reach for over-the-counter cold and cough medications, which have little to no effect on their symptoms, and they miss out on the opportunity to fight off the virus with food.

Americans turn to these medicines in astounding numbers. According to an article in the journal *American Family Physician,* one survey found that nearly a quarter of all adults in the United States had taken a cold or cough medication during the previous week.

Unfortunately, studies have found again and again that cold and cough medications don't work. At best, they may give you some relief from your symptoms, but they certainly won't shorten the duration of your illness. And although an antibiotic won't do anything to kick a viral cold or the flu, it's prescribed for 60 percent of patients who see their primary care doctors for these illnesses. The flu vaccine is recommended to help prevent the flu, and antiviral drugs can help you recover once you have it.

In the meantime, you have powerful cold and flu fighters right at your fingertips: immunity-boosting foods that can keep you healthy during fall and winter. Rather than running to the drugstore for a cold or cough remedy that doesn't work, run to the supermarket and pick up the ingredients to make healthful cold- and flu-fighting meals right in your kitchen.

Healing Foods for Colds and Flu

One reason adults have fewer colds than children do is that we build our immunity as we get older. But any time your immunity dips, you're at risk of catching a virus. One way to stay in tiptop shape is to eat a diet full of immunity-boosting foods.

★★★**Chicken soup** Chicken soup has been used as a cold remedy for centuries. Moshe ben Maimon (Maimonides), a 12th-century Egyptian Jewish physician, told his patients to eat chicken soup for respiratory symptoms, according to Stephen Rennard, MD, of the University of Nebraska Medical Center. In fact, Jews sometimes call chicken soup Jewish penicillin.

Not only does the soup provide the fluids you need to help fight off viruses, but studies have found that it reduces inflammation, which leads to colds. Dr. Rennard and his researchers collected blood from healthy volunteers. In the laboratory, after exposing the samples to several diluted variations of chicken soup, they watched the movement of neutrophils, the most common type of white cells in the blood that defend against infection. They found that the soup reduced the activity of the neutrophils, which they suspect lowers the activity in the respiratory tract that causes inflammation and cold symptoms. In other words, the soup can give you much-needed relief.

The researchers couldn't pinpoint a specific ingredient in the soup that made it an effective cold fighter, so they believe it's the combination of vegetables and chicken that soothes symptoms. The soup they made included a stewing hen or baking chicken, chicken wings, onions, a sweet potato, parsnips, turnips, carrots, celery, parsley, and salt and pepper. I recommend adding lots of garlic, ginger, and hot pepper.

If you're not well enough to cook, buy some chicken soup from the supermarket. Researchers found that even commercial soups were effective.

★★★**Citrus fruits and other foods rich in vitamin C** When researchers reviewed 21 studies that used 1 to 8 grams of vitamin C a day, they found that this antioxidant reduced cold symptoms by 23 percent, on average.

In one study done in the United Kingdom, 168 people received either a vitamin C supplement or a placebo twice a day for 2 months between November and February. Those taking vitamin C had significantly fewer colds or recovered from colds more quickly. And a group of six studies that examined runners, skiers, and soldiers

FOODS TO WATCH

Some foods can derail your efforts to sidestep a cold or the flu this winter. Here's what to pay attention to.

Too much caffeinated coffee, tea, or cola. Staying well hydrated helps boost your immunity and fight off a cold or the flu, but caffeine can dehydrate you. Be sure to keep caffeinated drinks to a minimum during cold and flu season.

More than one or two alcoholic drinks. In addition to causing dehydration, drinking too much alcohol lowers your immunity and makes you more likely to catch a virus. A glass of red wine or elderberry wine may help increase your immunity, but don't go overboard by drinking too much. Experts recommend that women stick to one glass of wine a day, while men should stop after two.

who were exercising in a subarctic climate showed that vitamin C lowered their risk of catching a cold by 50 percent.

Many experts suggest taking 1,000 milligrams of C a day, but it's always a good idea to get as many phytochemicals as you can from food. I prefer to get my vitamin C from as few pills as possible and enjoy eating the foods that provide it.

I recommend reaching for citrus fruits, bell peppers (especially red ones), broccoli, Brussels sprouts, butternut squash, cantaloupe, kiwifruit, papaya, strawberries, sweet potatoes, and tomatoes. In the summer, I like to add crushed cherries, another fruit that contains vitamin C, to my lemonade.

Of course, I can't close this discussion without mentioning my tropical friends camu camu and acerola, which put citrus fruits to shame as far as vitamin C is concerned. Camu-camu also packs antiviral, decongestant, and analgesic compounds, whch together will give any cold or flu bug a run for its money.

High amounts of vitamin C can cause diarrhea in some people, so if you notice this side effect, cut back on your supplement dose.

★★★**Elderberries** These small, dark berries contain more than a dozen antiviral compounds and flavonoids that stimulate the immune system to help ward off disease. They also contain anthocyanins, which help reduce inflammation and relieve the aches and pains of a cold or the flu.

Russell Greenfield, MD, a leading practitioner of integrative medicine and medical director of Carolinas Integrative Health, advocates treating flu with black elderberry, but he notes that Sambucol, an elderberry extract available in drugstores, is the only preparation that has been shown effective in clinical studies.

A small study published a few years ago showed that 93 percent of flu patients given Sambucol were completely symptom free within 2 days; those taking placebos recovered in about 6 days.

Dr. Greenfield is right about Sambucol being the only preparation proven effective in clinical studies, but that's because studies haven't been done on elderberry wine, juice, or jam. I argue that having a glass of the wine or juice or spreading the jam on your bread may be even more effective. Our ancestors have been eating elderberries for millions of years, so our bodies are programmed to grab those flavonoids when we eat them. Our genes also recognize the phytochemicals in elderberries that aren't present in Sambucol or the prescription drug zanamivir (Relenza), which treats the flu.

We won't know which is better at beating the flu—elderberries or Relenza or Sambucol—until they're compared in clinical trials. But if I had the flu, I'd try the food first, followed by the elderberry extract, and finally new pharmaceuticals like Relenza.

★★★**Garlic, onions, and leeks** If you want to increase the effectiveness of your chicken soup, add plenty of garlic and onions. Together they contain probably more than a dozen broad-spectrum antiseptic compounds and more than a dozen immunity boosters. They also help open the sinuses and keep vampires at bay. (I'm not kidding about the vampires; in our jungle hammock in Panama, those who ate the most garlic were less liable to be bitten by vampire bats.) Garlic contains one of the most potent broad-spectrum antibiotics among plants, called allicin, as do other members of the garlic family.

Like chicken soup, garlic and onions have been used for health for centuries. According to a Midrashic tale (an interpretation of the Hebrew Bible), a rabbi called Yehuda was walking to Jerusalem when he asked a boy if the Jerusalem water was clean enough to drink. The boy responded by saying, "Do not worry. There are plenty of onions and garlic." Perhaps the clever boy understood that garlic and onions were antiseptic and would reduce the level of pollution in the water.

Researchers have found that garlic specifically helps keep a cold at bay. In a Finnish study, 52 volunteers were given Nasaleze cellulose extract (a plant material) alone or with powdered garlic extract. They were told to spray it into each nostril once a day or three times a day if they developed an infection while traveling. After 8 weeks, those who received the combination of cellulose and garlic had significantly fewer infections than those who received only the cellulose.

In another study, 142 people were given either a placebo or a garlic supplement for 12 weeks between November and February. The volunteers who were given garlic reported a total of 24 colds, while those receiving placebos got 65 colds. And when the participants did get colds, the placebo group had them for significantly longer, the researchers said.

★★★**Ginger** Inside the shavings of a ginger root are chemicals called sesquiterpenes that specifically work against rhinoviruses, the most common family of cold viruses. Ginger also contains substances that suppress coughing and reduce pain and fever. It's even a mild sedative, which can help you rest when you're sick with a cold. I recommend adding a couple of tablespoons of shredded gingerroot to your teacup and pouring boiling water over it to make a soothing hot infusion.

★★★**Honey** The World Health Organization has cited honey as a potential remedy for colds because it coats the throat and relieves irritation. It also has antioxidant and antimicrobial properties, which help fight infections from viruses, bacteria, and fungi.

In one study, researchers at the Pennsylvania State University College of Medicine directed the parents of 105 children who had upper respiratory infections and a nighttime cough to give their kids either a spoonful of buckwheat honey (a dark

Feeding a Fever

The first question you may want to ask yourself when you're pondering fever remedies is, Do I even want to treat my fever? Nature may have equipped living creatures with this process long ago as a useful way to fight off infections.

Typically, a fever is a sign that a virus or bacterium has invaded your body and is trying to make itself at home. Your body is trying to get rid of the invaders, much as you might turn up the heat in your home to encourage lingering visitors to wrap up their stay. By reducing a garden-variety fever, you may end up prolonging your illness.

As a result, the literature isn't brimming with home remedies for fevers, but here are a few tips that may make you more comfortable or relieve your fever should you choose to go that route. Most of these remedies are intended for adults; a fever in a baby or toddler may be a more serious sign that may require a call to your doctor. Call the doctor for your own fever if it's over 103°F or lasts for more than 3 days.

Drink up. Your body loses more fluids when you're running a temperature, so be sure to drink plenty to replace them. Water is a good choice, or you may try some of the other fluids recommended below.

Stay warm. Drinking warm fluids can help keep you from becoming uncomfortably chilled and shivery when you have a fever. Drinking some tea or soup (warm or hot) is a good way to ward off the chills.

Sip a fever-relieving tea. According to my database, tea contains an antipyretic chemical (which means it lowers fevers) called alpha-spinasterol. Stir in some cinnamon (with antipyretic cinnamaldehyde) and ginger (with 6-shogaol and 6-gingerol). As an alternative, you can try licorice tea or goldenseal tea. Licorice contains a chemical called paeonol, and goldenseal has berberine and berberastine, which may be helpful.

Cook up my Beat-the-Heat Soup. Start with chicken noodle soup and stir in the following ingredients, all of which, according to my database, contain antipyretic chemicals: shallots (beta-sitosterol), basil (many ingredients, including menthol and alpha-bisabolol), and sweet bell peppers (eugenol).

Try fever-relieving snacks. Some good snack foods from my database contain salicylic acid, a cousin of fever-reducing aspirin. Try pumpkin seeds, raspberries, peanuts, or soybeans, all of which contain this chemical.

honey packed with antioxidants), a honey-flavored over-the-counter cough suppressant, or no treatment at all at bedtime. After just one night, the parents rated honey as the best cough relief remedy.

A warning, however: Don't give honey to children under 1 year of age. It can lead to infantile botulism, a condition in which the spores in honey germinate into bacteria in the bowel and become toxic. Taking a spoonful of honey at night also isn't something you or your kids should get into the habit of doing if you don't have a cough, because it could promote dental cavities. If you have diabetes, use caution when taking honey.

★★★**Water and tea** A common refrain from doctors when you're sick with a cold or the flu is: "Drink plenty of fluids." That's because drinking the recommended eight glasses a day helps your immune system function properly and keeps your throat moist so it's easier to clear away mucus. It also replaces fluid that's lost due to a fever. Drinking tea can pack a double whammy for a cold or flu virus. Not only does it help keep you well hydrated, it also contains compounds that help break up congestion and prevent the virus from multiplying.

Adding moisture to the air you breathe with a humidifier can also help with your symptoms.

★★★**Yogurt** A cool, creamy cup of yogurt can help stop a cold or flu virus in its tracks. When a virus invades your body, it multiplies, but yogurt that contains beneficial bacteria called *Lactobacillus reuteri* has been found to block the replication of the virus.

In one study, researchers gave 94 workers a supplement of *Lactobacillus reuteri*, while another 87 workers took a placebo. Those taking the supplement reported 56 percent fewer colds than the group taking the placebo.

As of now, there's only one brand of yogurt sold in the United States that contains these bacteria: Stonyfield Farm.

★★**Brazil nuts, seafood, and other selenium-rich foods** Just 1 ounce of Brazil nuts contains well above the daily value for selenium, a mineral that helps boost your immunity. In fact, the average Brazil nut contains about 70 micrograms of selenium, which is why I recommend these nuts as a top source. But most nutritionists will suggest delicious lobster, oysters, clams, crabs, tuna, and cod, which also contain selenium. Your choice may come down to taste, or possibly to what your body will tolerate. Some people are allergic to Brazil nuts, and some react to seafood. In studies done on mice, researchers found that a deficiency of selenium and vitamin E can make a flu infection more severe. And researchers in Britain have found that having enough selenium in your body increases the production of proteins called cytokines, which help remove the flu virus from your body.

★★**Caraway seeds** Caraway seeds scored well in my database search of foods that help with colds and coughs. The seeds are rich in limonene, which has flu-fighting properties. I would sprinkle some into any cold, cough, or flu tea I might be brewing.

★★**Grape leaves and red wine** Like the beneficial bacteria in yogurt, the resveratrol in red wine has been found to stop the flu virus from multiplying once it enters your system. Laboratory studies in Rome have found that polyphenols in the wine have a strong effect on the replication of the flu virus. If you're heading to the liquor store, you may want to pick up a bottle of pinot noir from California. University of Mississippi researchers found it to have the most resveratrol of the 11 wines they tested. You can get even more resveratrol from grape leaves, the red inner husks of peanuts, or the edible weed Mexican bamboo.

★★**Mushrooms** The mushroom, a time-honored tonic food and herbal medicine, has several pharmacologic properties, including boosting immunity. Traditionally, mushrooms were used to increase energy and support immune function, and modern scientific studies demonstrate that those effects are real. Mushrooms work by increasing the production of cytokines, which play essential roles in immune defenses against infection. Lately I've been adding more and more mushrooms and garlic to my cold-chasin' chicken soups.

★**Black pepper** Black pepper is one of the ingredients in chicken soup that makes it an effective remedy for congestion and cough. Asian Indians gargle with an infusion of black pepper to relieve a sore throat. Taking a mixture of black pepper, ground ginger, and a little vinegar helps increase the absorption of other medicines, whether they're over-the-counter cold medicines or herbal remedies.

★**Salt water or lemon water** Some doctors advise their patients to gargle with warm salt water to soothe a sore throat and relieve a cough. Drinking warm water flavored with fresh lemon juice and a little honey can have the same effect.

From the Herbal Medicine Chest

Here are some herbs that can help keep you healthy during cold and flu season.

American ginseng (Panax quinquefolius) This herb, which is different from Asian ginseng, has been shown to help keep colds and flu at bay. In one study, 279 people in Alberta, Canada, who had had at least two colds in the previous year, were given either two capsules a day of American ginseng extract or a placebo, beginning at the start of flu season and continuing for 4 months. On average, those taking ginseng had significantly fewer colds or colds of shorter duration than the placebo group.

When researchers tested Cold-fx, a standardized extract of American ginseng, with seniors, they found that it reduced the risk of developing a respiratory illness by 48 percent and the duration of symptoms by 55 percent.

We Americans don't treat ginseng as a food, but Asians often add it to soups (with pork more often than chicken).

Aniseed *(Pimpinella anisum)* The German Commission E, a government agency that evaluates the safety and efficacy of medicinal herbs, endorses aniseed for reducing phlegm. I recommend making an infusion by steeping 1 to 2 teaspoons of crushed aniseed in 1 or 2 cups of boiling water for 10 to 15 minutes.

Astragalus *(Astragalus propinquus)* This herb has been used to improve immunity in Traditional Chinese Medicine and is known for treating several viral illnesses, including colds and other upper respiratory infections, by decreasing inflammation and improving lung function. Americans rarely eat this Chinese answer to echinacea as an immune booster.

Echinacea *(Echinacea* spp.) Extracts of echinacea root have antiviral activity that fights the flu and other viruses and increases levels of properdin, a chemical in the body that strengthens immune defenses against viruses and bacteria. However, studies have been mixed about its effectiveness.

The National Center for Complementary and Alternative Medicine performed a clinical trial, published in the *New England Journal of Medicine* in 2005, that found that three echinacea root preparations, at a dose of 900 milligrams daily, failed to protect volunteers from the cold virus or reduce a cold's severity or duration. Other studies have had similar results. A Cochrane review stated that there's not enough evidence to conclude that echinacea can treat or prevent a cold.

Not all research, however, fails to show benefits. One meta-analysis published in 2007 by researchers from the University of Connecticut included 14 unique studies. They found that taking echinacea reduced the chances of getting a cold by 58 percent. It was also shown to shorten a cold.

I use echinacea because there's still good research that says it helps strengthen the immune system, but I don't view it as a miracle cure. It doesn't stop all colds.

Cold Sores

COLD SORES AREN'T REALLY SORES AT ALL. They're actually painful, fluid-filled blisters, and they're extremely contagious. They can be caused by exposure to different strains of the herpesvirus; type 1 herpes simplex used to be associated solely with cold sores and type 2 with genital outbreaks, but recent research shows that both types can cause both conditions.

Cold sores most often start with tingling in the affected area before blisters arrive 1 or 2 days later. They tend to appear on a lip, although they may develop on the chin, nostrils, or fingers as well. In rare cases, they appear on the gums or the roof of the mouth. Sores that appear anywhere else in the mouth, such as the inside of a cheek, are canker sores, which are ulcers and not contagious.

Over a period of a week to 10 days, the cold sore blisters break and ooze, then a yellow crust forms on the area and eventually falls away to reveal healthy skin underneath. Though the blister vanishes, the virus doesn't, and new outbreaks can flare up at unpredictable times—although colds, stress, and extreme weather conditions are frequent triggers.

Cold sores are uncomfortable and annoying, but they're not life-threatening. They typically disappear without treatment, and you need to visit a doctor for help only if they haven't healed after 2 weeks or they appear near your eyes. That said, you'll want to prevent future outbreaks or soothe discomfort if you have one now.

Healing Foods for Cold Sores

★★★**Fig** In addition to its proteolytic enzyme ficin, the biblical fig contains more than a half-dozen antiherpetic and a dozen antiviral compounds, plus many painkillers. If your fresh figs are still juicy, you might find some milk in the greenish skin; that's where most of the ficin is located. I'd periodically apply some grated green fig skin to my cold sore, then eat the rest of the fig.

★★**Beans** The herpes simplex virus doesn't function on its own. Like every other element in the human body, it works together with some things and competes with others. High tissue levels of the amino acid arginine, for example, help the virus replicate itself. The amino acid lysine, on the other hand, suppresses replication and helps with recovery from outbreaks, so it seems to make sense to up your intake of lysine-rich foods.

One way to do that is to look at your bean options. For example, 100 grams (about ½ cup) of lima beans, small white beans, kidney beans, or black beans provide 1.4 grams of lysine. The same amount of winged beans has 2.1 grams. In my *CRC Handbook of Phytochemical Constituents,* watercress and soy lead for lysine, followed by black bean sprouts and carob; lentil sprouts; lamb's-quarters and winged bean seeds; spinach and velvet beans; pea and pumpkin seeds; and asparagus, butterbeans, Chinese cabbage, faba beans (broadbeans), fenugreek, parsley, and tepary beans, in that order.

Keep in mind, though, that lysine doesn't cure herpes; it merely reduces the risk of outbreaks and speeds recovery time.

★★**Chile peppers** The active ingredient in hot peppers—the stuff that gives them their heat—is called capsaicin, and strangely enough, when it's diluted and added to a cream, it can be applied to the skin to block pain signals from the nerves under the surface.

For cold sores, apply a capsaicin-based cream, either a commercial brand or one you make by combining powdered red pepper with white skin lotion until the mixture turns pink. Dab it onto affected areas that aren't near your eyes. Be sure to wash your hands thoroughly afterward to avoid irritating other parts of your body, and discontinue use if you experience any irritation, especially on your lips.

★★**Clove** The excellent *Encyclopedia of Common Natural Ingredients* identifies clove oil as a strong medicinal for fighting both herpes simplex strains. Thai studies demonstrate this effect. In another study, clove oil, when combined with the antiherpes drug acyclovir (Zovirax), helped keep the herpes virus from replicating—at least in the test tube.

★★**Garlic** One study, published in the journal *Planta Medica,* found that garlic fights a number of viruses, including herpes simplex types 1 and 2. Garlic contains a number of active compounds, but the researchers weren't able to determine which are responsible for what protection, so your best course of action is to add freshly chopped or minced garlic to pasta or pizza or use whole cloves in a tossed salad. You can also make a cup of garlic tea by boiling a few cloves in water, straining out the garlic, and adding a bit of honey and lemon juice to cut the garlic bite.

★★**Oregano** I was surprised when the mint we call oregano emerged as a top scorer for cold sores, almost twice as high as melissa (lemon balm), which has a more extensive folk history and a documented reputation as a herpes treatment. Both melissa and oregano are loaded with analgesic, antiherpetic, and antiviral compounds. This has the makings of a recipe for Cold Sore Tea—equal parts melissa and oregano, brewed with cinnamon, clove, and/or peppermint to taste.

★**Milk and cheese** A cup of 2 percent milk also has a better than 2:1 ratio of lysine to arginine, with 57 milligrams of lysine. There's no FDA recommendation for the amount of lysine you should include in your diet, but since this amino acid also aids in calcium absorption, you get a twofer by drinking milk. An ounce of Swiss cheese has 73 milligrams of lysine and only 26 milligrams of arginine, for an almost 3:1 ratio. Other cheeses—such as mozzarella, Parmesan, and Romano—have similar totals and ratios.

★**Pork** The king of lysine may be pork, which boasts 3.7 grams in a single broiled, boneless loin chop. If you choose ground pork, 3 ounces has nearly 2 grams of lysine, and one center slice of cured ham contains almost 0.5 gram. Even a pork hot dog contains 853 milligrams. No matter how you slice it, pork provides a lot of lysine—and it goes awfully well with the beans mentioned on the previous page.

★**Starfruit, papayas, apricots, apples, pears, and figs** Besides adding more high-lysine foods to your menu, eating foods that have a high lysine-to-arginine ratio may help you avoid herpes outbreaks. Foods that fall into this category include starfruit (70 milligrams of lysine vs. 19 milligrams of arginine in a medium fruit, for a 3.5:1 ratio), papaya (a 2.5:1 ratio), apricot (2:1), apple (2:1), pear (almost 2:1), and fig (almost 2:1).

★**Strawberries, oranges, cantaloupes, grapefruit, and other vitamin C–rich foods** All of these foods pack plenty of C, which can help boost immunity. At least one study found that bioflavonoids, commonly found in colorful fruits and vegetables, and ascorbic acid, which is one type of vitamin C, were helpful for reducing outbreaks caused by the herpesvirus. Black currants, guavas, and kiwifruit provide lots of vitamin C, along with the fruits listed above. If you want to turn to veggies instead, reach for red and green bell peppers and broccoli.

If you're feeling adventurous and have a good source of less conventional foods, you might also try some bitter melon, emblic seeds, cashew apple, vine spinach, or Cherokee rose, all of which are high in C.

Constipation

YOU CAN LEARN A LOT ABOUT AVOIDING CONSTIPATION FROM COWS. They eat tons of roughage, drink gallons of water, and have incredible regularity. I've been a high-fiber freak since hearing the late Denis Burkitt, MD, a respected British surgeon, say in his usual picturesque fashion: "Your turds should splat like a cow's." Not the most pleasant topic, I know, but it's true.

During his lifetime of work in East Africa, Dr. Burkitt noted that people in non-industrialized societies eat very high-fiber diets and rarely experience constipation. And then there are Americans, who probably wouldn't need to spend nearly $140 million a year on over-the-counter laxatives if we ate right. We eat lots of meat, dairy, and fatty foods—the perfect formula for constipation. Cheeseburgers and fries, ribs and chicken, and greasy pizza offer little or no fiber. No wonder more than four million Americans have chronic constipation! If you're among them, the first thing you should do is fiber-check your diet.

Fiber Power

There are two kinds of fiber, soluble and insoluble, and neither is absorbed by your digestive tract. Soluble fiber forms a sticky gel that acts like a protective coating inside your bowel. Insoluble fiber soaks up water as it passes through, helping to bulk up, weigh down, and soften your stools—all the better for moving them down and out more quickly and easily, allowing you to strain less.

Both kinds of fiber are important for preventing constipation because together, they help sweep things along from your stomach, through your intestines, and out. And a high-fiber diet can aid in preventing a host of other digestive disorders, including hemorrhoids, diarrhea, irritable bowel syndrome, and diverticular disease. When it comes to digestion, fiber is king.

Fiber-rich fruits and vegetables are best for preventing and relieving constipation. Fruits highest in fiber include apples, apricots, avocados, guavas, raspberries, and strawberries. Artichokes, Brussels sprouts, and peas top the high-fiber vegetable list.

Michael Murray, ND, a natural medicine expert and author of *The Encyclopedia of Healing Foods,* suggests eating fresh radishes if you're constipated. Radishes contain a variety of chemicals that help improve digestion (in addition to keeping your gallbladder healthy and protecting against cancer).

If you have chronic constipation, try eating five fruits and five vegetables every day—but start gradually. Eating a lot more fiber than your body is used to can bring on cramping and gas. Begin slowly by adding more fiber to your diet over the course of several weeks or months.

Go for Whole

There's a whole-grain buzz going on, and for good reason. Foods made with whole grains—grains that haven't had their bran and germ removed by milling—are great sources of fiber. Many food companies are making whole-wheat versions of favorite products, including pasta, crackers, tortillas, and even cookies.

For those of you who prefer white bread, many bakeries now offer whole-grain versions of white bread, which traditionally contains very little fiber. Even diehard Wonder Bread fans can now get this favorite in whole-grain white or whole-grain wheat.

All of these products are easy to find; simply look for "whole" on food labels. For true whole-grain items, one of the first three ingredients should be listed as whole. The most fiber-rich whole grains include barley, buckwheat, bulgur, cracked wheat, millet, oats, and rye. Oats, for example, are high in both soluble and insoluble fiber, so whole-grain oat products pack an excellent fiber punch. Bulgur, which is wheat in its whole form, is one of the healthiest foods you can eat. Studies show that besides being extremely high in fiber, bulgur may also help prevent colon and breast cancer as well as heart disease and diabetes.

The Water-Fiber Link

When it comes to efficient bowel function, water and fiber go hand in hand. Your stools absorb a lot of water, and when they don't get enough, they get hard and dry and more difficult to pass. When you're eating more fiber to combat constipation, water is a must to really get things moving.

Italian researchers studied two groups of constipated people—those who ate about 25 grams of fiber a day and drank water to their liking (not enough, by the way) and those who ate the same amount of fiber but drank about 2 quarts of mineral water each day. The study found that although daily fiber consumption certainly helped relieve constipation in both groups, the group that drank more water experienced even better results.

To help prevent constipation, drink six to eight full glasses of water a day. This may sound (and feel) like a lot, but it's what you need to stay regular. If you don't care to drink that much water, make up the difference with soups and high-fiber juices—or eat lots of watermelon and cucumbers, which are nearly 100 percent water by weight.

A good rule of thumb is to measure out 2 quarts of water every morning and make sure it's gone before you go to bed. Another trick is to drink two glasses of water a half hour before breakfast. This primes your system by flushing out wastes and getting it ready for food. A colleague of mine swears by this "clockwork" routine each morning.

Healing Foods for Constipation

Many foods are high in fiber and can help prevent and relieve constipation. Try these top picks.

★★★**Apples** If you're constipated, apples are an excellent choice because they contain both kinds of fiber. Insoluble fiber is found in the skin, and studies have found that apple peel also has powerful antioxidant activity, even inhibiting the growth of cancer cells. But that's not all; it also helps lower your cholesterol and in turn your risk of heart disease and stroke.

The insoluble fiber in apples is good roughage and great for relieving constipation. It also helps prevent other digestive disorders, such as diverticular disease and possibly even colon cancer. (Wait, there's more.) Pectin, a particular type of soluble fiber in apples, appears to reduce the amount of cholesterol produced in your liver. Apples are a power food, no doubt about it.

If you're in need of a good cleanout, try eating three or four small apples a day until your constipation clears up. Be sure to eat them with the skin, and if possible, go with organic apples to avoid ingesting pesticides.

★★★**Beans** Beans are also superfoods. They have lots of protein, minerals, and disease-fighting antioxidants. But they're even more special because they're high in both soluble and insoluble fiber, which makes them great ammo against constipation.

Black beans contain 6 grams of fiber per serving. Chickpeas, kidney beans, and lima beans have about 7 grams, and black-eyed peas top out at 8 grams per ½ cup. All of these varieties are extremely versatile. Add them to soups, salads, casseroles, dips—you name it.

To be fair, beans do have a dark side; they're not called the musical fruit for nothing. So here's a trick. Spice up your beans with fresh or ground ginger (yet another natural laxative), which has been shown to help reduce gassiness. In fact, any herb that soothes your digestive tract (carminatives) can help, including allspice, basil, caraway, cinnamon, cloves, coriander, dill, fennel, garlic, lemon, nutmeg, onion, oregano, peppermint, rosemary, sage, tarragon, and thyme, to name a few.

FOODS TO WATCH

Certain foods and food practices don't help constipation.

Cheese. By now, it's well known that cheese is the food that binds, along with other dairy items like ice cream and milk. These foods have little or no fiber and contain an insoluble protein called casein, which slows digestion and worsens constipation. Steer clear of the dairy case if you struggle with constipation.

Tea. Contrary to some beliefs, tea isn't a natural laxative. Tea is rich in tannins, which can help if you have diarrhea because they help bind stools and hold back bowel movements. If you're constipated, avoid drinking tea.

Separated oils. If I had chronic constipation, I'd try not to eat oils that have been removed from their sources, such as vegetable, olive, and soy oil. For example, flaxseed is an excellent source of fiber, but flaxseed oil has almost none. Separated oils form a film in your stomach that makes it difficult to digest certain foods, which can back up in your colon and large intestine. Go for oils from actual food sources like avocados, olives, nuts, and fish.

Machine-squeezed juices. In order to work for constipation, fruit and vegetable juices must retain their fiber. Prune juice does this best, and some juice experts say apple-pear juice makes a good laxative, too. For vegetable juice, try asparagus and potato. However, a powerful juicing machine can squeeze out most of the fiber, so either use a simple blender or hand-squeeze your juices and drink them immediately to get the most benefit.

★★★**Berries** Besides being delicious, berries are a great solution for constipation. They have large amounts of fiber, and the type they contain also helps prevent bile acid—a chemical your body uses for digestion—from being converted into a more dangerous, possibly cancer-causing form.

Elderberries top the list, packing a powerful 5 grams of fiber in a ½-cup serving. Blackberries are next with more than 3 grams per serving, and raspberries come in third with 4 grams. Blueberries and strawberries are good, too. When it comes to berry juice, mulberry and boysenberry juices are gentle laxatives.

★★★**Flaxseed** Also known as linseed, flaxseed is very high in fiber and rich in beneficial omega-3 fatty acids, both of which are helpful for constipation. Three tablespoons of flaxseed has about 3 grams of fiber. It has a sweet, nutty taste and can be added to almost anything; it's great in salads, cereals, casseroles, and breads.

Whole flaxseed provides little benefit, though, because your digestive tract is unable to crack open the hard shells that surround the seeds (which is where all the benefits are). Go for ground or crushed flaxseed for easier digestion, pleasing flavor, and crunch.

Also, don't fall for common claims that flaxseed oil is just as good for you. While the oil has some nutritional benefits, it doesn't offer the fiber you need to help with constipation.

If you try flaxseed for regularity, be sure to drink plenty of water—eight full glasses a day to keep all that bulk moving through your digestive tract.

★★★**Prunes** Prunes are the oldest and most effective food remedy for constipation. They contain three ingredients to help keep you regular. First, they're very high in fiber, with 3 grams in just three prunes. Second, they have a compound called dihydroxyphenyl isatin, which stimulates the contractions in your intestines necessary for regular bowel movements. Third, prunes contain a natural sugar called sorbitol, which, like fiber, soaks up large amounts of water in your digestive tract to keep things moving.

Give and Take

Some foods can act as both a natural laxative and a stool-binding aid, depending on what your body needs. Here are some common foods known to be amphoteric, which means they can work in either way—plugging you up if your bowels are loose or loosening you up if you're constipated.

Apples	Coffee
Bananas	Milk
Berries and currants	Psyllium

Remember that some foods may constipate one person but not another. Milk, for example, can be extremely constipating for some, while it gives others diarrhea. Sometimes it just comes down to eating too much of a certain food that otherwise wouldn't give you trouble.

Spice It Up—And Out

Certain herbs and spices can help with constipation by making foods easier to digest (and taste better, too). These are the best.

Asafetida (an Indian spice with an
   onion-garlic flavor)

Basil (the seeds, not the leaves)

Coriander

Cumin

Fennel

Ginger

Ground red pepper

Parsley

Turmeric

Most fruits generally contain less than 1 percent sorbitol. Prunes, however, have about 15 percent—another reason they're such a potent natural remedy for constipation. They're also much more pleasing to the palate than a laxative from the drugstore.

Other dried fruits—such as raisins and figs—also do wonders for relieving constipation. Raisins contain a compound called tartaric acid, which acts as a natural laxative. Figs are an excellent source of fiber, providing about 5 grams in just three dried or fresh fruits.

★★**Dark leafy greens** A salad tossed with various dark leafy greens is a good choice to combat constipation. Throw in a few handfuls of apple slices, raisins, blackberries, red cabbage, and toasted flaxseed, and you have the makings of a digestive dream. Dark greens are a great source of omega-3's, which help keep your bowels moving beautifully.

Good greens to choose include kale, Swiss chard, endive, dandelion greens, beet greens, turnip greens, purslane, chicory, and spinach. When it comes to color, the darker the better. The deepest hues offer the biggest benefit.

Dandelion in particular is more than just a backyard weed. It has long been regarded as an effective natural laxative that increases bile flow into your large intestine, which helps prevent constipation. Dandelion greens can be found in popular "spring mix" salad combinations in many restaurants and supermarkets.

★★**Ginger** Long known for its many healing properties, ginger is a tasty way to deal with constipation. This spice contains chemicals that stimulate your digestive system by increasing the wavelike muscle contractions (peristalsis) that move food through your intestines.

There are many ways to get the health benefits of ginger, which comes in a variety of forms, including fresh, dried, crystallized, candied, pickled, and powdered. Fresh ginger is best, with crystallized coming in second. When buying fresh ginger, look for firm roots that have smooth skin and a spicy smell. Pickled ginger, often found in Asian restaurants and served with sushi, is just as beneficial as fresh. Candied ginger can be sweet to nibble on and is handy for baking. Seasoning meats and vegetable stir-fries with fresh ginger is a good option, too.

And then there's ginger ale. Although some varieties aren't made with real ginger and often contain unhealthy additives, soda made with the real thing is available and is a refreshing option. One brand, Reed's Ginger Brew, is made with real ginger (up to 25 grams in one variety) and other natural ingredients—like apple, raspberry, pineapple, and honey—that are also constipation fighters.

★★**Honey** Honey contains large amounts of fructose, a sugar that can act as a natural laxative by helping draw water into your bowels and soften your stools. Honey is higher in fructose than almost all other foods. If I were constipated, I'd substitute honey for artificial sweeteners. Drizzle it over fresh berries to get double the digestive benefits.

★★**Rhubarb** The stalks of rhubarb have long been used in folk medicine to relieve constipation. Rhubarb is a member of the buckwheat family (many other members of this family are also good sources of fiber). A half cup of rhubarb stalks contains large amounts of insoluble fiber—the kind you need to keep your bowels moving regularly.

It's important to know that you should eat only the stalks because the leaves contain very high levels of toxins called oxalates that can cause stomach irritation and kidney problems. My friend Ronald L. Hoffman, MD, director of the

Grocery Store Get-and-Go

To get things moving, here's an easy food remedy to try.

½ cup applesauce

½ cup unprocessed bran (Kellogg's All-Bran cereal)

¼ cup 100 percent prune juice

Stir the ingredients together and have it with your evening meal. Repeat as needed.

Hoffman Center for Holistic Medicine in New York City and author of *Seven Weeks to a Settled Stomach,* suggests this rhubarb constipation-relief recipe: Chop three stalks of fresh rhubarb (removing and discarding the leaves), combine in a blender with 1 cup of apple juice, a quarter of a peeled lemon, and 1 teaspoon of honey, and puree until smooth. Drink as needed to get things moving. If you find this thick drink too tart, add other fruit juices. Remember that rhubarb's laxative action can be pretty powerful, so it may be better to try less potent food remedies first.

★★**Squash** Researchers have just begun to discover the incredible healing potential of this vegetable, particularly winter squashes such as acorn, butternut, and Hubbard. When it comes to digestion, the fiber found in dark yellow and orange winter squash can be particularly helpful with constipation. Pale summer squash, on the other hand, is lower in fiber and not as beneficial.

★**Coffee** Besides keeping you on schedule, a cup of coffee in the morning can keep you regular, too. The caffeine in coffee signals your large intestine to contract, keeping your bowels awake and working. However, drinking too much coffee removes more fluids from your body than it puts in, and when used addictively, caffeine prevents your bowels from maintaining their natural rhythm. If you drink coffee, try to limit yourself to less than five cups a day.

From the Herbal Medicine Chest

Tiny psyllium seeds are very high in fiber and the main ingredient in many over-the-counter laxatives. They contain a type of fiber called mucilage, which absorbs a great deal of fluid in your gut. This makes the seeds swell, adding bulk to your stools to help trigger the urge to go. Psyllium seeds need water to work, so be sure to drink plenty if you decide to try them.

If you have allergies or asthma, don't use this herb. Some allergic reactions to psyllium have been reported, including a few cases of serious asthma attacks from inhaled psyllium seed dust.

We have a psyllium relative in the Green Farmacy Garden, a weed picturesquely called the white man's footprint (or the common plantain), whose seeds I've used instead of psyllium on the rare occasions when I've gotten off my high-fiber diet and needed help. These seeds work just as well. I add milk and stevia and eat the mixture like All-Bran cereal.

Corns

SOME HISTORIANS SPECULATE THAT THE FIRST SHOES were created when early man wrapped animal skins around his freezing feet during the Ice Age. Necessity is the mother of invention! I suspect that a few months after that, one of those first shoe wearers developed the first case of corns.

Corns—and closely related calluses—are thickenings of the outer layer of skin. They develop as part of your skin's defense against rubbing, pressure, and other irritations. Generally, corns are caused by wearing the wrong shoes. This is probably why I've never been bothered by them, given my penchant for going barefoot.

According to the American Podiatric Medical Association, 5 percent of Americans are bothered by corns and calluses. Among women who wear high heels, it's much higher: 29 percent. Most of them just suffer in silence, never seeking professional help.

A small corn or callus may not cause you any problems, except perhaps making you frown when you slip on a pair of sandals. A larger corn, however, can cause pain and even difficulty walking. That's bad news, because as the ancient Greek philosopher Socrates claimed, "When our feet hurt, we hurt all over."

Fortunately, there are some food remedies that may help corns, and ironically, *corn* syrup is one of them!

If your corns prove too hardy for these self-care tips, see a podiatrist. And see one *before* trying these remedies if you have diabetes, lack sensation in your feet, or have bad circulation in them.

Healing Foods for Corns

★★**Corn silk** Corn silk is one of the best sources of allantoin, a keratolytic (corn-dissolving) compound. Boil corn-on-the-cob with the silk in place, then save the silks and the cooking water. Let the water cool a bit before soaking your feet for about 15 minutes. You might "tenderize" your corn first with fig milk or corn syrup (see next page). You also can make a poultice from the cork silk and apply it directly to your corn.

★★**Garlic** Russians apply raw garlic to corns for 12 to 18 hours at a stretch. If you want to try this remedy, crush or slice a fresh garlic clove and apply it directly to the corn, avoiding the surrounding skin. Cover it with a bandage, leave it in place overnight, and wash off the garlic in the morning. Blisters should form, but repeat as necessary until the corn disappears.

Science backs this up. Researchers in Iran treated nine people who had one or two corns each with a lipid extract of garlic twice a day for 10 to 20 days. The corns of seven of the people went away completely, and the corns of the other two showed marked improvement.

Here's an important caution, however: Never apply raw garlic to an infant or child's skin. It can cause serious burns.

★**Black tea** Brew yourself a big pot of strong black tea. Pour a cup to drink, then sit back and soak your corn in the rest of it for 30 minutes each day for a week or two. The tannic acid in tea dissolves corns.

★**Castor oil** Aha, that's not a food, you may be thinking. Well, the oil made from castor beans is sold in supermarkets, and you can drink it, so that's close enough in my book. My mother used to give it to me as a laxative whether I needed it or not. To try castor oil on your corns, dip a cotton ball in the oil and place it on your corn. Secure it with a piece of surgical tape, put on a sock to keep the oil from staining your sheets, and wear it overnight. *Note:* Don't put castor oil on broken skin.

★**Corn syrup** To soften the hard skin of a corn, apply a bit of corn syrup and wrap it with gauze.

★**Lemon** Peruvians apply lemons to their corns. Even here in the United States, an age-old food remedy is to apply a piece of lemon peel (white side down) to a corn. Hold it in place overnight with surgical tape or a bandage. You can remove it during the day, but repeat the application each night for seven nights. Or you could dab some lemon juice straight on your corns.

★**Salt** Salt is a great natural foot scrub, and for good reason. It removes dead skin, so it's logical that it may help get rid of corns. Mix up a salty solution of 3 parts salt to 1 part water. Soak your feet in water for 10 to 15 minutes, apply the exfoliating scrub, and then rinse.

★**Sugar** Sugar is also a common ingredient in foot scrubs. Make a solution of 3 parts brown sugar to 1 part water. Soak your feet for 10 to 15 minutes, then apply the scrub and rinse.

★**Vinegar** Here's another home remedy that's worth a shot. Saturate a piece of white bread with ¼ cup white vinegar. Let stand for 30 minutes, apply the poultice to the corn, and cover with a piece of gauze to keep it in place overnight. By morning, the vinegar should have dissolved the thick skin so you can peel the corn right off. If necessary, repeat this process for a few nights.

Coughs

IT'S HARD TO GET THROUGH YOUR DAY when you have a persistent cough, and getting through the night can be even harder. To make matters worse, a cough from a cold can linger for as long as 3 weeks. It's the most common reason people see their doctors, accounting for an estimated 29.5 million visits to office-based doctors a year in the United States, according to the American College of Chest Physicians.

It's no surprise that Americans spend billions of dollars on over-the-counter cough medications. When you're feeling that terrible, you need relief! Unfortunately, I have to be the bearer of bad news here. Those colorful bottled syrups sitting on the drugstore shelf don't work. Studies have found that dextromethorphan, the most common cough ingredient in over-the-counter cough suppressants, isn't any more effective than a placebo.

In 2006, the American College of Chest Physicians recommended that Americans stop using over-the-counter cough syrups for bronchitis, and because an overdose of cough medicine can injure or even cause death in children, over-the-counter cough suppressants should *never* be given to anyone under age 15.

Now it's time for some good news. There are plenty of plant-based remedies that can help quiet your cough. If it's particularly persistent even after trying home remedies, it's a good idea to get a medical evaluation. Coughs are often caused by colds, but a chronic cough could mean something more serious. A study by Mayo Clinic researchers found that chronic cough was a sign of sinusitis in more than a third of the patients they studied. The top three causes of chronic cough, according to the researchers, were allergies, acid reflux, and sinusitis.

Healing Foods for Coughs

Here are foods that work specifically to relieve a cough, but if yours is caused by a cold or the flu, bronchitis, or sinusitis, see those chapters for more remedies.

★★★**Chicken soup** If your cough is due to a cold, eating chicken soup helps you stay hydrated, improves your immunity, provides antioxidants that your body needs to help fight the virus, helps clear mucus from your system, and reduces inflammation. In a study by researchers at the University of Nebraska Medical Center, chicken soup reduced the movement of neutrophils in blood, which they think lowers activity that causes inflammation and cold symptoms in the respiratory tract.

★★★**Cloves** This spice, popular in Sri Lanka and northern India, scores well in my database search for relieving coughs. Asian Indians suck on cloves when they have a tickling cough. The reddish-brown spice consists of dried flower buds and is sold as whole or ground cloves.

★★★**Garlic** Garlic is an important healing food that shouldn't be overlooked if you have a cough. Chris Deatherage, ND, a naturopath in rural Missouri, recommends combining garlic with hydrotherapy to treat coughs, colds, fevers, flu, pneumonia, strep throat, and yeast infections. He advocates fever therapy, in which he has patients take a hot bath for 25 minutes to create a fever of 102°F. While they soak, they drink carrot juice that contains echinacea and raw garlic. If the patients are very sick, he tells them to take three cloves of garlic in 4 to 6 ounces of carrot juice every 2 hours.

Dr. Deatherage isn't the only one who recommends garlic. Jill Stansbury, ND, of the National College of Naturopathic Medicine in Portland, Oregon, tells her students to combine garlic with "lung herbs," such as yerba santa and coltsfoot, to treat a cough.

★★★**Ginger** Ginger is a popular folk remedy that helps suppress cough, reduce pain and lower fever. In addition, it contains chemicals called sesquiterpenes that

FOODS TO WATCH

Depending on what's causing your cough, some foods can make it worse. Keep these foods in mind when you're looking for relief.

Foods that trigger acid reflux. Acid reflux can cause a chronic cough, so it's a good idea to avoid foods that trigger your heartburn if you have a condition called gastroesophageal reflux disease (GERD). These may include alcohol, chocolate, acidic foods, and high-fat foods.

Fatty and sugary foods. Foods that are low in nutrition won't help you avoid the illnesses that cause a cough, such as a cold, the flu, bronchitis, and sinusitis. Be sure to pack your daily diet with immunity-boosting healthy foods instead of fat- and sugar-laden choices.

Dairy products. Dairy foods may increase mucus buildup in your airways, which will make your cough worse. Avoiding them may help.

fight rhinoviruses, the most common of the cold viruses. I add ginger to chicken and other soups, and I make tea by pouring boiling water over fresh ginger shavings.

★★★**Honey** Honey is a powerful healing agent that's used in cultures all over the world. When it comes to coughs and colds, honey coats your throat and helps relieve irritation. It also has antioxidant and antimicrobial properties that help fight infections from viruses, bacteria, and fungi.

Researchers at the Pennsylvania State University College of Medicine recently asked the parents of 105 children to treat nighttime coughs due to an upper respiratory infection with either buckwheat honey (a dark honey with an abundance of antioxidants), a honey-flavored over-the-counter cough suppressant, or no treatment before bed. According to the parents, honey was the most effective of the three treatments.

Be sure not to give honey to children under 1 year of age because of the risk of infant botulism, caused by a type of spore that can contaminate honey through contact with dirt and dust. The spore can cause serious breathing problems and even death. Also keep in mind that honey may promote dental cavities, so use itonly as needed. And if you have diabetes, keep an eye on your blood sugar while taking honey, as it may have a tendency to rise.

★★**Black pepper and chile peppers** The black pepper in chicken soup is part of the reason it helps a cough and congestion. Asian Indians also gargle with a black pepper solution to relieve a sore throat.

Hot peppers can help relieve a cough by dilating blood vessels, reducing congestion and helping to clear mucus. Irwin Ziment, MD, of the UCLA School of Medicine recommends eating a chile pepper a day.

★★**Chamomile tea** This tea is packed with compounds that will help a cough or cold, the flu, or bronchitis, particularly if the chamomile comes from Rome or Hungary. As you're boiling the water, inhale the aroma of the chamomile flowers and carefully direct the steam from the tea toward you after you pour in the water. Inhaling the steam and drinking the tea can both help.

★★**Dark chocolate** An ingredient in chocolate called theobromine can help stop a cough in its tracks.

Researchers from the National Heart and Lung Institute in London performed both an animal and a human study on theobromine. In a study with guinea pigs, the animals were exposed to citric acid for 3 minutes to make them cough. Then they were treated with theobromine or codeine and exposed to citric acid again an hour later. The theobromine was effective at stopping coughs for up to 4 hours.

In the human study, 10 volunteers received capsaicin to induce coughing and then took either theobromine, codeine, or a placebo at three different times. It took a third more capsaicin to cause a cough after participants took theobromine than after they took a placebo.

Researchers said theobromine suppresses vagus nerve activity, which is responsible for coughing. What's more, theobromine had no side effects.

Dark chocolate or cocoa has the highest amounts of theobromine, but keep in mind that the content varies based on the cocoa beans used. The researchers gave the people in their study 1,000 milligrams of theobromine, which is quite a bit more than the 184 milligrams in a 1.45-ounce Hershey's Special Dark chocolate bar. Some researchers have said that 1.76 ounces of dark chocolate can contain up to 519 milligrams of theobromine.

Another thing to keep in mind is that chocolate is high in fat and calories. The 1.45-ounce Hershey's bar has 218 calories and 13 grams of fat.

★★**Fresh fruit and soy** Researchers compared the diets of 49,140 men and women in China with symptoms of coughing and phlegm and found that eating fruit and soy foods was associated with fewer symptoms. Another study found that the fiber you get from fruit improves the health of your lungs while reducing phlegm and coughing episodes.

In addition to fiber, the researchers think flavonoids, which are found in soy foods and fruits such as apples and pears, may also improve lung function. Many fruits, such as oranges and strawberries, also contain vitamin C, an antioxidant that has been shown to reduce cold symptoms by an average of 23 percent.

My advice is to make all kinds of fruit a part of your daily diet, including oranges, grapefruits, apples, pears, grapes, melons, kiwifruit, pineapple, peaches, plums, apricots, and berries.

★★**Horseradish** If you can bear the heat, eat horseradish or other hot foods such as hot mustard or wasabi several times a day. It will liquefy phlegm and help to relieve a cough.

★★**Lemon** Christopher Hobbs, a fourth-generation California herbalist and author of several books on herbal medicine, suggests a formula that I think is worth taking two or three times a day for a cough. Add 2 teaspoons of organic lemon rind, 1 teaspoon of sage, and ½ teaspoon of thyme to boiling water and steep for 15 minutes. Then add the juice of half a lemon and 1 tablespoon of honey. Remember to use organic lemon rind because the pesticides used on citrus fruits is extremely hard to wash off.

★★**Peppermint** Inhaling essential oils such as peppermint is known to help you breathe more easily when you have a stuffy nose from a cold, the flu, or a sinus infection. But peppermint can also help with a cough. Gargling with peppermint tea, sucking on peppermint lozenges, and using peppermint tablets that dissolve in your mouth (called troches) will help soothe a sore throat and stop a cough.

A caution, however: Never ingest peppermint oil. While it's safe to inhale, it's toxic and should never be ingested. In addition to peppermint, eucalyptus, fennel, menthol, and thyme used in these ways may also help with a cough. Another good choice is products made of tolu balsam, which comes from balsam trees in the Amazon. You can purchase them on the Internet, but they're very expensive.

★★**Pineapple juice** In his book *Alternative Medicine: The Definitive Guide*, Burton Goldberg suggests drinking pineapple juice and honey to curb a cough. Pineapples contain bromelain, an enzyme that's thought to act as an anti-inflammatory and help relieve sinus infections. Adding honey to the drink activates the bromelain.

★★**Plum paste** If you have a dry cough, Goldberg also suggests using umeboshi plum paste, a puree of ume plums from Japan. It can be used as a spread, in salad dressing, or on sushi.

★★**Sage** You may use it to flavor meats or Thanksgiving stuffing, but eating sage is also a good way to fight a cough. People in Hungary use this herb medicinally for that purpose. Sage extract is antiseptic and contains flavonoids that inhibit histamine.

★**Elderberries** These berries have been praised by naturopaths for their effectiveness against coughs, colds, Epstein-Barr syndrome, fever, and allergies. They contain two ingredients that work against the flu virus. While eating elderberry jam or drinking elderberry wine is always an option, you can also find the herb in over-the-counter drops or chewable tablets called Sambucol.

★**Onions** Onions have traditionally been applied in poultices to treat pneumonia, croup, and other ailments, and it's even been used to make a homemade cough syrup. Some people also seem to really benefit from eating onions. In 1995, I addressed more than 100 physicians at Flower Hospital in Toledo, and one physician told me that several decades earlier, a Lebanese patient with tuberculosis had been staying in a sanitarium. After the patient found a load of discarded onions, he ate and enjoyed several a day, and within a month, he was well.

Interestingly, an onion-scented herb from Panama and Peru called petiveria has a folk reputation for treating pneumonia. The world-famous father of ethnobotany, the late Richard Evans Schultes, PhD, told how Amazonian Indians take petiveria leaves, mashed with lemon juice and a drop of kerosene, for pneumonia.

From the Herbal Medicine Chest

Adding a couple of herbs to your daily defense against a cough can bring even more relief. If your cough is caused by bronchitis, a cold or the flu, or sinusitis, see those chapters for more herbal remedies.

Aniseed (*Pimpinella anisum*) Aniseed has been endorsed by Germany's Commission E, a government agency that evaluates the safety and efficacy of medicinal herbs, to remove phlegm and suppress coughing. I recommend trying a tea made by steeping 1 or 2 teaspoons of crushed aniseed in 1 cup of boiling water for 10 to 15 minutes, then straining. You may want to try drinking a cup in the morning and another in the evening.

Licorice (*Glycyrrhiza glabra*) Licorice contains a compound called glycyrrhizin that helps your body fight viruses and bacteria. It has long been recommended for coughs, bronchitis, and asthma. For cough, it helps soothe mucous membranes. You can buy licorice as a standardized herb and add it as a sweetener to the aromatic teas mentioned in this chapter. Another option is to make a tea with 1 teaspoon of dried root in 1 cup of boiling water.

There are a few caveats when using licorice. Because long-term use can lead to headaches, lethargy, sodium and water retention, loss of potassium, and high blood pressure, don't take it regularly for longer than 6 weeks, and don't take it if you're pregnant or nursing or if you have severe liver, kidney, or heart disease or high blood pressure. You should also avoid it if you're taking a diuretic.

Plantain (*Plantago major*) This herb (not the tropical fruit) contains silicic acid, which helps boost your resistance to infection.

Slippery elm (*Ulmus rubra*) The FDA considers slippery elm a safe, effective herb for soothing a cough. It contains mucilage, which suppresses coughing and soothes the throat. You can make a tea with the dried herb or buy throat lozenges that contain it.

Cuts and Scrapes

By NATURE OF BEING HUMAN, we've all sustained more than a few cuts and scrapes in our lives, and I've certainly had more than my fair share. But whether it's a paper cut, a slip with a pairing knife, or a gravel-filled brush burn after a fall from a bike, cuts and scrapes can literally be a pain.

For severe cuts or puncture wounds, you must see your doctor—no food remedy is going to help you. Immediately after getting a cut or scrape, the first thing to do is clean it with soap and water. If the cut is more than ½ inch long or deep enough to show the yellow layer of fat under the skin, it needs stitches within the next 24 hours. In the meantime, you can put a bandage on the wound and apply ice to keep the swelling down. You also want to pay a visit to a healthcare professional if:

- The wound won't stop bleeding
- The cut area is inflamed and tender or discharging pus
- You have multiple cuts or scrapes
- You have a fever or swollen lymph nodes
- You have a cut on your face or other prominent area of your body
- Cinders, gravel, or another substance is embedded in the wound

In the case of minor cuts and scrapes, however, foods—when eaten or used topically—can help speed healing or support the immune system by killing germs.

Healing Foods for Cuts and Scrapes

Unfortunately, there's nothing you or I can do to prevent cuts and scrapes except be a little more careful. You can, however, make sure your nutritional status is up to snuff to keep your body at its ultimate healing potential. Nutrients such as protein, vitamin C, and zinc help build new skin, and if you don't get enough of them, wounds will take longer to heal.

★★★**Cloves** The oil made from the dried flowers of this tropical tree is an aromatic staple of dentists' offices. Not only does it have a calming, pleasant, spicy scent, it is also rich in eugenol, a chemical that has both painkilling and antiseptic properties. I wouldn't hesitate to apply clove oil on a cut to prevent infection. Its antibiotic spectrum is remarkably broad; it's even active against some strains of drug-resistant *Staphylococcus* bacteria.

★★★**Garlic** Garlic is one of nature's best antibiotics. An Ethiopian study looked at garlic's antibacterial effects on wound infections and found it to be an effective remedy. I suggest you try taping a crushed glove over a cut or scrape. If it starts to irritate your skin or make the wound more painful, take it off right away.

Garlic isn't alone in its antibacterial powers; all the closely related species, including chives, leeks, onions, ramps (wild leeks), and ramsons (wild garlic) contain the major antiseptic compound allicin or its precursor alliin. Thanks to some enzymatic magic, allicin antiseptic is released when you nick the bulb. Be careful, though—it can burn a bit, like some of your grandmother's antiseptics did.

★★★**Thyme** As one of the richest sources in my garden of the potent aromatic antiseptic thymol, thyme is next in line after clove and garlic as my choice for an herbal broad-spectrum antiseptic. Jean Valnet, MD, a French physician who used topical, oral, and inhaled applications of essential oils, claimed that thyme essence destroyed some skin-threatening bacteria, including anthrax and bacillus. And thyme has been successfully used topically for burns and skin and muscular problems, as outlined in Valnet's 1964 book, *Aromatherapie*.

★★**Citrus fruits** Studies have shown that vitamin C, either consumed in food or used topically, helps repair wounded skin. This vitamin is necessary for the formation of collagen, the tissue that holds skin cells together. It also helps promote proper immune function and acts as an antioxidant, all of which helps heal wounds. Conversely, when you don't get enough vitamin C, collagen weakens, and your cuts and scrapes heal more slowly. No matter what kind of wound you have—or even if you are wound free—you should aim to get at least 500 milligrams of vitamin C a day (which is eight times the recommended daily intake) from fruits and vegetables. If you are older or smoke, try to get closer to 1,000 milligrams. In addition to loading up on C-rich citrus fruits, you can boost your levels by eating more strawberries, broccoli, cantaloupe, tomatoes, bell peppers, and potatoes.

Jim LaValle, ND, a pharmacist, naturopathic physician, and founder of the LaValle Metabolic Institute in Cincinnati, suggests you mix a few tablespoons of powdered vitamin C with ½ cup of aloe gel (both are available at most health food stores) in a spray bottle. Shake it well to dilute the vitamin C and then spray it right onto the wound a few times a day; it works well. But never take aloe gel internally.

A specific vitamin C–rich food that may work topically to prevent infection in a cut or scrape is the orange. In Chinese medicine, oranges are placed on wounds to draw out toxicity or heavy metals. Carolyn Dean, MD, ND, and Chinese medicine guru Jeffrey Yuen tout oranges for their power to draw toxins from the body. Personally, I would prefer camu-camu, when in season. This Amazonian fruit is the world's richest source of vitamin C, and it has antiseptic properties besides. It is hard to find, though.

★★**Cranberries** Native Americans used astringent cranberry poultices to pull toxins from arrow wounds. Dr. Dean and Yuen say that cranberries work for wound healing because they contain hippuric acid, which may have antibacterial properties.

★★**Honey** Need a Band-Aid for your wound? You can use honey instead—it dries to form a natural bandage! It also has antibacterial properties, and studies show it speeds wound healing. An analysis of nearly two dozen studies done in New Zealand revealed that honey works to clean a cut or scrape and prevent infection. In one study, 50 women with infected C-section or hysterectomy incisions received applications of either honey or topical antiseptics every hour. The honey group's infections cleared up in about 6 days—8 days sooner than those in the group receiving the topical antiseptic. And if that weren't convincing enough, honey also reduces swelling and helps minimize scars. Although I've never used honey as a topical treatment for wounds, I have seen Indians in Panama and Peru use it quite successfully. To get the best results, I would follow the method used by the New Zealand researchers: Drizzle some honey on a sterile piece of gauze, apply it to the wound, and change the dressing once a day.

★★**Pineapple** Highly technical studies in Germany suggest that the proteolytic enzyme bromelain in pineapple stimulates wound healing. On my tropical trips, I might wash with pineapple juice before applying freshly cut garlic to cleanse a wound in the unforgiving tropical humidity. I'd drink a cooling beverage from this fruit and eat some garlic as well to boost my immune system.

★★**Spinach** Spinach helps speed wound healing because it's an excellent source of zinc, a trace mineral that helps organ tissue—including the skin—grow and repair itself. In a study done at the University of Texas Shriners Hospital for Children, zinc injections accelerated wound healing in adult rabbits. A British review called topical zinc "underappreciated" for wound healing. And a Turkish study revealed that the severity of traumas was associated with decreases in blood levels of certain trace elements, zinc included. Most Americans don't get enough of this important mineral from sources like spinach, and if you experience slow wound healing, it may be a clue that you're one of them. Eating more zinc to meet—or exceed—the recommended daily intake (15 micrograms) just may help your cuts and scrapes heal faster. In addition to spinach, nutritionists list oysters, wheat germ, sesame seeds, pumpkin seeds, low-fat yogurt, parsley, collards, Brussels sprouts, cucumbers, string beans, endive, prunes, and asparagus as rich in zinc.

★★**Tea** When applied topically, the tannins in tea appear to help treat open wounds. A Russian study showed that an oil extraction from tea leaves accelerated the healing process in wounds. And John Boik, PhD, an acupuncturist and author of the power-packed book *Cancer and Natural Medicine,* tells us that flavonoids may stabilize collagen. Tea contains many flavonoids as well as catechins, which stimulate collagen synthesis. I would try applying a black or green tea bag to a wound to help speed healing.

★★**Tofu** Although only about 10 percent of the body's protein is found in the skin, when your body tries to heal itself after a cut or scrape, your protein needs can double. The amount of additional protein you need depends on the severity of the wound, but you should add at least a few extra servings of a rich plant source of protein such as tofu (a 4-ounce serving has more than 9 grams of protein).

Or try this idea from Dr. LaValle: Get a protein drink made from brown rice powder or whey powder. Dr. LaValle particularly likes whey powder for wound healing because it improves immunoglobulin antibodies that help fight bacteria. If you're not a vegetarian, you can boost protein with fish, poultry, eggs, or lean meat. You can also add shredded cheese to vegetable dishes or stir some nonfat dry milk into milk, cereal, soup, or gravy.

From the Herbal Medicine Chest

Patients with scars and slow-healing cuts have often found calendula preparations helpful in healing wounds that have frustrated contemporary physicians. Nineteenth-century housewives boiled calendula flowers, soaked them in alcohol, or simmered them in melted lard to make washes or ointments for minor wounds. In front of my local supermarket, you can see potted calendula, alias pot marigold, on sale when spring gardening fever begins.

A calendula tea can be an effective topical treatment for wounds when used as a poultice. The late herbalist Varro Tyler, PhD, noted that calendula is approved by Germany's Commission E, a government agency that evaluates the safety and efficacy of medicinal herbs, for promoting wound healing with local application. I suggest pouring a cup of hot water over 1 to 1.5 grams of dried calendula petals and steeping for 10 minutes. Then pour the mixture onto a cloth and apply it to the wound. Calendula may be even more effective when incorporated into creams and gels. I've used a calendula cream with good results while traveling in the Amazonian rainforests.

Dandruff

DANDRUFF IS A CONDITION IN WHICH DEAD SKIN CELLS are shed from the scalp in amounts large enough to become noticeable as flakes on the scalp and clothing. It can also cause itching. To the chagrin of many image-conscious kids, the condition—like acne—often begins in the teen years and then waxes and wanes throughout life. People often find that it's less severe in warmer months.

Although dandruff may look like a dry skin condition, it's actually just the opposite. Experts believe that it's caused by a type of yeast called *Malassezia ovalis*, which is lipohillic (loves oil), so if your scalp is oily, you're more likely to develop a white-fleck problem.

Healing Foods for Dandruff

Fortunately, your pantry and fridge offer quite a few remedies that can help stop the shedding. But you'll have to exercise a little patience. David H. Kingsley, PhD, a board-certified tricologist (hair and scalp specialist) in New York City, says that normal skin turnover time is about 28 days. When you have dandruff, the process is faster, but you'll still have to wait at least 2 to 3 weeks to know if a remedy is working. On the other hand, if something hasn't worked in a month, it's probably not going to.

★★★**Honey** A study conducted in the United Arab Emirates found that honey can stop the itching and scaling of dandruff within 1 week. Participants diluted crude (unpasteurized) honey slightly with warm water (9 parts honey to 1 part water) and applied the mixture to their scalps every other day for 4 weeks. Each application consisted of gently rubbing the honey into the scalp for 2 to 3 minutes, leaving the mixture on for 3 hours, and rinsing it off with warm water. The patients' itching and scaling eased, and they enjoyed an additional benefit—their hair loss slowed down.

★★**Barley** Researchers have discovered that a zinc deficiency can lead to dandruff, so it wouldn't hurt to add some zinc-rich foods such as pearled barley and kidney beans to your diet.

★**Apple cider vinegar** This remedy helps control dandruff by balancing the pH (acidity vs. alkalinity) on the surface of the scalp. Warm the vinegar in the microwave or a saucepan on the stove, then soak a small towel in it and lay it on your hair for 1 hour. Finally, wash it out well with a mild herbal shampoo.

FOODS TO WATCH

Back in the 1960s, researchers in Britain noticed that people who had seborrheic dermatitis (one cause of dandruff) ate significantly more sugar than people who didn't have it. So, logically, if I had this condition, I'd eliminate sugar from my diet to see if it helped clear up the scaly patches.

Because dandruff is associated with oily skin, foods that may make your skin oilier may also make dandruff worse. Hair and scalp specialist Dr. David Kingsley suggests avoiding hard cheeses such as cheddar, oily/fatty foods, and chocolate.

★**Lemon** Squeeze a fresh lemon, massage a few tablespoons of the juice into your scalp, and rinse well with water. Repeat once a day until your dandruff is gone.

This remedy works in essentially the same way as apple cider vinegar. The skin of the scalp is slightly acidic, with a pH of about 5.4, but it can become more alkaline from either hair care products or its own secretions. Bringing it back to normal acidity may help relieve your dandruff.

★**Olive oil** Oil may help loosen dandruff scales. Warm a bit of olive oil on the stove or in the microwave and test it carefully with your hand to be sure it's not too hot. Massage it into your scalp and leave it on for 20 minutes, then brush your scalp with a hard-bristled hairbrush and rinse well with water. Repeat twice a week. Dr. Kingsley cautions, however, that scratching the skin can stimulate cell turnover, so try it for a week, but if it makes your dandruff worse, stop.

★**Salmon** One of the symptoms of a deficiency of vitamins B_6 and B_{12} is seborrheic dermatitis, which is a cause of dandruff. If I were bothered by this condition, I'd eat more salmon, beef, and beef liver, which are all good sources of both vitamins. (If you have circulatory problems or heart disease, you may want to forgo the meats and stick with the salmon. Or choose vegetarian sources of B_6, such as members of the cabbage and spinach families.)

★**Salt** Folk wisdom suggests that simple table salt may decrease dandruff. Fill a cup with warm water and dissolve 3 tablespoons of salt in it. Massage the solution into your scalp, then rinse well with water.

★**Yogurt** Here's an old folk remedy you may want to try. A thick coat of plain yogurt applied to your scalp can ease itching and treat dandruff. Cover the yogurt with a towel, leave it on for 20 minutes, then rinse well with warm water.

From the Herbal Medicine Chest

Tea tree oil has been used as a natural remedy for a variety of skin complaints. In fact, studies have found it nearly as effective as over-the-counter medicines in treating fungal and yeast infections of the skin, nails, and scalp, including dandruff.

In one Australian study, participants who shampooed their hair each day with a shampoo containing 5 percent tea tree oil showed a 41 percent improvement in their dandruff compared with just 11 percent improvement in the people who used a placebo treatment.

You might mix a few drops of tea tree oil with your own herbal shampoo when you wash your hair. But don't take tea tree oil—or any essential oil, for that matter—internally. They are extremely concentrated and can be poisonous.

Depression

WHEN I WROTE *THE GREEN PHARMACY* BACK IN THE 1990S, I rarely experienced any kind of depression, except perhaps seasonal affective disorder. These days, however, I get a bit maudlin at times that are supposed to be happy, like Thanksgiving and Christmas. Even at my New Year's party, picking bluegrass music in a room lit by a small artificial Christmas tree with white lights, I felt little joy. As a matter of fact, I found it kind of gloomy! I almost misted up when the 79-year-old bass player (that's me), 76-year-old lead vocalist and guitarist, and 75-year-old mandolin player sang what tends to be a tear jerker at our age: "All the good times are o'er." So I guess I'm learning something about mood problems firsthand.

Here's what I've learned through research: Depression comes in many flavors and levels of intensity. People can experience major depression, which prevents them from performing their normal activities. They may struggle with seasonal affective disorder (called SAD, fittingly enough), which leaves them feeling down during the winter months, when the days are shorter. They may have bipolar disorder, in which they go through cycles of feeling depressed and agitated, or a milder form of chronic depressive disorder called dysthymia.

Different factors can contribute to your risk for depression, ranging from genetic predisposition to losses in your personal life. During depression, chemicals that carry messages in the brain—called neurotransmitters—don't seem to be present at the proper levels.

If you feel really depressed, have suicidal thoughts, or find yourself pondering death a lot, you need to see a medical professional quickly. But if you just feel a little blue more often than you'd like to, some foods can help boost your mood. Perhaps if I had been sucking on a licorice stick or filling my plate with saffron rice or some of the other foods in this chapter, I wouldn't have been so mournful while ringing in the new year.

Healing Foods for Depression

★★★**Fish oil** The longer the nights and the darker the days become as my part of the world moves toward midwinter, the more I head for the fish oil. For updates on the wonders of fish oil, I turn to Jerry Cott, PhD, a psychopharmacognocist at the National Institute of Mental Health, who's on top of the antidepressant literature about it. He tells me there have been at least eight clinical studies on omega-3 fatty acids (the active ingredients in fish oil) and depression.

In 2006, the *Journal of Clinical Psychiatry* ran a meta-analysis (a study that combines and interprets the results of an entire group of other studies) reviewing the evidence on omega-3's for depression and other mental disorders, written by a committee assembled by the American Psychiatric Association. Grouped together, the results show that omega-3's are useful for both depression and bipolar disorder. Research has found that major depression and bipolar disorder are 30 to 60 times more common in countries whose populations eat less fish. In Iceland and Japan, where people consume lots of seafood, there's less seasonal affective disorder— those winter blahs—than you'd expect.

The best way to get your omega-3's is from fatty fish. And I suppose that sipping fish oil—if you're up to the challenge—is one way of feeding yourself those omega-3's, too. That's the way I get it, though I can't say that it's the most savory beverage. And Mrs. Duke keeps fish-oil capsules in the refrigerator.

The meta-analysis cited above recommends eating fish at least twice a week, and if you have a mood disorder, consuming a gram of the fatty acids eicosapentaenoic acid (EPA) and docosahexaenoic acid (DHA) daily. Taking 1 to 9 grams in supplement form may be helpful, but any dose over 3 grams a day should be taken under your doctor's supervision, as too much fish oil can lead to bleeding disorders. Running a distant second are the vegetarian sources of omega-3's. Nearly all of them contain only alpha-linolenic acid (ALA), which the body must convert into DHA before using it. They include chia, chiso, flax, and walnut, with the last being the tastiest but not as high in ALA.

★★**Beans and seeds** Many beans and seeds are good sources of folate, which may make them helpful in treating depression. In 1962, a researcher went on a low-folate diet for 18 weeks and found that he became forgetful, irritable, and unable to sleep. That's not a good mental state for doing research, but it does describe the way many people with depression feel. Since then, folate has become a nutrient of interest to scientists investigating diet and depression.

Folate, also called folic acid and vitamin B$_9$, is thought to play a role in creating the brain chemicals dopamine, serotonin, and norepinephrine. If you run low on folate, you may also run low on these neurotransmitters. In addition, a deficiency of folate can cause a rise in your body's homocysteine levels, and studies have linked high homocysteine with depression.

A 2007 meta-analysis from the United Kingdom pooled the results of 11 studies and found that low folate was associated with at least a 42 percent increase in the risk of depression. I can't promise that getting more folate will ease your depression, but if you're running low on the nutrient, every little bit may help.

The recommended daily intake for folate is 400 micrograms. Here are some foods that will easily help you reach that amount, with their folate content given in micrograms.

½ cup black-eyed peas—180

½ cup lentils—180

1 avocado—164

½ cup sunflower seeds—160

½ cup pinto beans—148

½ cup chickpeas—140

½ cup lima beans—136

½ cup spinach—132

½ cup lima beans—128

½ cup kidney beans—116

A mixed bean soup with black-eyed peas, chickpeas, lentils, lima beans, and pinto beans could easily provide more than the recommended daily amount.

★★**Chocolate** Of the 300 compounds in chocolate, many are brain-altering chemicals that can help fight depression, including phenylethylamine and anandamide. Phenylethylamine is a cerebrostimulant, somewhat similar to amphetamine. Some people are highly sensitive to even small amounts of phenylethylamine, which is naturally present in our brains. In high enough doses, it can bring about reduced fatigue, exhilaration, and a sense of general well-being.

The other compound, anandamide, binds to the same receptors in your brain that are activated by smoking or ingesting marijuana. I've read that the professor who first discovered anandamide in pigs' brains named it from the Sanskrit word Aananda, which means bliss.

In addition, chocolate contains caffeine, theobromine, and theophylline, which are stimulants. These give you a bit of energy when you eat chocolate. I wouldn't recommend that you overindulge—chocolate is full of fat—but when you feel depressed, having a little just may lift your spirits a bit.

★★**Saffron** Saffron is a traditional Persian remedy for depression, so it's not surprising that much of the recent research into this golden reddish spice's effect on depression has come from Iran.

In a 2007 study from the University of Tehran, researchers gave 40 people with depression either 30 milligrams of saffron in capsule form or fluoxetine (Prozac) each day for 8 weeks. The two were similar in effectiveness. In a study from the previous year, also from Tehran, 40 depressed people took either 30 milligrams of saffron daily or a placebo for 6 weeks. Those who received the saffron had significantly improved symptoms compared to the placebo group. Yet another study, from 2004, found that saffron's effectiveness was similar to that of the antidepressant imipramine (Tofranil).

One problem with using saffron for depression that researchers frequently point out is its price. It's said to be the most expensive spice available, and I've seen a gram-size jar selling online for $10. But when you do the math, your $10 jar would give you 33 "doses," at 33 milligrams each, of the stuff—and I suspect it tastes better than any antidepressant!

★★**Seafood** Be sure to leave room on your plate for foods rich in vitamin B_{12}, such as cereal and certain types of seafood. One 2002 study found that people with B_{12} deficiency were 70 percent more likely to experience severe depression than those with ample blood levels of B_{12}.

The following foods are some of the best choices for getting more B_{12} into your diet, with the amount in each measured in micrograms. Men and women need 2.4 micrograms daily.

½ cup canned clam chowder—12

3 ounces steamed king crab—10

1 cup raisin bran cereal—6

1 blue-crab cake—3.6

3 ounces lamb loin—2

★★**Turmeric** This spice, like saffron (both have been identified as the "saffron" of the Bible), has undergone a lot of solid research into its effects on depression. There are 10 studies relating to turmeric and depression, and 11 on curcumin (a compound in turmeric) and depression. A 2008 Chinese study concluded that turmeric's anti-depressant activities involve the same system in the brain that uses serotonin.

★★**Walnuts** In the garden, I often ask my classes and tours to tell me the best source of serotonin, an important chemical messenger in the brain. Then I give them a clue: This brain food looks like a brain, and in more superstitious times, something that looked like a brain would be used to treat the brain. Yes, I'm talking about the humble walnut.

Walnuts are rich in serotonin. A few years ago, I asked more than a dozen scientists if dietary serotonin could increase cerebral serotonin. Finally I received a nice but negative reply from Dr. Cott, who told me it couldn't because the liver breaks down the chemical too quickly. However, quite by accident, I later heard a radio interview with Michael Gerson, MD, author of *The Second Brain*, who noted that the digestive tract is lined with serotonin receptors, and they would transmit the "message" long before the serotonin was broken down. So walnuts may be good for depression after all.

Walnuts are also a source of omega-3's. As a result, I think it couldn't hurt to toss back a few of these nuts on a regular basis if you're feeling down.

★**Floral teas** A cup or two of chamomile tea may help lift your spirits. It contains two antidepressant compounds (caffeic acid and quercetin) and an anti-stress compound (apigenin), so it may alleviate depression in several ways. Certified lactation consultant Sheila Humphrey, RN, notes that melissa, a.k.a. lemon balm or the "gladdening herb," can help in overcoming postpartum depression. "A couple of cups of fragrant lemon balm tea can lift the spirits, and so can lavender and rose teas," she says.

★**Garlic and onions** Although they're not often associated with depression relief, these odoriferous bulbs have components that may be useful in improving your mood and fighting the associated symptoms of insomnia, fatigue, and anxiety. Onions also contain isorhamnetin and kaempferol, which can act as monoamine oxidase inhibitors, an older form of medical antidepressant.

★**Ginger** This flavorful root has been used as a folk remedy for treating depression. It contains caffeic acid, melatonin, and quercetin, which may enhance mood, and components such as borneol and camphor, which act as stimulants.

★**Inositol-rich foods** Foods like soy, carob fruits, tea leaves, rice, peas, and lentils score high for inositol. This substance, which, according to the National Cancer Institute, is important for nerve and brain function, is a type of sugar. It may have anti-depressant activity, although this is still under investigation. My doctor, Ken Singleton, MD, a specialist in chronic Lyme disease, recommends inositol for the anxiety and compulsiveness that sometimes accompany Lyme and other tickborne diseases. An antidepressant soup made with rice, edamame, peas, and lentils would provide substantial quantities of inositol. Thicken or spice it up with antidepressant omega-3's such as walnut or flaxseed oil if you don't like fish oil, and add some saffron and turmeric.

★**Oregano** While you're raiding your spice cabinet, sprinkle some oregano on your foods. The caffeic acid, quercetin, and rosmarinic acid it contains may help with depression, and other components may relieve fatigue and anxiety and serve as monoamine oxidase inhibitors.

★**Sunflower seeds** Growing happily beside each other in my Green Farmacy Garden are evening primrose, perhaps best source of the natural antidepressant tryptophan; St. John's wort, with several antidepressants with actions similar to Prozac's; and sunflowers, reportedly a good source of the antidepressant phenylalanine. Of these, only sunflower seeds can be found on the shelves of your supermarket. Why not coat them with chocolate (with its anandamide and phenylethylamine) or carob (with its myoinositol) and flaxseed or walnut oil with its antidepressant omega-3's? Without added sugar, this could be a great healthful snack and a food farmaceutical for depression.

From the Herbal Medicine Chest

In *The Green Pharmacy*, I wrote that no plant in my database had more antidepressant compounds than licorice, yet it lacked a folk history. A trip to the computer shows me that licorice still outweighs any of the other herbs I checked out, so I still consider it a very useful tool for treating depression. Licorice contains numerous compounds that act as monoamine oxidase inhibitors, a type of antidepressant medication. Monoamine oxidase is an enzyme that breaks down the neurotransmitters norepinephrine, serotonin, and dopamine. Inhibiting the enzyme keeps levels of these neurochemicals higher in your brain.

If I were depressed, I'd brew up a tasty tea with some licorice (the herb, not the candy). Don't drink more than three cups a day, and for no longer than 6 weeks; long-term use can lead to headaches, lethargy, sodium and water retention, loss of potassium, and high blood pressure. Steer clear of alcohol; smoked and pickled foods; and medications, including hay fever and cold remedies, diuretics, tryptophan, tyrosine, and amphetamines, while you're drinking the tea. Don't use it at all if you're pregnant or nursing or if you have severe liver, kidney, or heart disease or high blood pressure.

Diabetes

ANYONE CONTENDING WITH DIABETES OR PREDIABETES (also called impaired glucose tolerance) knows that keeping blood sugar under control is a crucial and ongoing challenge. Fortunately, many foods and herbs can help you, and of them, cinnamon gets my biggest gold star.

My longtime friend, herbal enthusiast Roy Upton, uses cinnamon regularly to help control his type 2 diabetes. Roy is president of the American Herbal Pharmacopoeia, a national organization that advocates for the safe and responsible use of herbal medicines, so he knows his stuff. After he read about a number of US Department of Agriculture studies conducted by Richard Anderson, PhD, and colleagues, Roy started using cinnamon himself, both to help his body make better use of insulin and to rev up his metabolism to help keep his weight under control.

Incidentally, Mrs. Duke also uses cinnamon to help with her prediabetes. It's been almost a year since our primary physician diagnosed her as prediabetic. On my advice, she started taking cinnamon and turmeric. At her next checkup, she was out of the prediabetic range and back into the normal range. The physician just laughed when she said she did it with herbs: He doesn't believe in herbs.

By the way, there are two types of diabetes—type 1 and type 2. Most of the advice in this chapter applies to type 2. In type 1, the immune system destroys the cells in the pancreas that manufacture insulin, a hormone that helps the body use sugar to produce energy. In type 2 diabetes, the body either doesn't properly use insulin or the pancreas doesn't make enough. In either case, unhealthy levels of sugar build up in the body instead of providing energy. Over time, excess blood sugar causes damage in many areas of the body, causing conditions such as kidney disease, nerve damage, blindness, and circulatory disease. So it's imperative to keep blood sugar under control. That's why, if you have diabetes, paying attention to what and when you eat is so important.

Type 2 diabetes typically develops later in life in people who are sedentary and overweight. Conversely, keeping your weight down can help prevent type 2 diabetes, and losing weight may even help reverse prediabetes. So, if you have type 2 diabetes or have been told you are prediabetic, you may also want to also pay attention to all the foods and herbs detailed in the Overweight chapter.

People with diabetes will find plenty of healing products on the spice shelf and in the produce section of the supermarket. In fact, there are more than a hundred plants that can help. Here are some of my favorites.

Healing Foods for Diabetes

★★★**Chromium** Here's some trivia for you: Chromium accounts for 6 percent of mineral supplement sales in the United States, in part because manufacturers tout it for treating diabetes. The quality of research on chromium for this condition isn't great, but it's still worth adding chromium-rich foods to your diet.

A 2007 meta-analysis—a study that pools the results of other studies—found that in people with type 2 diabetes, chromium supplementation improved their levels of hemoglobin A1c (a common indicator of long-term blood sugar control) by 0.6 percent, which is a nice improvement, since a 1 percent drop has been associated with a 20 percent lower risk of heart attack or stroke. Chromium does its work by making your body more sensitive to insulin, which then takes up glucose from your blood.

Again, better studies need to be done, and so far the government hasn't made any daily dosage recommendations, so don't go overboard with the supplements. Good food sources include blackstrap molasses, eggs, liver, chicken, cornflakes, and oysters.

There are plant foods that provide this mineral as well. Surprise: The richest source in my USDA database is roselle, the red in red zinger tea. Other good sources include dandelion, oats, stevia, lemongrass, peach, juniper, and barley.

★★★**Cinnamon** What's not to like? It smells good. It tastes good. And even a bit added to your food has medicinal value. One study found that as little as ½ teaspoon of powdered cinnamon a day may help decrease blood sugar levels and other risk factors in people with diabetes.

It's worth taking a closer look at this study, done by Dr. Anderson. Sixty Pakistani participants with type 2 diabetes, none of whom were using insulin, were randomly divided into six groups. One group took 1 gram of cinnamon per day, a second group took 3 grams, and a third group took 6 grams. The other three other groups were given placebo capsules.

In volunteers taking as little as 1 gram—less than ½ teaspoon—per day for 40 days, the results were amazing. They had about a 20 percent improvement in blood sugar, cholesterol, and triglyceride levels. There seemed to be no advantage to taking more than that amount. Significantly, the volunteers' blood sugar levels started climbing again when they stopped taking the cinnamon.

A half teaspoon a day isn't much. You can sprinkle some on your morning oatmeal. And apple butter is made with cinnamon, so you can put a big glob on any hot cereal as an alternative to sweetener, spiking it with more cinnamon if desired. Cinnamon toast is one of Mrs. Duke's favorites, especially on blah mornings. Just sprinkle a bit of cinnamon on top of whatever you spread on your toast. Use a cinnamon stick to stir your cocoa or cut a raw apple into slices and sprinkle them lightly with cinnamon for a snack that also provides fiber.

★★★**Fiber** Normally, the body does a pretty good job of keeping blood sugar within the normal range after a meal (70 to 145 mg/dl). But when you have diabetes, your blood sugar is apt to climb. The experts call this a postprandial glucose excursion, but you can think of it as your blood sugar zooming up a great big hill. The idea is to eat so that after a meal or snack, your blood sugar level stays steadier. Fiber can help.

Fiber makes your stomach release food more slowly and causes the rest of your digestive tract to release nutrients into your system more gradually. As an added benefit, beans, fruits, vegetables, and whole-grain foods that pack lots of fiber are also good sources of vitamins and minerals. They contain chemicals that dampen inflammation and reduce the damaging effects of free radicals (rogue oxygen molecules), which are of particular concern to people with diabetes.

A 2004 meta-analysis found that people with diabetes who ate moderate-carbohydrate, high-fiber diets had 21 percent lower post-meal blood sugar. They also had 7 percent lower total cholesterol and 8 percent lower low-density lipoprotein ("bad") cholesterol. People who ate high-carbohydrate, high-fiber diets had 14 percent lower fasting blood sugar and post-meal blood sugar and a significant decrease in their hemoglobin A1c.

The authors of this paper recommend getting 25 to 50 grams of fiber daily. Before you start dreading the idea of spooning powdery fiber supplement into your drinks all day, take a look at some foods (with fiber amounts in grams) that can help you easily get more than 40 grams of fiber.

Baked product containing 1 cup buckwheat flour	12
1 pear	10
1 cup canned chili	9
½ cup black beans	7.5
1 cup whole wheat spaghetti	6

There you go—more than 44 grams! How easy was that? No supplements, and no eating bowl after bowl of bran cereal.

★★**Bay leaf** Dr. Anderson's studies show that as little as ⅛ teaspoon of bay leaf can triple your insulin efficiency. It's a snap to get that much—or should I say that little? You don't have to make gourmet or "from scratch" recipes either. Just adding a couple of pinches of powdered bay leaf when you're heating canned soups or sauces will enhance the taste while doing you a lot of good. Or you can add a couple of whole bay leaves, but be sure to fish them out before eating, since they have sharp edges and can get stuck in your throat.

★★**Chicory** If you live in the South, you know all about chicory. There's a good chance you drink roasted chicory in your coffee. But if you don't live in the South, you owe it to yourself to learn about chicory. It may be a little harder to find outside of Dixie, but it's worth the effort.

The major component in chicory, one of the earliest and most widely used coffee substitutes, is inulin. Chicory and other inulin-containing herbs, such as Jerusalem artichoke, dandelion, and endive, can all be roasted or scorched and used as coffee substitutes. But you don't have to do this yourself; you can buy coffee mixed with chicory or plain roasted chicory to brew into a tasty beverage.

Studies have shown that chicory can help stabilize blood sugar levels. Dare I say that inulin modulates insulin? That's what the science seems to indicate.

★★**Fenugreek** Studies show that this spice, popular in Indian and Middle Eastern cuisines, can actually help your body produce more insulin. A chemical in the herb (4-hydroxyisoleucine) acts directly on the beta cells in the pancreas to encourage insulin secretion.

"It is now well documented from a number of studies that adding fenugreek seeds to the diets of diabetic patients or animals results in a significant fall in blood glucose and improvement in glucose tolerance," writes an author reviewing fenugreek in a 2005 issue of the *International Journal of Food Sciences and Nutrition*. In one study, 17 of 21 people with type 2 diabetes who took 15 grams of fenugreek daily had a decrease in blood sugar with no change in their insulin levels. In another study, diabetic volunteers took fenugreek seeds for 3 weeks, which resulted in improved blood sugar and less excess thirst and urination.

★★**Green beans** Studies done in India have shown that green beans (string beans) can lower blood sugar in lab animals with diabetes. Now, I've never needed any encouragement to eat my green beans. I'm perfectly capable of standing out in the garden and chomping them fresh from the vine. In fact, if I had to choose one veggie dish as my absolute favorite, it would green beans cooked with onions, with some diced raw onions added after cooking.

★★**Magnesium** People with diabetes—especially those with poor blood sugar control—are often low in magnesium. Studies have shown that getting more of this mineral in your diet may help your body produce more insulin and use it more efficiently, improve your cholesterol, and maintain healthier blood vessels.

A 2006 meta-analysis published in the journal *Diabetic Medicine* combined the results of nine studies and found that an average of 12 weeks of magnesium supplementation was associated with lower fasting glucose levels and increased high-density lipoprotein ("good") cholesterol. The average supplement dose was 360 milligrams.

The recommended daily intake for magnesium is 400 to 420 milligrams for men and 310 to 320 milligrams for nonpregnant women. It's not hard to get that much in a healthful diet; here are some foods with a good supply of the mineral, measured in milligrams.

½ halibut fillet	170
1 cup boiled spinach	157
1 ounce pumpkin seeds	151
1 cup white beans	134
1 oat bran muffin	89

★★**Onions and garlic** Important elements of the Mediterranean diet, onions and garlic can be used to prevent or treat type 2 diabetes. Raw onion bulbs have long been used to treat diabetes in Asia, Europe, and the Middle East, and there's some scientific validation for this treatment. Onions improve metabolism in people with diabetes, thanks in part to a couple of chemicals it contains (allylpropyldisulfide and S-methylcysteine sulfoxide). Studies have also shown that garlic helps lower blood sugar levels and prevent cardiovascular complications associated with diabetes, and it stimulates the beta cells in the pancreas to secrete insulin.

I don't need to tell you that there are all kinds of delicious ways to enjoy both onions and garlic. My bottom-line advice here is simply to look for more ways to include both in your cooking. Or eat them raw if you can. Some people find them tough to tackle raw, but you get more of the active ingredients this way.

★★**Turmeric** This spice, from which Indian curries and American mustards derive their yellow color, has a long tradition of use in treating diabetes. Research has shown that the active components—curcumin and tetrahydrocurcumin—possess anti-diabetic, anti-inflammatory, and antioxidant activity. In lab animals, these substances helped lower levels of blood sugar, increase insulin levels, and protect against kidney damage.

You don't have to confine this spice to curries, however. Any time you make rice, you can add ¼ to ½ teaspoon of turmeric to the cooking water, which will turn the rice a lovely yellow color without significantly altering the taste. When making rice dishes, Hispanic cooks sometimes use commercially prepared packets of annatto, a yellow coloring agent, to create the look of saffron, a dearly expensive spice. The problem is that this product often contains high amounts of sodium in the form of salt and MSG. You can get that same appealing color without the sodium by using a small amount of turmeric.

You can also add a bit of turmeric to potatoes and vegetables like cauliflower.

★★**Vinegar** Long ago, diabetes was diagnosed by the sweetness it gave to urine. (I certainly hope those doctors were paid well.) In the more recent past, before the invention of blood sugar–reducing drugs, folks used vinegar as a home remedy for diabetes—and it's still useful today. The acetic acid in vinegar makes your stomach empty more slowly, which helps you feel fuller after eating and causes your body to slow its absorption of carbohydrates. Therefore, your blood sugar rises more gradually.

Studies have shown that adding just a spoonful or two of vinegar to white bread or white rice (which normally takes your blood sugar zooming on one of those excursions I mentioned) lowered blood sugar after consumption by at least 25 percent and more than doubled participants' sense of fullness after eating. An easy and very palatable way to sneak some vinegar into your meals is to mix a few spoonfuls with a little olive oil—and maybe stir in some crushed walnuts—and use as a salad dressing.

★**Almonds** If you're having trouble with your blood sugar, I say nuts to you! That is, maybe you should eat some nuts. In a 2007 Canadian study, researchers gave nine healthy volunteers a "meal" of white bread to be eaten either alone or with 1, 2, or 3 ounces of almonds. Eating the almonds reduced the blood sugar surge from the bread, and they worked in a dose-dependent manner: the more almonds eaten, the greater the effect. I wouldn't recommend stuffing yourself with them—they're calorie dense—but eating a few may be a good way to precede or end a meal.

★**Blueberries and bilberries** It may seem contradictory that blueberries made this list. They are, after all, pretty sweet. But the benefits of their phytochemicals may outweigh the detriments of their sugar content. I recommend them mainly for the prevention of retinopathy, which is damage to the retina that can develop in people with diabetes. Unless you live in the West, you probably don't have access to bilberries, but if you do, they deliver the same beneficial nutrients.

★**Buckwheat** The next time you join friends or family for breakfast at your local pancake restaurant, order the buckwheat pancakes rather than the regular ones. They taste pretty good, and they can help lower your blood sugar. Go easy on the syrup, though.

★**Cloves** Mom alleviated many of my toothaches long ago with a drop of clove oil applied directly to the tooth. But cloves can help more than a toothache. They contain eugenol, a substance that can stimulate insulin production. People with insulin-dependent diabetes can safely use reasonable doses of clove (500 milligrams has been shown effective) to increase the efficiency of their insulin. Try steeping a few whole cloves in your regular cup of tea.

★**Dairy foods** This tidbit should make your next cool glass of milk taste even more refreshing. A 2007 review of earlier research showed a relatively consistent association between low vitamin D levels and dairy intake and the presence of type 2 diabetes. Up to half of American teens and adults may be low in vitamin D, one of whose important jobs in your body is to work hand in hand with calcium. The authors speculate that the rising numbers of diabetes cases in this country may be due in part to Americans' low levels of calcium and vitamin D.

Some research suggests that in people with prediabetes, vitamin D and calcium supplementation may help prevent the condition from progressing to full-blown type 2 diabetes. Make room in your diet for plenty of low-fat milk, yogurt, and other dairy products. Beside dairy, other sources of D include salmon, mackerel, and sardines.

★**Prunes** Recent USDA studies suggest that the mineral boron may help reduce the amount of insulin required to manage blood sugar levels. Prunes are the most readily available rich source of dietary boron; others include plums, strawberries, peaches, cabbage, asparagus, and tomatoes. Prunes are also a good source of fiber.

★**Tea** The caffeine in coffee and tea can help rev your metabolism and keep your weight under control. But research shows there are several reasons to favor tea over coffee if you have diabetes.

In one study of lab animals with diabetes, green tea extract helped prevent cardiac dysfunction, reduce LDL cholesterol and elevate HDL, reduce triglyceride levels, and control weight gain.

In a 2007 study published in the *Journal of the American College of Nutrition*, participants consumed a set amount of sugar along with either plain water, caffeinated water, or black tea. Two hours later, the people who drank tea had significantly lower blood sugar levels and higher insulin levels.

Based on my read of the chemicals involved, you can substitute black tea for green and get the same benefits. And here's yet another way to use cinnamon: Sprinkle a little in your tea, add a bit of stevia as a sugar substitute, and enjoy!

From the Herbal Medicine Chest

For years, I've suggested that anyone who enjoys licorice can benefit from using it as a sweetener in place of sugar. Lo and behold, scientific studies over the past few years have suggested that this would be a helpful practice for preventing or decelerating the onset of metabolic syndrome, a combination of health conditions that increases your risk of heart disease, stroke, and diabetes.

The studies in question used fairly high amounts of licorice tincture (ethanolic extract). You might try using a small piece of natural licorice root, which is available in many health food stores, to sweeten coffee or tea. I'm not a big fan of its taste, but by all means give it a try and see if it appeals to you.

Diarrhea

COMMON, RUN-OF-THE-MILL DIARRHEA just happens now and then. We've all had our bouts of it. Diarrhea usually occurs when bacteria and viruses get into our digestive systems or when certain foods we eat aren't completely digested and end up fermenting in our intestines. Our bodies then react by pulling in pools of water, causing unpleasantly loose stools.

Most diarrhea lasts only a day or two, but when it continues beyond a few days, it can deplete large amounts of fluids and essential nutrients from the body.

Go for Bland

Until diarrhea runs its course, stick with bland foods such as the following, which won't aggravate your already irritated colon.

Applesauce   Soda crackers

Bananas   White bread

Noodles   Rice

A bonus: The fiber in these gentle foods absorbs water in your large intestine and helps add bulk to your stools.

If you've heard recommendations to drink fruit juice, flat cola, and diluted sports drinks during and after bouts of diarrhea, that's why; doing so helps replace lost sugars and minerals. Replenishing your body after the draining effects of diarrhea is key.

There are a number of natural approaches to clearing up a bout of diarrhea, all of which contain one or more of three active ingredients: tannins, pectin, and mucilage.

Tannins are the chemicals that give some foods their astringency, that is, their ability to bind up and contract tissue. They adhere to the protein layer of inflamed mucous membranes (i.e., an irritated intestine in the case of diarrhea) and cause it to thicken, which slows absorption of toxins and hinders secretion.

Pectin is a type of soluble fiber that adds bulk to your stools and soothes your digestive tract. The "pectate" in the over-the-counter antidiarrheal medicine Kaopectate contains pectin.

Mucilage is another potent type of fiber. It soothes your digestive tract and adds bulk to your stools by absorbing water and swelling considerably.

Ironically, the two fiber types are amphoteric, firming stools when they're too loose and softening them when they're too hard.

Healing Foods for Diarrhea

A number of foods can be helpful in battling diarrhea. Here are some to try.

★★★**Apples** Both the skin and the pulp of apples are rich in pectin, which is why apples and applesauce are common folk remedies for diarrhea. Apple pectin also helps treat constipation because it acts as a gentle stool softener. As they say, eating "an apple a day" can do wonders for keeping you regular.

★★★**Tea** One of the most astringent natural remedies for diarrhea is conventional tea in traditional teabags. The next time you have diarrhea, try a nice cup of tea— just plain, without any other herbs or spices added. It's rich in tannins, which help bind stools and hold back bowel movements.

★★**Bilberries and blueberries** These berries work well against diarrhea because they are rich in both tannins and pectin. Dried, not fresh, bilberries and blueberries are best. And studies suggest that eating blueberries may reduce your risk of colon cancer to boot.

★★**Carob** Nearly 30 years ago in Panama, I had an acute attack of salmonella after handling some turtles. My Panamanian doctor prescribed powdered carob for the serious diarrhea, and it seemed to work. But not until 1995 did I read about a 1989

FOODS TO WATCH

Certain foods can raise havoc with your bowels. If you have chronic diarrhea, try reducing or eliminating these foods from your diet.

Dairy foods. Dairy items contain a natural sugar called lactose, which many people have a hard time digesting (lactose intolerance). However, many people with lactose intolerance can eat yogurt, which is naturally lower in lactose than other dairy foods.

Prepared foods. If you love to eat in restaurants, try to avoid ordering menu items that are typically prepared early in the day and reheated later on. Foods such as lasagna and quiche, for example, are more prone to bacterial contamination than foods that are made fresh and served hot.

Fruit juice and honey. These contain a natural sugar called fructose, which, when eaten in large amounts, can move into the large intestine undigested. This can cause it to ferment and bring on unwanted gas and diarrhea.

Sugarless gum and candy. Sorbitol, an artificial sweetener found in sugarless gums and candies, can be hard to digest. Like fructose, it can ferment in the intestine and cause diarrhea. Other artificial sweeteners—such as mannitol, xylitol, erythritol, and D-tagatose—can cause problems, too. If you have frequent bouts of diarrhea and happen to eat or chew lots of "sugarless" or "sugar-free" items, try switching to the regular kind instead.

Vitamin C. Although the health benefits of vitamin C are incredibly plentiful, and it can actually protect the digestive tract by boosting immunity against nasty bacteria, too much can cause diarrhea. Large doses of C—especially 500 to 2,000 milligrams of dietary supplements taken regularly—may bring on gastrointestinal problems.

study, published in the *Journal of Pediatric Gastroenterology and Nutrition*, involving 41 infants with bacterial or viral diarrhea. Children given 1.5 grams (per kilogram of body weight) of carob powder had diarrhea for only 2 days. Normalization of bowel movements, body temperature, and weight, as well as cessation of vomiting, all occurred more quickly with carob.

★★Carrots Cooked carrots seem to soothe the digestive tract and control diarrhea. They also provide nutrients that are lost during an attack. Interestingly, folks who live in the Appalachian Mountains cook their beans with a small whole carrot—a natural way to reduce the sometimes unpleasant effects of fiber-rich foods, such as gas and bloating.

★★Garlic, onions, and leeks Eating foods known as prebiotics—indigestible food elements that stimulate the growth of "good" bacteria in the digestive tract—can be helpful in preventing diarrhea. Natural sources of prebiotics include garlic, onions, and leeks (which are also antiseptic). Eating lots of these flavorful foods can boost the immune system and ward off diarrhea-causing bacteria. And according to studies in India, garlic's link to good bacteria in the intestines also improves digestion and enhances absorption of minerals, a helpful bonus during and after a nasty case of diarrhea.

★★Pomegranate This biblical fruit is often used to treat diarrhea. It's the seeds, full of tart yet sweet astringent juice, that help to bind and dry up your bowels. The husk, rarely consumed directly, may have even more binding tannins; it's sometimes blended into pomegranate juice, so sipping this juice is a good option.

From the Herbal Medicine Chest

These herbs can help prevent or clear up diarrhea.

Agrimony (Agrimonia eupatoria) This herb is high in stool-binding tannins. Try using 2 or 3 teaspoons of agrimony leaves to make a tea.

Fenugreek (Trigonella foeum-graecum) The seeds of this herb contain up to 50 percent mucilage, which absorbs water in the intestine and swells. Don't use more than 2 teaspoons of fenugreek at a time, or you may experience abdominal distress.

Psyllium (Plantago ovata) Psyllium is also high in mucilage, which makes it useful for treating diarrhea by adding bulk to stools. If you have allergies or asthma, however, use this herb with caution.

Diverticulitis

OUR ANCESTORS ATE LOTS OF FIBER and had healthy colons to show for it. But as the American diet began moving toward processed foods in the early 1900s, fiber consumption faded, and so did our ability to avoid digestive disorders like diverticulitis.

Diverticulitis involves little pockets or pouches known as diverticula that form in the wall of the colon. These pouches can become plugged with bits of digested food or little seeds. If they then become inflamed or infected, an array of unpleasant symptoms can occur, including chronic lower abdominal pain, cramping, gas, bloating, and alternating bouts of diarrhea and constipation.

Diverticulitis can be a particularly miserable condition, but it's rare in parts of the world where diets remain rich in fiber, such as Africa and Asia. In the United States, unfortunately, it has become far too common. Today, about 10 percent of Americans over age 40 and about half of people over age 60 have diverticulosis—a precursor of full-blown diverticulitis ("-itis" means inflamed or infected).

Pockets Full of Pain

So how do those nasty little colon pockets happen? Again, the answer is in the diet. People who most often develop diverticulitis often have what expert nutritionist Andrew Weil, MD, professor at the University of Arizona College of Medicine in Tucson, calls a less than healthy lifestyle. These folks tend to eat very little fiber and often experience constipation and difficult bowel movements with hard stools. All the pushing and straining to "go" causes the walls of the colon to become weak and develop diverticula. These pockets then trap food particles that ferment and decay, causing all kinds of gastrointestinal trouble.

The good news: Diverticulitis is quite preventable if you eat right, and high-fiber foods are the secret to keeping your colon healthy. Eating lots of fruits, vegetables, beans, and whole-grain cereal and bread every day is the trick. And drink lots of water, which is important to keep all that great fiber moving on through. Remember: If you're avoiding constipation, you're avoiding diverticulitis.

However, if you have a diverticulitis attack, you'll want to scale back on fiber to give your colon time to heal. Try a low-fiber diet and clear liquids for a few days. Then ease yourself back into fiber by eating 5 to 15 more grams of fiber each day to let your colon slowly readjust.

Healing Foods for Diverticulitis

★★**Apples** An apple a day may keep the diverticular doctor away. Consuming soluble and insoluble fiber (a 10-ounce apple can have 6 grams of fiber), which keeps the digestive system working well, may prevent both constipation and its sequel, diverticulitis. My good friend James Joseph, PhD, also champions the colorful apple for diverticulosis in his book *The Color Code*.

★★Chamomile It smells like apple, and chamomile (called *manzanilla,* or "little apple," in Spanish) may be as helpful as the apple. Super phytotherapists Simon Mills and Kerry Bone, in their book *Principles and Practice of Phytotherapy,* describe chamomile more for prevention than for cure.

David Hoffman, a British-trained medical herbalist, suggests sipping on chamomile or peppermint tea throughout the day as an anti-inflammatory approach. He regards peppermint as an antacid. You might think that the salicylates (aspirin-like compounds) in chamomile would be contraindicated for diverticulitis, but Hoffmann says it has a specific value in diverticulitis as well as colon trouble in general. Loaded with the COX-2 inhibitor apigenin and several calming compounds, chamomile may also ease the pain of an attack. Its anti-inflammatory action is especially welcome in the digestive system, where the infusion releases soothing oils. His recipe suggests infusing 2 teaspoons of herb for 5 to 10 minutes in water that has reached a boil and drinking it after meals.

★★Flaxseed In their beautifully illustrated book, *Natural Geographic Desk Reference to Nature's Medicine,* Steven Foster and Rebecca L. Johnson recommend flax (and I'd add crushed flaxseed) as a safe and gentle laxative for chronic constipation, diverticulitis, and irritable bowel syndrome. Commission E, the expert panel that decides on the safety, effectiveness and dosage of medicinal herbs for the German government, approves using 1 to 3 tablespoons of crushed (not whole, as the seeds can get stuck in the diverticula) flaxseed two or three times a day—with lots of water—to treat diverticulitis. Flaxseed is very high in fiber, the key to a healthy colon. Equally important, it's a good vegetarian source of alpha-linolenic acid (ALA), one of the omega-3 fatty acids.

In *The Omega-3 Phenomenon*, by Donald O. Rudin, MD, and more recent publications, omega-3's in proper ratios with omega-6's can probably help more than 50 ailments, including diverticulitis. Most of us have bad omega-3 to omega-6 ratios, and since it seems clear that omega-3's can help with inflammation, restoring the balance between the two may help prevent diverticular flare-ups. Other good sources of ALA include chia, chiso, hemp, inca peanut, and walnut seeds.

★★Hempseed Beside me, I have a can of Nutiva (shelled hempseed, rich in omega-3's), which comes from Sebastopol, California. The label says that 2 tablespoons (19 grams), the recommended serving, contains 5,360 milligrams of omega-6's, 1,500 milligrams of omega-3's, and 3 milligrams of gamma-linolenic acid. The seeds are tasty with cereals, salads, and soups. I calculate that the shelled seed cost $13 a

FOODS TO WATCH

Seeds and foods with seeds can be particularly troublesome if you have diverticulitis because they can get stuck in the diverticula and irritate your colon, especially during an attack. Here are a few to avoid.

Seeds:

Poppy seeds

Sesame seeds

Sunflower seeds

Foods with seeds:

Pomegranates

Strawberries

Raspberries

Tomatoes

Popcorn kernels can cause trouble, too, so your best bet is to steer clear of this snack food.

pound. My fish oil runs closer to $20 per pound, so you do the math. You can order the product online from www.nutiva.com.

★★**Peppermint** While so far this plant only has folkloric evidence for its effectiveness in treating diverticulitis, it has approval for dyspepsia from the German Commission E, a German government agency that evaluates the safety and efficacy of medicinal herbs. With more than a dozen anti-inflammatory compounds, painkillers, and sedatives and a half dozen carminatives, peppermint has good phytochemical rationale. As mentioned earlier, David Hoffman recommends sipping the tea for diverticulitis.

★★**Prunes** Prunes have lots of fiber and are considered the most effective food remedy for constipation, the biggest risk factor for diverticulitis. They also contain a substance called dihydroxyphenyl isatin, which stimulates the contractions in your intestines that you need for regular bowel movements. Prunes contain a natural sugar called sorbitol, which, like fiber, soaks up large amounts of water in your digestive tract to keep things moving.

Robert's Formula

During an attack of diverticulitis, several herbs called demulcents can be used to coat and soothe the walls of the large intestine and help heal swollen, irritated tissues. Robert's Formula is an herbal combination known to be very good for gastrointestinal irritation. The mixture contains herbs such as slippery elm, marshmallow root, and geranium. Echinacea and goldenseal may also be included to help boost the immune system. The formula can be found at some health food stores; the herbal ingredients vary.

★★**Thyme** As a rich source of fiber, plus dozens of analgesic, anti-inflammatory, and antispasmodic compounds, thyme seems like a good choice for your antidiverticulitis arsenal. Try using it to season sauces, soups, and salads.

★★**Turmeric** It's strange to think that spicy Indian food would help with diverticulitis, but it does. Turmeric, the main ingredient in curry, is truly a powerful anti-inflammatory that's been used as a natural medicine for thousands of years. India's traditional Ayurvedic doctors used it for all kinds of swelling, and it's believed to have a number of gastrointestinal benefits, including reducing the swelling of colon pockets in diverticulitis.

Curcumin, the most active ingredient in turmeric, has great medicinal power. Jonny Bowden, PhD, a nutrition and health expert and author of *The Most Effective Natural Cures on Earth*, praises curcumin for its enormous power as an anti-inflammatory and says it's a great help for swollen and inflamed diverticula. If you have diverticulitis, I suggest eating more curry loaded with turmeric.

★★**Wheat bran** Wheat bran has long been seen by doctors and nutritionists alike as the safest, cheapest, and most effective way to prevent and treat constipation and therefore diverticulitis. Neil Painter, MD, the British researcher whose groundbreaking 1972 study suggested that diverticular disease might be due to a dietary fiber deficiency, estimated that wheat bran contains five times more fiber than whole-wheat bread does, making it a fiber power food. You can't go wrong with wheat bran.

When I use it, I sometimes take a slippery elm and peppermint tea, sweetened to a syrup-like consistency, with 15 grams of bran flakes in it. To make the syrup, bring a handful of slippery elm bark and two handfuls of fresh peppermint barely to a boil in just enough water to cover. Take the mixture off the heat and thicken it with honey. Then refrigerate it and use as needed with the wheat bran flakes.

From the Herbal Medicine Chest

Wild yam can help relieve the pain and inflammation of diverticulitis. It's antispasmodic (to reduce wavelike cramping) and anti-inflammatory (to reduce swelling), which makes it useful for treating the gastrointestinal woes that often accompany diverticulitis. It's also been shown to help calm irritable bowel syndrome.

Wild yam is a perennial vine plant that grows in wild in moist, wooded areas. It's not the same vegetable as the "yams" sold in supermarkets, which are members of the sweet potato family and not true yams. The herb can be found in health food stores.

California herbalist Kathi Keville, author of *The Illustrated Herb Encyclopedia* and *Herbs for Health and Healing*, has a good formula.

2 parts wild yam (antispasmodic and anti-inflammatory)

1 part valerian (relaxes and soothes the digestive tract)

1 part black haw (antispasmodic)

1 part peppermint (antispasmodic and anti-inflammatory)

If I had diverticulitis, I might use a couple of tablespoons of this herbal mixture brewed in a quart of water.

Dry Mouth

TO SOME, DRY MOUTH MIGHT SEEM LIKE A HEALTH PROBLEM along the same line as "two left feet" or "itchy trigger finger." But xerostomia—the medical name for dry mouth—is a real condition that may have serious consequences.

In addition to a feeling of dryness, xerostomia might bring on thick or stringy saliva, cracked lips, bad breath, a sore throat, and sores at the corners of your mouth. A dry mouth might affect your sense of taste since you don't have the saliva needed to thoroughly chew and process food. More seriously, since saliva washes away food particles and plaque from teeth, a dry mouth can lead to increased plaque, tooth decay, and gum disease.

On an average day, a healthy adult produces roughly 3 pints of saliva, but as you age the saliva glands start to be less productive and your sense of thirst changes so that you're less aware of your body's thirst for fluids. In addition to this natural drying, many medications—particularly antihistamines, medications for high blood pressure, and drugs that treat depression and anxiety—dry out the mouth as a side effect. Chemotherapy and nerve damage can also cause dry mouth, along with controllable behaviors such as snoring, breathing through your mouth, and smoking.

Depending on the cause, you might be able to alleviate dry mouth in different ways: see a doctor about the snoring so that you can breathe easily at night and not through your mouth; stop smoking (which will simultaneously improve many other aspects of your health); or get switched to a different medication or an adjusted dose of the current medication.

A couple of medications are meant to stimulate saliva production, but rather than turn to them, let's see what else we can do. Chewing gum and sucking on hard candies are obvious ways to get more saliva flowing, but choose sugar-free options or else your actions will be counterproductive: producing more saliva to wash away bacteria, while coating your teeth with sugar to feed and produce more of them! You might consider placing a humidifier in your bedroom at night to add moisture to the air.

Healing Foods for Dry Mouth

★★★**Water and other nonsweetened drinks** This might be the most obvious food solution for dry mouth, but I thought I'd mention it just the same. Keep a water bottle with you, and place a glass of water by your seat or bed, so that you can sip at all times. Having water readily accessible will undoubtedly encourage you to drink more. As with the gum and hard candy, choose drinks that don't contain sugar.

If you can stand the cold, you might instead want to suck on ice cubes for the slow release of water and the stimulation of your saliva glands.

★★**Hard cheese** As you'll notice later in this chapter, I push pudding and sauces rather than gummy foods. As a result, you might be surprised to see hard cheese on the list of food suggestions.

A short explanation: Saliva normally has a pH level between 6.5 and 7.4, and with water—the most neutral of substances—having a pH of 7, you can see that

FOODS TO WATCH

> They say that two glasses of wine is max for us men if we want to be healthy.
>
> Alcohol is a real dehydrator–three glasses will give me a dry mouth.

saliva ranges only from mildly acidic to mildly alkaline. When xerostomia reduces the amount of saliva that you produce, the pH level of your mouth's environment drops, making your mouth more acidic and increasing the chance of developing dental caries—that is, the destruction of the tooth enamel on the level of microbes.

Believe it or not, a study in the *American Journal of Dentistry* looked at the effectiveness of hard cheese on saliva production in patients undergoing radiotherapy—one of the potential causes of xerostomia—and found that patients who ate cheese had more rehardening of their enamel than patients who had their saliva production artificially stimulated. In fact, the enamel rehardening in the cheese eaters was nearly at the level of study participants who weren't undergoing radiotherapy at all.

★**Chile peppers** I put chile peppers here instead of cayenne because technically the hot pepper contains more capsaicin than the cool or bell pepper and because the hotter the pepper, the more capsaicin it contains. While it seems illogical to take a hot pepper for dry mouth, capsaicin stimulates salivation, as well as other watery exudates, lachrymation, and sweat.

★**Gravies, sauces, broths, and dressings** Along the same lines as the previous advice, add toppings to your dishes to increase the amount of liquid that makes up your meals. Instead of chicken, for example, you might have chicken soup, which will add broth to your diet. Boil down berries to create a fruit glaze for a piece of pork. Try to avoid using dressings and gravies with lots of fat or sauces with added sugars so that you'll get the benefits of added liquid without adding other complications to your diet.

★**Pudding, yogurt, fruit sauces, and ice cream** In case you needed a warning, do not mix the items listed above into a single dish or else your stomach will be very unhappy. These items are all examples of foods that have a high percentage of liquid in them, and the liquid should make them easier to eat than dry foods such as crackers, potato chips, granola, and nuts. Do not, however, use this as an excuse to go nuts with the amount of ice cream you eat.

Earache

IF YOU WERE A CHILD AT SOME POINT IN YOUR LIFE—and I'd wager that you were—then you probably suffered through at least one ear infection in your youth. According to the National Institute on Deafness and Other Communication Disorders, three out of four children have had an ear infection by the time they turn 3 years old.

Most instances of earache come from one of two types of ear infection: acute otitis media—*otitis* means "inflammation of the ear" and *media* means "middle"—or otitis media with effusion. In the first case, the inner ear is infected or swollen, and fluid and mucus become trapped in the ear. In the second case, the infection has cleared up, yet fluid remains trapped in a child's ear, laying the groundwork for new infections.

Ear infections usually come about when a virus gives you a cold, which then swells and blocks the eustachian tubes—passageways that connect the middle ear to your nose and equalize pressure within your ear by moving fluid through it. Eustachian tubes in children are thinner and shorter than those in adults and are more easily blocked; blockages keep your ears from being able to adjust to different air pressures.

Another possible cause of earaches is your adenoids. These tissues, which are located behind your ears near the eustachian tubes, produce cells that help you fight infection. If they become infected on their own—as sometimes happens during strep throat or tonsillitis—they swell and block the eustachian tubes. If this happens frequently, a doctor might recommend an adenoidectomy, in which the adenoids are removed to keep pressure off the eustachian tubes.

If fluid builds up behind the eardrum—something doctors can detect with hearing tests since the fluid causes temporary hearing loss—then the patient might undergo myringotomy, in which small tubes are placed inside the eardrum to let the fluids drain out. The tubes fall out on their own after a few months, and ideally the eardrum will stay a dry zone from that point on.

Earaches can also be caused by severe ear wax, tooth infection, water retained in the ear from swimming or bathing, pressure changes due to changes in altitude, arthritis of the jaw, or temporomandibular joint syndrome. Smoking has also been shown to cause ear infections in children.

Despite the mention of adenoidectomies and myringotomies, in most cases doctors don't have to do anything to rid patients of ear infections because most clear up on their own after only a few days. Sometimes, such as when a child is under 6 months of age or has had several infections within a month, a doctor will prescribe antibiotics.

So where does food come into the picture? It turns out that avoiding certain foods—namely peanuts, tree nuts, milk, eggs, wheat, soy, fish, and shellfish—may help prevent earaches. They're common causes of food allergies, and anyone (especially children) who eats foods to which they're allergic will get congested. Congestion will create more fluids, which can block the eustachian tubes and lead to ear infections.

In one study, a researcher tested 104 children with recurring ear infections for food allergies and found that 81 of them were allergic to some item they normally ate, with one-third allergic to milk and another third allergic to wheat. At the researcher's request, the parents withheld those foods for 4 months, and 70 of the children were much improved.

At the end of that period, the parents began feeding the forbidden foods to their children once again, and within 4 months 66 of those 70 children had redeveloped clogged middle ears.

It might take some experiments on the dinner table to determine what your child might be allergic to, but if that research time leads to better aural health, then it's time well spent.

As for actual food remedies, I have one that you might consider.

★**Garlic** My friend Paul Strauss, an Ohio-based herbalist, reports that Asian Indians mix garlic in olive oil as an earache treatment. It makes sense to me since garlic has antibiotic and immune-boosting properties. Now you wouldn't want to try this if you have a perforated eardrum. You can always add more garlic to your cooking, though I suspect that the more direct route of dripping the garlic oil directly into the ear canal will be more effective.

Erection Problems

IF YOUR ERECTIONS DON'T ALWAYS MEASURE UP, you've got lots of company. In several community surveys, 20 to 46 percent of men ages 40 to 69 self-report some degree of erectile dysfunction, according to the National Institute of Diabetes and Digestive and Kidney Diseases (NIDDK), one of the National Institutes of Health. Erectile dysfunction (or ED, defined as the repeated inability to raise or sustain an erection adequate for intercourse and ejaculation). More than a million men are currently under treatment for the condition with either prescription medications; penile implants; or a hormone called prostaglandin E, which the patient injects into the base of his penis. Ouch!

Doctors once believed erection problems were mostly psychological. Now experts agree that while some may have a psychological basis, most are due to physical causes. Having diabetes or heart disease can increase problems with ED, as can taking certain drugs for diabetes, hypertension, and depression. Erectile problems may also occur after heart or prostate surgery or an injury to the pelvic area. Basically, anything that reduces blood flow and deprives the penis of oxygen can lead to ED.

Although you may have no control over some physical causes, you'll certainly want to stay on top of any chronic diseases you may have, such as diabetes or heart disease. Without that, no one food or herb has a chance of helping consistently. Lifestyle factors also play a role. Factors that make the problem worse include smoking, drinking too much alcohol, not getting enough sleep, eating a poor diet, and gaining too much weight. Fortunately, these are all things you can change.

One study, published in the *Journal of the American Medical Association*, found that obese men with erectile dysfunction perked up their performance just by losing weight and getting more exercise. The more they exercised and lost weight, the more their erections improved. At the end of the study, about a third of the men no longer had erectile dysfunction.

What if you suspect your ED is psychological rather than physical? Performance anxiety or depression, for example, can cause it. To find out, try the test suggested by Andrew Weil, MD, a professor at the University of Arizona College of Medicine in Tucson. This simple test will tell you if you're having normal spontaneous erections during sleep. If you are, chances are that no physical problem is preventing you from functioning normally.

To do the test, wrap a strip of postage stamps around the shaft of your penis before you go to bed. If the strip is intact in the morning, you didn't have an erection during sleep, and you may have a physical problem. If the strip broke during the night, the problem may well be psychological. This test isn't foolproof, but it's a good place to start.

Whether you think the problem is physical or psychological, the next logical step is to discuss the results with your doctor. But before you go sticking needles into your penis, you might give these food remedies a try.

Healing Foods for Erection Problems

★★★**Fava beans** Think beans aren't sexy? Think again. With an age-old reputation as an aphrodisiac, the fava bean is said to have incited the ancient Roman poet Cicero to passion.

While they haven't been scientifically examined specifically for their potential as a remedy for ED, fava beans are our best food source of the compound L-dopa, which helps make dopamine, a neurotransmitter in the brain associated with pleasure, movement, emotion, and motivation. L-dopa is widely studied for its use in treating Parkinson's disease, and as a result, we've learned that large amounts of it may cause priapism, a painful, persistent erection. But don't let this put you off favas. Research suggests L-dopa causes priapism in no more than 3 percent of people, and, in any case, you'd have a tough time eating enough favas to cause the problem.

I suspect that a big serving of fava beans—8 to 16 ounces—just might contain enough L-dopa to help turn a dysfunction into a function. Try them Mediterranean-style, with a little pancetta, chopped onions, extra-virgin olive oil, and black pepper. If the beans seem to help, try sprouting them. The sprouts contain almost 10 times more L-dopa, and it's easier to eat 2 grams of sprouts than a pound of beans.

★★**Garlic** Popping a garlic appetizer before a hot date may sound like a bad idea if your goal is to remain kissable. But for the more ambitious, the odorous herb may also provide erectile benefits, according to both folk traditions and science.

In India, garlic has a long folkloric history as an aphrodisiac. When holy men prepared food in their temples, they were forbidden to use garlic and other alliums for fear they would lead to passionate encounters.

Recent research on heart disease prevention and treatment suggests that garlic may positively affect blood flow. Allicin, a chemical in garlic, has been shown to produce hydrogen sulphide, which has a relaxing effect on blood vessels. This may also help prevent ED, according to a study at the National University of Singapore.

If you're going to experiment, I recommend sharing the garlic with your partner so neither of you will notice the scent. For an ideal combo, prepare a candlelight dinner of oysters in garlic sauce with a little parsley to help freshen the breath. Share a glass or two of red wine (generally better for the blood vessels than white). And for a potential extra boost, chase it with a dose of ginseng.

★★**Pomegranate** Along with this trendy fruit's many other benefits, drinking antioxidant-rich pomegranate juice may improve erectile function in men with mild to moderate ED. It wouldn't hurt to try it with breakfast or instead of a soda at lunchtime to see if it works for you.

In a randomized, placebo-controlled, double-blind, crossover study, researchers at the Male Clinic in Beverly Hills looked at 53 men with mild to moderate erectile dysfunction over a 6-week period. Those who drank pomegranate juice were more likely to have improved scores on the International Index of Erectile Function and to report an improvement on Global Assessment Questionnaires. Although this study was small and the findings were not statistically significant, the researchers suggest that larger studies and longer time periods may achieve better results.

Also, unlike grapefruit juice, pomegranate juice is safe to drink even if you're taking prescription drugs. Previous animal and in vitro studies hinted that pomegranate juice may inhibit CYP3A, an enzyme that allows the body to metabolize drugs. But in 2007, researchers at Tufts University School of Medicine published a study in the *Journal of Clinical Pharmacology* that debunked the earlier research. It was the first study to test pomegranate juice for drug interactions in humans.

Both studies used POM Wonderful juice, which is widely available across the country.

★**Pumpkin** As if you needed more motivation to enjoy a pumpkin pie fresh out of the oven, this treat tops the list of foods with arousing aromas most likely to spice up a man's sex life. You don't even have to eat it to feel the effect, according to one intriguing study. Alan Hirsch, MD, neurological director of the Smell and Taste Treatment and Research Foundation in Chicago, found that many patients who had lost their sense of smell also lost interest in sex. That piqued his curiosity about the power of scents to boost desire. To see which, if any, aromas could provoke a sexual response, Dr. Hirsch asked a group of 31 men to sit in a laboratory with their penises attached to a machine that measures blood flow. Then he had the men sniff 30 odors.

Here's what he found: The men responded sexually (with increased penile blood flow) to all of the scents, proving the theory that it doesn't take much. But the hands-down winner for most arousing smell (it increased penile blood flow by 40 percent) was the mingled scents of pumpkin pie and lavender. Runners-up were doughnuts with black licorice (32 percent) and pumpkin pie with doughnuts (20 percent).

From the Herbal Medicine Chest

In Asian countries, where it also goes by other names, such as silver apricot or white nut, ginkgo often appears in recipes. In the United States, it's best known as an herb that improves blood flow to the brain, but few people know it may also boost blood flow to the penis.

In small studies, researchers produced good results with 60 to 240 milligrams daily of a standardized ginkgo extract. In one 9-month study, 78 percent of men with erectile dysfunction due to atherosclerotic clogging of the penile artery reported significant improvement with no side effects. Atherosclerosis is the same disease that clogs the blood vessels that supply the heart, leading to heart attacks.

Ginkgo extracts are available at many health food stores and herb shops. The active compounds in ginkgo leaves are too dilute to do much good, so standardized extracts concentrate it: A 50:1 extract means that 50 pounds of leaves were used to produce 1 pound of extract. You can try 60 to 240 milligrams a day, but don't take more than that because in large amounts, ginkgo may cause diarrhea, irritability, and restlessness. Also, check with your doctor before using ginkgo if you're taking a blood-thinning medication such as coumadin (Warfarin). And give it time; if it's going to work, it will do the trick in about 6 months.

Fatigue

ABOUT HALF OF ALL ADULTS WHO SEEK MEDICAL TREATMENT list fatigue among their symptoms. It's not surprising that fatigue is so common when you consider all the issues, big and little, that can cause it. Stress. Too much work. Too little sleep. Boredom from not having anything to do. Too much exercise. Depression and other medical conditions, including anemia and underactive thyroid. Most of us will probably encounter at least one of those difficulties at some time during our lives.

In addition, a million people feel the effects of a more chronic type of fatigue, fittingly called chronic fatigue syndrome (CFS). This condition can make you feel so tired that you have difficulty maintaining a normal routine. People also have symptoms such as trouble with thinking, tender lymph nodes, muscle aches, and difficulty sleeping. CFS has no known cure, but some medications and moderate exercise may help with symptoms. Although the legitimacy of this diagnosis has long been controversial, the medical community is beginning to accept it more broadly.

One simple way to help keep your energy going through the day is by picking your foods wisely. Eating sweet foods causes a jolt of blood sugar, which signals your body to release insulin. That makes your blood sugar levels drop, resulting in fatigue. A better idea is to eat so that you can avoid a lot of blood sugar ups and downs during the day. Instead of doughnuts and candy bars, eat whole-grain carbohydrates combined with some protein. Try whole-wheat toast with cream cheese or peanut butter for breakfast and a sandwich with grilled chicken for lunch.

Other tactics for boosting your energy level may include getting more sleep, practicing stress-relieving strategies such as meditation, and adding some of the following foods to your daily fare.

Healing Foods for Fatigue

★★**Cinnamon and ginger** Since I like cinnamon, with its energizing cinnamaldehyde, and ginger, with its fatigue-fighting zingerone, I would combine these two spices with several herbs that are high in cineole, a gentle stimulant, to make a Synergic Cineolade. Mix up a drink containing cinnamon, ginger, nutmeg, peppermint, and spearmint and give yourself a refreshing pick-me-up. This is more of a quick-fix energizer that's probably best taken occasionally for acute fatigue rather than frequently for chronic fatigue.

★★**Crucifers** People with chronic fatigue tend to come up short on B vitamins, especially vitamin B_6. So increasing your consumption of B-rich foods may be helpful. For B_6, the best plant sources can be found in the cabbage/cauliflower/cress family, with cauliflower, watercress, and spinach at the top of the list. Other good sources include avocadoes and bananas. As a point of reference, the recommended daily intake of B_6 is 1.7 milligrams for men and 1.5 milligrams for women.

★★**Fish** The omega-3 fatty acids found in fish like salmon may be helpful in reducing the fatigue that comes with CFS (and may also help alleviate the depression that can accompany the condition). If I had chronic fatigue, I'd probably eat several servings of fish each week. Walnuts and flaxseed are also good sources of omega-3's, so it may be wise to enjoy those on a regular basis, too.

★★**Garlic** Research has shown that garlic can help animals endure longer bouts of exercise, and in humans, it reduces symptoms of physical fatigue and fatigue due to cold. It's easy to add garlic to sauces or sauté it with foods (such as shiitake mushrooms). Or just chop a few cloves and sprinkle them on a piece of toast with margarine.

★★**Mustard greens** Having low levels of the brain chemical dopamine has been linked to fatigue. An amino acid called tyrosine is a precursor—or type of building block—of dopamine, so eating tyrosine-rich foods may help get your dopamine flowing. In my research, mustard greens top the tyrosine charts. Other good plant sources include velvet bean seeds, bean sprouts, soy, oats, peanuts, and watercress. Make room for these foods in your diet, and they may help take the edge off your fatigue.

★**Cereal** One possible cause of fatigue is anemia, the most common form of which is iron-deficiency anemia. About one out of five women are iron deficient (the problem is much less common in men). If you're a woman of reproductive age, menstruation may be the culprit. Your doctor can diagnose this problem and may recommend iron supplements.

Adult men need 8 milligrams of iron daily. Women up to age 50 need 18 milligrams daily and 8 milligrams a day after that. You can get plenty of iron in 100 percent iron-fortified cereal, soybeans, beef chuck roast, and dark turkey meat.

In addition, I've read that sprouting legume seeds may be a rich source of heme iron, which is the more absorbable form people typically get from meat, fish, and poultry. If you're a vegetarian, it may be worth your while to learn how to sprout legumes, which is a simple process that involves rinsing and soaking.

FOODS TO WATCH

Caffeine has a well-deserved reputation as a stimulant. Why else would workplaces keep a coffee pot and soda machine in the break room? But using these drinks chronically as a pick-me-up can actually leave you feeling more fatigued. If you're a habitual caffeine user and you're feeling sluggish, try minimizing your coffee and soda intake or avoiding them entirely.

But be careful not to suddenly stop drinking these beverages if you're a regular consumer—caffeine withdrawal can also cause fatigue, as well as headache, depression, and difficulty concentrating. Over a period of a few weeks, gradually substitute water, decaffeinated tea, or my Synergic Cineolade for your usual caffeinated drink until you've weaned yourself off the buzz.

★**Citrus fruits** Research has found that people who get at least 400 milligrams of vitamin C daily feel less fatigue than people who get less of the vitamin. In addition, taking in plenty of vitamin C when you're fighting chronic fatigue may help your immune system work better and improve your endurance.

Nutritionists often suggest orange juice, strawberries, pineapple, and cantaloupe as great fruit sources of vitamin C, but if you have a taste for the exotic, you can find far richer sources. My tropical friend camu-camu—so far available in the United States only from Internet sources—may be the richest edible source of C on the planet. The cherry-like fruit grow on trees in the Amazon. Other unusual foods rich in vitamin C include bitter melon, rose hips, and pokeweed shoots.

★**Oats** Some—though not all—studies have found that magnesium deficiency is common in people with chronic fatigue, and supplementation has helped improve symptoms. If you want to boost your magnesium naturally, the following foods will help: oat bran, semisweet chocolate, cornmeal, tomato paste, and Brazil nuts.

In addition, purslane—which many people overlook as a common weed—contains nearly 2 percent magnesium on a dry-weight basis. Green beans, poppy seeds, and cowpeas are also good sources. I've been known to mix up a pot of Magnesisoup with high-magnesium vegetables like diced purslane, green beans, cowpeas, spinach, and nettle, with poppy seeds added for flavor.

★**Shiitake** These smoky-tasting mushrooms, available in supermarkets as a food, have long been used for medicinal purposes in China, and they may be useful in reducing the effects of CFS. Good ways to enjoy them include adding them to soups or sautéing them with onions and garlic.

Fibromyalgia

FIBROMYALGIA SYNDROME IS AN ONGOING CONDITION that causes widespread muscle and joint pain, fatigue, and poor sleep. Its trademark symptom is the emergence of multiple "tender points" in areas such as the neck, spine, shoulders, and hips. Other symptoms can include morning stiffness, fatigue, increased headaches or facial pain, irritable bowel syndrome, depression, anxiety, impaired concentration and memory, and an inability to perform multiple tasks. All of that would cramp anyone's style, including mine.

Because there are no specific laboratory tests to identify fibromyalgia, it was once thought to be a psychosomatic disorder—that is, it was "all in your head." Most experts now recognize it as a distinct medical condition, although some still believe that it's more psychological than physical. This belief may be due to recent research showing that people with fibromyalgia have abnormal pain perception thresholds compared to healthy people, people with depression, and those with chronic fatigue syndrome.

The most recent estimates, published in a 2008 issue of the journal *Arthritis and Rheumatism,* show that a whopping five million Americans—the vast majority of them women—have fibromyalgia. That means that at any given moment, nearly 1 in 60 Americans are coping with distress that can dramatically affect their quality of life and even become totally incapacitating.

Unfortunately, effective pain relief is hard to come by. In a national survey conducted in 2005 by researchers from Stanford University School of Medicine, 50 percent of respondents reported that pain medications were ineffective.

If you have fibromyalgia, you may be particularly resistant to these medications. Doctors have long noted that even strong opioids such as morphine have little effect on fibromyalgia.

In a 2007 study published in the *Journal of Neuroscience,* researchers from the University of Michigan may have identified the reason. After using positron emission tomography (PET) to scan 17 women with fibromyalgia and 17 women without the condition, they found that women with fibromyalgia had pain receptors in their brains that were less able to bind with opioids. When this binding process doesn't work properly, it means that these drugs will have little or no effect on pain.

What may give you better results, however, is losing weight—at least if you're overweight or obese. In a 2006 study published in the *Journal of Psychosomatic Research,* overweight fibromyalgia patients who lost just 4.4 percent of their body weight experienced significant improvements in mood, pain, and quality of life.

Healing Foods for Fibromyalgia

To help prevent fibromyalgia—or at least manage pain—a number of food remedies may prove useful. Although we don't yet have solid results from any studies, the National Fibromyalgia Association has posted anecdotal reports that a raw food diet consisting of uncooked organic fruits, vegetables, nuts, and seeds can help reduce the joint pain, fatigue, depression, tender spots, and cognitive problems associated with fibromyalgia. Although I'm not aware that such a diet has been scientifically tested, the recommendation makes sense because whole, uncooked foods contain higher amounts of natural enzymes and perhaps anti-inflammatory and antioxidant compounds. If you're considering such a radical change in your diet—which would be difficult to maintain—be sure to consult a healthcare professional or nutritionist first to make certain that you get a proper mix of proteins, fats, and carbohydrates. Here are some specific foods to try.

★★★**Buckwheat** Malic acid is essential for normal muscle function. One preliminary trial found that the combination of 1,200 to 2,400 milligrams of malic acid plus 300 to 600 milligrams of magnesium could reduce muscle pain in people with fibromyalgia when taken for daily 8 weeks.

Your body makes some malic acid; the rest comes from food. Though "malic acid" comes from *malus,* the genus name for apples, you'd need to eat about three apples a day to get the recommended amount. On the other hand, buckwheat is a top-notch source, as are mangoes, apricots, and figs (more on them in a bit). So my suggestion is to help yourself to a breakfast of buckwheat pancakes, perhaps topped with sliced mangoes or apricots.

If you'd rather eat the apples, your best choice is a Granny Smith; in fact, it's the malic acid that gives them their tart taste.

★★★**Fig** Besides malic acid, figs contain ficin, a proteolytic enzyme that can help reduce pain in many "-itis" (inflammatory) conditions, including fibromyalgia. I was surprised when I saw that fig scored better than all of the fruits and veggies that I investigated for fibromyalgia.

★★★**Spinach** Many leafy greens are rich in magnesium, a mineral that promotes energy production and cellular function. One cup of cooked spinach, for example, contains 157 milligrams of magnesium, almost 40 percent of the Daily Value. If I had fibromyalgia, I'd try to get more leafy greens in my diet—especially spinach, but also green beans, avocados, almonds, Brazil nuts, sunflower seeds, barley, quinoa, and amaranth. Even dark chocolate supplies a decent amount of magnesium.

★★**Chile peppers** Chile peppers contain a pungent substance known as capsaicin, which is number one among my painkillers. When applied topically to your tender points, capsaicin temporarily depletes substance P, a chemical in nerves that transmits pain sensations. Without substance P, pain signals go silent. Dozens of studies show that capsaicin can temporarily relieve many painful conditions, including fibromyalgia. It's even more potent than prescription COX-2 inhibitors.

You can buy a commercial topical capsaicin cream and apply it to your tender points three or four times per day or, as an inexpensive alternative, you can mash a fresh chile pepper and rub it on your skin.

No matter which route you choose, you may experience a burning sensation the first few times you use capsaicin, but it usually subsides with repeated use. Just be sure to wash your hands thoroughly after using it. If you get any in your eyes, nose or mouth, it may be even more painful than your tender points.

Although capsaicin is best used topically, it may be helpful to add more whole peppers, pepper-derived hot sauce, and cayenne to your diet. Another option is taking a cayenne tincture (0.3 to 1 milliliter) three times a day. You also can make an infusion (tea) by stirring ½ to 1 teaspoon (2.5 to 5 grams) of cayenne powder into 1 cup of boiling water, letting it steep for 10 minutes, and taking 1 teaspoon mixed with water three or four times daily.

★★**Ginger** Ginger contains high amounts of the digestive enzyme zingibain—as much as 2 percent by weight. Zingibain has powerful anti-inflammatory properties. According to some experts, it's even more powerful than the bromelain in pineapple or the papain in papaya. Ginger also contains at least four natural COX-2 inhibitors, and unlike prescription versions such as celecoxib (Celebrex), it doesn't produce any serious side effects.

It's easy to get enough ginger in your diet to help reduce pain. You can take it in an herbal tea by steeping three or four fresh slices in a cup of boiling water. If you prefer, you can get medicinal doses in tinctures or capsules. Personally, I prefer ginger as a liberal and tasty addition to my meals. You can get adequate doses by sprinkling ½ teaspoon of powdered ginger into your foods or simply by eating an ounce (6 teaspoons) of fresh ginger every day. If you're in a hurry, you might try New Chapter's product, Zyflamend. That way, you'll get several other edible COX-2 inhibitors—turmeric, oregano, rosemary, green tea, and holy basil.

FOODS TO WATCH

Arachadonic acid is a pro-inflammatory substance that is implicated in many chronic conditions, including fibromyalgia. Try to reduce your consumption of foods rich in arachadonic acid, such as beef, lamb, pork, and chicken. Recently I learned that eggs are particularly bad. The National Fibromyalgia Association also reports that many patients have obtained relief by eliminating all sugar from their diets for 1 month. I can do that with stevia, but like most people, I don't like its taste as much as I do that of sugar. You may also benefit from reducing or eliminating caffeine, alcohol, fried foods, red meat, and highly processed foods from your diet, as all of these tend to irritate tender muscles and stress out the immune system.

★★**Turmeric** This yellow curry spice is a rich source of curcumin, a strong antioxidant that protects against free radical damage. Curcumin contains natural pain-relieving COX-2-inhibitors, which makes it an attractive, side effect–free alternative to prescription COX-2 inhibitors. It also reduces inflammation by reducing histamine levels and possibly by stimulating the adrenal glands to produce more cortisone, one of the body's natural anti-inflammatories. Lately, I've had two students who switched from Celebrex to either curcumin or curried celery (see my Curried Celery COX-2 Inhibitor recipe on page 286) and thought it was a good tradeoff.

Human studies of curcumin have found that it can reduce the pain and stiffness associated with rheumatoid arthritis as well as help relieve postsurgical inflammation. I prefer consuming whole foods rather than supplements because I believe many phytochemicals working together offer more healing power than you would get from individual components. I often add liberal amounts of curry to rice and other dishes and would consider adding other anti-inflammatory foods such as pineapple and papaya. You can also make tea with turmeric.

Unfortunately, it's difficult to get medicinal doses of curcumin from your diet alone. According to naturopaths, you would need to consume 250 to 500 milligrams of pure curcumin a day between meals, which translates into 5 to 25 teaspoons of dried turmeric per day. That's an awful lot. I would recommend adding as much turmeric as possible to your diet to help prevent pain and, as an exception to my usual whole-foods rule, taking turmeric supplements—standardized to 90 to 95 percent curcumin—to help relieve acute pain. Ayurveda, the traditional healing art of India, recommends cooking turmeric with milk to enhance absorption, so you might try adding milk and freshly ground black pepper (to enhance absorption) to my curried celery recipe.

★**Pineapple** This exotic fruit is rich in a number of substances that can help people with conditions such as fibromyalgia. Foremost among these is bromelain, a proteolytic enzyme that helps reduce swelling and inflammation in many painful "-itis" (inflammatory) conditions. Its anti-inflammatory effects are so profound that the German government has approved its use for healing after injuries and surgical procedures. Pineapple also contains high amounts of manganese, which is essential for the formation of collagen, the tough, fibrous protein that builds connective tissues such as bone, skin, and cartilage. You can get 100 percent of the Daily Value for manganese (2 milligrams) from just a cup of fresh pineapple chunks or pineapple juice. Pineapple is also a rich source of vitamin C, another necessity for collagen formation, and it contains more of this important vitamin than apples, cranberries, or tomato juice. A cup of fresh pineapple chunks contains 24 milligrams, or 40 percent of the Daily Value for vitamin C. To get maximum antioxidant punch, try "Gold" pineapple, which is imported from Costa Rica and contains four times as much vitamin C as other varieties.

Unfortunately, recent research suggests that levels of bromelain in fresh pineapple and of papain, a related enzyme in fresh papaya, may be too low to relieve a bad episode of fibromyalgia. While I would encourage enjoying these fruits—either whole or as juice—you'll probably need to take supplements to get seriously effective levels. Still, you may want to take the fruit juices along with the pills, to get the benefit of compounds that work with bromelain. Naturopaths suggest taking anywhere between 250 and 500 milligrams of bromelain three times a day. In human studies, a daily dose of up to 2,000 milligrams has not been shown to be harmful.

From the Herbal Medicine Chest

Some older, double-blind, placebo-controlled studies suggest that oral SAMe, at a dosage of 800 milligrams a day for 6 weeks, may be effective for reducing pain, fatigue, and stiffness and for improving mood.

More recent evidence shows that there may be even more promising approaches. One of them is D-ribose (Corvalen), a main component of the body's main energy source, adenosine triphosphate (ATP). In a 2007 study published in the *Journal of Alternative and Complementary Medicine*, researchers gave 5 grams of D-ribose to 36 patients with fibromyalgia, chronic fatigue syndrome, or both three times daily for 25 days. The patients reported a dramatic 45 percent boost in energy levels and improvements in sleep patterns, mental clarity, and pain. Although D-ribose is commonly found in foods, especially foods high in RNA (ribonucleic acid), such as brewer's yeast, the concentration is probably too low to be of therapeutic value. You can, however, purchase it in supplement form.

An even more adventurous approach—the Myers' Cocktail—also shows promise, but it's not for the faint-hearted. Since 2001, the Integrative Medicine Center at Griffin Hospital in Derby, Connecticut, has been administering the cocktail, an intravenous solution containing calcium; vitamins B_5 (pantothenic acid), B_6, and B_{12}; and other essential nutrients, to its fibromyalgia patients. The early results have been so promising and free of serious side effects that the National Center for Complementary and Alternative Medicine is funding an ongoing randomized, controlled trial to test the effectiveness of the cocktail.

Flatulence (Gas)

HAVING GAS COULD BE A REASON TO FEEL GOOD ABOUT YOURSELF. A strange thought, I know, but gas is often a telltale sign of a healthFUL diet. If you eat lots of fruits and vegetables, little meat, fewer fats, and plenty of indigestible carbohydrates (especially beans), chances are that you're eating all the right stuff—and have the gas to prove it. A healthful diet, one full of fruits and vegetables, has the makings of some pretty forceful "wind."

Gas results when food breaks down in your digestive system. Some foods, such as those that are high in fiber, produce more gas than others (especially when they're added to your diet too fast). Beans and other plant foods that are high in two specific carbohydrates—raffinose and stachyose—are particularly big gas producers. Your intestine doesn't produce the enzymes necessary to digest these carbohydrates, so they just sit there until bacteria ferment them, a process that produces gas.

Having gas is natural. Most people who complain about having too much actually produce an amount that digestive system specialists (gastroenterologists) would say is perfectly normal. But just because it's normal doesn't mean it's welcome. Aside from presenting the obvious social challenge, gas often brings bloating and cramps to the party as well. Having gas can't be completely prevented, but you can significantly reduce the problems that come with it.

Any herb that soothes the digestive tract and minimizes gas is called a carminative. Below area few of the best.

Healing Foods for Flatulence

★★**Dandelion** It's rarely sold in the supermarket, but in the field right behind my grocery store you can find dandelion blooming pretty much the year round. It scores high in my evidence base for flatulence, having been approved by Commission E (a German government agency that evaluates the safety and efficacy of medicinal herbs) as a carminative. I see that they specified using the above-ground parts of the plant. However, I know—even if they don't—that the root is rich in flatugenic inulin, the same compound that led to the nickname "fartichoke" for the flatugenic Jerusalem artichoke.

★★**Ginger** Many cultures have taken advantage of ginger's antiflatulence properties for thousands of years. The ancient Greeks used ginger wrapped in bread after large meals to prevent all kinds of digestive repercussions, including gas. Eventually, they just added ginger to the bread dough and gingerbread was born. In the 19th century, barkeepers in English pubs put ground ginger in small containers so patrons could sprinkle the herb into their beer, creating ginger ale.

Beans, Deflated

To eliminate bean-induced flatulence, try soaking beans in water overnight, then discard the water and cook the beans in new water. It's an age-old antigas strategy. Here are more helpful deflating remedies from local cultures and around the world:

Appalachian. The Appalachians suggest cooking beans with a small, whole carrot.

Chinese. According to Albert Leung, PhD, a pharmacognosist (natural product pharmacist) and author of *Chinese Healing Foods and Herbs*, the Chinese soak their beans in water with wormwood added.

Mexican. People in Mexico cook their beans with a dash of wormseed or epazote, a type of pigweed. This may be difficult to find, but it's just as well. If eaten in large quantities, it can be poisonous.

FOODS TO WATCH

Here are some big gas producers to avoid:

Beans It's no secret that beans, being high in fiber and nondigestible carbohydrates, have the most gas-producing potential. Those that can make the most "wind" are English peas, soybeans, and black-eyed peas. Lima beans, pinto beans, and black beans come in a close second.

Dairy foods If milk and cheese seem to cause you a lot of gas, you may be lactose intolerant. This means you have trouble digesting milk sugar (lactose). Try cutting down on dairy foods for a week or two to see if that helps. You can also use Lactaid, a commercial product that contains the enzyme that digests lactose.

Sweets Natural or not, sweeteners from honey, fruits, and juices (fructose) as well as artificial sweeteners in sugarless gums and candies (sorbitol, xylitol, mannitol) can be hard to digest, resulting in large amounts of gas.

Inulin That's the gas-maker in Jerusalem artichoke.

Fruit Eating fruit at the end of a meal promotes gas by causing fermentation on top of all the other food, which can bring on lots of gas. Fruit is important for a healthy diet, so it's not right to cut it out just because of a few gas bubbles. If you suffer from flatulence, try to eat fruit first thing in the morning or as a bedtime snack after your dinner has had a chance to digest a bit.

The medicinal part of ginger is the rhizome, an underground stem of the plant that's often mistaken for the root. This stem is ground up and used in many Chinese herbal prescriptions. Ayurvedic doctors call ginger "the universal medicine."

Ginger is a particularly helpful digestive aid because it helps to relieve not only gas but also bloating and cramps. It works by settling the intestine and removing gas from the digestive tract. Try spicing your beans with a teaspoon of ground ginger to reduce their gaseous effects.

A helpful remedy comes from Vasant Lad, BAMS, MASc, director of the Ayurvedic Institute in Albuquerque, New Mexico. Lad says that a teaspoon each of grated fresh ginger and lime juice taken right after you eat can prevent excess gas.

★★**Other assorted herbs** These carminative herbs are also concentrated in gas-relieving chemicals:

Allspice	Dill
Caraway	Fennel
Cardamom	Nutmeg
Cinnamon	Peppermint
Cloves	Sage
Coriander	Thyme

Michael Murray, ND, natural medicine expert and author of *The Encyclopedia of Healing Foods*, suggests concocting an effective, flavorful mixture of ginger, cardamom, cinnamon, and coriander to spice and tame gas-producing foods.

Food Allergies

TO MANY PEOPLE, SHRIMP ARE A TASTY TREAT. You can eat them batter dipped, fried, boiled, or handed to you chilled on a serving tray with cocktail sauce at a party. For other people, however, they can be deadly. Nearly 4 percent of adults—and up to 8 percent of kids under age 3—have food allergies. The most common food allergens are shellfish (including shrimp), nuts, fish, and eggs. The most troublesome foods for kids are eggs, milk, and nuts—including peanuts, which are actually legumes.

A food allergy, which is an immune response, isn't the same as an intolerance, which has nothing to do with the immune system. Many people with lactose intolerance, for example, can still handle limited amounts of food made from cow's milk. With food allergies, however, your immune system overreacts to even the smallest amounts of certain components—usually proteins—in particular foods. This can lead to itchy hives, both on the skin and in the mouth and throat, or to an anaphylactic reaction with symptoms such as lowered blood pressure, wheezing, vomiting or diarrhea, and often a potentially fatal loss of consciousness.

As a result, it's wise to take food allergies very seriously. I don't know of many foods you can eat to protect you if you're allergic to a particular item. The first and best advice is to avoid whatever triggers your allergic reaction. However, I can offer a few tips on exactly how to go about avoiding troublesome foods as well as a few food remedies that may help reduce your symptoms.

Healing Foods for Food Allergies

★★**Citrus fruits** Foods rich in vitamin C—such as citrus fruits and strawberries—may help with food allergies. This vitamin may work as a natural antihistamine, neutralizing the action of the body chemicals, called histamines, that play a role in allergic reactions. I've seen references to vitamin C showing antihistamine effects in lab studies. Again, if I had significant food allergies, I wouldn't trust these to totally protect me, but they may help. Avoid any foods containing vitamin C if you're allergic to 'em.

★**Yogurt** I've read that eating foods containing *Lactobacillus* bacteria may be helpful in controlling food allergies. A study back in 1997 found that giving *Lactobacil-*

Educate Your Palate

Much of the challenge with food allergies lies in learning how to avoid problematic foods. This isn't as simple as it seems, but here are a few tips that may help.

Avoid similar triggers. If a particular food sets off your allergies, be wary of similar foods since they may also trigger a reaction. For example, if you're allergic to shrimp, you may need to avoid crab and lobster, too. If you're allergic to one type of nut that grows on a tree, such as walnuts, you may have problems with almonds and other tree nuts. This is called cross-reactivity. If you're allergic to foods that seem similar but are of different families, such as chestnuts (tree nuts) and peanuts (legumes), it's called coincidental reactivity. If you have a food allergy, talk to your doctor about other foods you should avoid.

Read those labels. If you use reading glasses, take them with you to the supermarket. Before you put an item into your cart, carefully peruse the tiny print of the ingredient list. Do this even for familiar processed foods, since their ingredients may have changed since the last time you ate them.

Manufacturers don't always use familiar words to describe ingredients. If you're allergic to milk protein, avoid foods containing lactalbumin, casein, lactoglobulin, and lactulose. If you're allergic to egg proteins, avoid albumin, albumen, and meringue. If you're allergic to soy, steer clear of miso, MSG, soybean oil, hydrolyzed vegetable protein, and lecithin. That's just the tip of the iceberg for words that point to potential allergens, and traces of troublesome ingredients can lurk in lots of processed foods. Your allergist should be able to provide you with more comprehensive advice on words to look for on labels.

lus GG to infants with a cow's milk allergy and eczema could be a useful treatment. This approach may help reduce inflammation in your gut and help create a "barrier" in your digestive system to keep your body from absorbing food allergens. You can easily find yogurt and milk containing *L. acidophilus,* and these bacteria are also available in special liquid and capsule form. Obviously you should avoid any of these products if you're allergic to any of the ingredients.

★**Apples** A flavonoid called quercetin keeps certain cells in your body, called mast cells, from releasing histamine during allergic reactions. It also reduces the production of inflammatory compounds called leukotrienes, which are much more powerful than histamine. Quercetin is easy to find; it's in apples, tea, garlic, and onions.

★**Chamomile or green tea** Chamomile can trigger reactions in those who are allergic to it, but if you're not, you may benefit from the wide array of antihistaminic compounds it contains. It also has linoleic acid and quercetin, which may have anti-anaphylactic properties. Green tea also contains linoleic acid and quercetin, and, like chamomile, it contains an antihistamine called apigenin. If you have food allergies, enjoying these teas regularly may be helpful.

★**Ginger** Years ago, I reported how Terry Willard, an herbalist who joined me on one of my trips, made his own medicine for a food allergy. Suffering with hives one day, he simmered ½ pound of ginger in a gallon of water for 5 minutes in a nonaluminum pot and added it to his hot bath. After steeping himself for a while, he sponged off with chamomile tea. "It worked every time," he said. I think he would have fared even better by also *drinking* some chamomile/ginger/green tea for some of its antihistaminic contents.

Ginger contains a variety of antihistaminic compounds, including quercetin. The quercetin, plus citral and linoleic acid, may have properties that reduce the risk of anaphylaxis.

Fungal Infections

MOST OF US FEAST ON FUNGI REGULARLY. Mushrooms are a fleshy type of fungus, and wine, cheese, and certain breads are all the result of fermenting fungi. And you can thank these "lowly" organisms for helping make lifesaving antibiotics like penicillin.

Unfortunately, the news is not all good. Some fungi can cause yeast infections or forms of ringworm such as athlete's foot and jock itch. You can treat those specific infections with a nutritional arsenal of food (for yeast infections and athlete's foot, see those chapters).

Some health conditions can invite chronic fungal infections, such as a weakened immune system, diabetes, and HIV/AIDS. Certain medications can also make fungi feel welcome. Antibiotics, for example, kill harmful bacteria but also reduce the helpful bacteria that keep fungi in check. Most mild fungal infections respond well to over-the-counter medications, though some of those medications can have serious side effects. In addition, experts are becoming more concerned that the overuse of these products will lead to drug-resistant fungi. That's why I think a nutritional approach to treatment and prevention is best. Some botanicals contain more than a dozen antifungals, which are less likely to cause resistance than a single antibiotic.

Healing Foods for Fungal Infections

★★★**Caraway** The aromatic fruit and seeds of the caraway plant have long been used throughout the world as a curative. Caraway contains a laundry list of fungicides, which explains why it's so effective against mycosis (a scary name for any condition caused by fungus). Most of the medicinal properties of caraway come from its volatile oil, which is available in enteric-coated supplements. You can also purchase powdered caraway fruit to make a tea. However, flavoring meat and breads with caraway seeds is a tastier way to fight fungi.

★★★**Celery** It wasn't until the 1700s that people began appreciating the culinary merits of celery. Prior to that, the Romans wore wreaths of celery to ward off various ills, such as hangovers. Fortunately, today we know that you needn't sacrifice your dignity to enjoy the medicinal properties of this pleasant vegetable.

Celery is naturally resistant to pathogens during storage because it contains a melting pot of fungicides, with more than two dozen already identified. If you're prone to fungal infections or currently battling one, eat a celery stalk a day to keep those microbes in check.

★★★**Garlic** If I were to find myself on a deserted island with nothing but a fungal infection to keep me company, I would seek out garlic or its wild relatives to treat my irritated skin. Come to think of it, I would reach for garlic even if I were living right next to a drugstore. That's because garlic has shown itself to be one of the most powerful antifungals in the natural world. Laboratory research suggests that garlic kills yeast, the fungi that cause vaginal and oral infections, on contact. In a study at Loma Linda University in California, animals with yeast infections were given either a placebo or a formula made with aged garlic extract. After 2 days, those in the garlic group were completely fungus free, while the animals given the placebo were still infected. This pungent herb may also prevent future infections. Garlic appears to stimulate immune system cells called neutrophils and macrophages, which help your body battle infection.

To treat and prevent yeast infections, try eating from several cloves to an entire bulb of garlic a day, says Paul Reilly, ND, a naturopath and an adjunct instructor at Bastyr University in Seattle. I have trouble getting one down chewed. I tried swallowing a whole clove once, but you lose the garlic's medicinal power if you don't break the bulb's skin, so you have to chew, crush, slice, or mash it. Raw is best, but some of its strength remains even when it's baked, microwaved, or sautéed.

★★**Chamomile** Don't let the relaxing effects of this "sleepy time" herb fool you. It contains some highly charged components that ease bacterial and fungal irritations of the skin. Chamomile has over two dozen antiseptic compounds, the most powerful of which are bisabolol, chamazulene, and other cyclic ethers.

The best way to put chamomile to work is to use the spent tea bag as a poultice and apply it directly to fungal infections on the skin.

Add cinnamon to marinades, soups, meat rubs, and batter or have a breakfast of cinnamon toast and cinnamon tea and start the day with an antimicrobial punch.

★★**Cinnamon** Along with almost every other spice, cinnamon was used to preserve foods back in the days before refrigeration. Most spices are good antiseptics and were probably used for their antifungal properties as much as for their flavor. Cinnamon contains more than two dozen antiseptic compounds, many of them fungicidal. It's especially lethal against food-borne bacteria such as *Escherichia coli*. In fact, cinnamon's antimicrobial abilities are so powerful that some food manufacturers are experimenting with cinnamon-infused packaging to prevent invasions of dangerous microbes.

★★**Turmeric** Is there anything turmeric can't do? It's shown to protect the heart, aid digestion, prevent ulcers, and ward off fungus. Turmeric compounds have significantly inhibited the growth of various strains of fungi in lab studies. While turmeric isn't an antifungal superstar (yet), it contains at least 20 fungicidal compounds.

You can make your own medicinal drink with a teaspoon of powdered turmeric stirred into a cup of warm milk. Or include turmeric in your diet the traditional way—sprinkle it on your food. It has a pleasant taste, but don't overdo it; large amounts taste bitter.

★★**White tea** The immune-stimulating benefits of green tea are fairly well accepted by both the medical community and the lay population. In some studies, however, the lesser known white tea beats green at disarming bacteria and viruses and killing yeast cells. Laboratory research conducted at Pace University in New York City has consistently shown that white tea extract inactivates various species of yeast that cause urinary tract infections, peritonitis, and pneumonia. The researchers also found that adding white tea extract to toothpastes and mouthwashes enhances their microbial effects.

White tea is made with immature tea leaves that are picked shortly before the buds have completely opened. These leaves are closer to their natural state than other tea leaves, which may explain the power behind white tea's antifungal punch. Based on the results of these studies, the researchers suggest drinking up to two cups of white tea a day for overall microbial protection.

From the Herbal Medicine Chest

Tea tree oil is one of the most powerful antiseptics that the natural world has to offer. It can even kill some drug-resistant fungi and is especially detrimental to the growth of the organisms that cause chronic thrush, athlete's foot, and vaginitis. In one study at the University of Glasgow, researchers exposed 301 yeasts from the mouths of cancer patients with oral fungal infections to the oil and found that it inhibited all of them (including 41 that are resistant to the antifungal medications fluconazole and itraconazole). Based on these findings, the researchers believe that tea tree oil merits further study for immunocompromised patients. However, do *not* apply tea tree oil to your mouth, and keep it away from children. When swallowed, even small amounts can be fatal.

For skin infections, apply a few drops of oil to the affected area three times a day. The oil can irritate skin, so you may want to dilute it first with an equal amount of vegetable oil. If you experience any discomfort, stop using it. I advise using tea tree oil for vaginal infections only as a last resort since vaginal tissues are especially sensitive. If you decide to use it, talk to your doctor first.

Gallstones and Kidney Stones

STONES OF ANY KIND BELONG ON THE GROUND, not in your body, but unfortunately, some of your internal organs can be very good at making them—especially your kidneys and gallbladder. In fact, it's not terribly unusual for individuals to form stones in *both* of these organs. Here's a quick rundown of how this happens.

Gallstones: Too Much Cholesterol

Gallstones may form when you have too much fat and cholesterol in your diet. Gallstones are small lumps or nuggets that develop in your gallbladder—the organ that stores the bile (also known as gall) that your body uses to digest fats in your small intestine. Bile is normally a liquid that contains cholesterol, protein, and fat. However, too much cholesterol or calcium salts in bile can cause them to clump together, just as it can clog your arteries and cause heart disease, high blood pressure, and stroke.

Gallstones that stay in your gallbladder typically don't cause any symptoms. But if these little stones start moving around, particularly into the bile ducts—the tubes that carry bile in and out of the gallbladder—you can expect some excruciating pain in your upper or middle abdomen on the right side. The pain may come and go.

Women are three times more likely than men to develop gallstones because estrogen concentrates more cholesterol in bile. The risk for gallstones also increases if you're older or overweight. Doctors today usually treat gallstones with laparoscopic surgery or, sometimes, bile acid drugs that dissolve the cholesterol in the stones.

Kidney Stones: Too Much Mineral

When certain minerals become too concentrated in your urine, crystals of calcium salts and other minerals that are usually flushed out when you urinate start to build up and resemble hard, rough little pebbles. As a kidney stone attempts to leave your kidney, it doesn't go as smoothly as urine does—not even close. The narrow tubes (ureters) that easily carry liquid have a much harder time moving a solid mass on through, and this causes intense, often fluctuating waves of pain through your lower back, sides, and pelvic area.

Kidney stones affect mostly middle-aged and older men. Unlucky guys! The pain of passing a kidney stone is said to be as close as a man can get to experiencing the pain of childbirth. These stones usually aren't treated, and the pain can be controlled with medication as they're passing. In the past, a stone that wouldn't pass constituted a surgical emergency. Today, a noninvasive procedure called lithotripsy can break up the stone with pulverizing shock waves to help it move on out.

Calcium Conflict

Doctors used to think that too much calcium in your diet contributed to gallstones and kidney stones. This is because both of these types of stones are linked to calcium buildup in either the gallbladder or the kidneys, often from taking calcium supplements. Recently, however, studies have found that people who get plenty of calcium from their diet are actually the least likely to get gallstones and kidney stones. Scientists believe that calcium from food instead of from a pill is the key. Dietary calcium has shown to lower the amount of cholesterol in the gallbladder and kidneys, reducing the risk for stones.

Water 'Em Down

Water is an essential part of helping every system in your body work well, and its role in preventing gallstones and kidney stones is certainly included. Drinking plenty of water flushes your liver and dilutes the bile that thickens and causes gallstones. The more water you drink the less concentrated your urine is, which prevents crystals from forming and developing into stones. Experts agree that drinking six to eight glasses of water a day is your best bet. Here's a trick: Measure out 2 quarts of water every morning and make sure it's gone before you go to bed.

Healing Foods for Gallstones

To ward off gallstones, experts recommend eating a low-fat, low-cholesterol diet. For more protection, these healing foods could help:

★★**Beet greens** During a gallbladder attack, eating beet greens can help ease the pain. Beet greens are very high in minerals, vitamin A, and betaine, a compound that both stimulates the production of bile and dilutes it at the same time. Betaine also causes the muscles around the gallbladder and bile ducts to contract, which helps move things through. Other good sources of betaine include the edible weed called lambsquarter and the marshmallow. Coincidentally, the marshmallow may be a better recommendation than the beet, containing four times as much betaine. Linda White, MD, author of *Rodale's Herbal Drugstore*, recommends this mucilaginous herb to soothe the urinary tissues.

★★**Dandelion** This backyard "weed" increases bile flow in your gallbladder and improves how your body processes fat and cholesterol. Dandelion greens can be found in popular "spring mix" salad combinations. Drinking several cups of dandelion tea each day has been shown to prevent gallbladder attacks.

★★**Fiber** Dietary fiber hinders stone formation by reducing the concentration of cholesterol in your bile. You can lower your risk for gallstones with a high-fiber diet. Fiber from fruits, vegetables, whole grains, and bran binds with bile salts (part of bile) and cholesterol in your intestines, preventing your body from absorbing them. In addition, fiber absorbs lots of water, which softens your stools. Water-soaked stools absorb fat, and less fat in your system can help prevent gallstones. Even better, a 2004 Harvard study found that a high-fiber diet is just as protective against gallstones even when other risk factors are involved.

★★**Globe artichoke** (as distinguished from the Jerusalem artichoke) According to Mills and Bone, the globe artichoke was used traditionally for urinary stones and the related oliguria. They say that it stimulates bile flow and inhibits cholesterol synthesis.

★★**Radishes** Radishes contain a variety of chemicals that help improve digestion, and they increase the flow of bile. Michael Murray, ND, a natural medicine expert and author of *The Encyclopedia of Healing Foods*, suggests eating fresh radishes to maintain a healthy gallbladder. Both the root and the juice of the plant have medicinal benefits.

★★**Turmeric** Commission E, the German agency that evaluates the safety and efficacy of medicinal herbs, considers turmeric, the main ingredient in curry, to be an effective herb for treating gallstones. Turmeric contains curcumin, a compound shown to fight gallstones because it thins out bile. This effect, in turn, helps prevent gallstones from forming and dissolves any that have already formed. If I had gallstones, I would eat lots of Indian dishes loaded with curry made with turmeric.

★★**Vegetables** Eating a lot of vegetables is a good way to prevent gallstones. According to Dr. Murray, vegetable proteins have preventive properties to fight the formation of gallstones. A Harvard research team has also found that proteins in vegetables seem to block gallstones.

★**Bilberry and blueberry** These fruits are crushed with the roots and steeped in gin and consumed as a diuretic, of value for kidney stones.

★**Fish** Studies at John Hopkins University School of Medicine suggest that fish oil may slow down gallstone formation. Certainly, fish omega-3's can lower cholesterol. So can alpha-linolenic acid. Good sources of alpha-linolenic acid include chia,

FOODS TO WATCH

In addition to eating a low-fat, low-cholesterol diet loaded with fiber, fruits, and veggies, here are some specific foods and diet practices that may help limit your risk of developing gallstones or kidney stones:

For gallstones:

Coffee. Coffee, both regular and decaf, can stimulate gallbladder contractions. If you have gallstones, refrain from drinking java until they're dissolved.

Eggs. Studies have shown eggs to cause a gallbladder attack in 93 percent of people with gallstones.

Sugar. A study done in the Netherlands suggests that eating a diet high in sugar can almost double your risk for gallstones.

Not enough fat. An extremely low-fat diet allows bile to sludge up in your gallbladder. You need some fat in your diet, just not too much.

Whole dairy foods. Animal proteins, such as those found in whole or high-fat dairy products, have been shown to increase the likelihood of gallstones.

For kidney stones:

Meats. Animal protein has been found to increase the concentration of calcium in urine, and more calcium can mean more stones.

Oxalate-rich foods. People who are prone to kidney stones tend to absorb higher levels of dietary oxalates. If you're prone, try to avoid oxalate-rich foods, such as beans, beets, blueberries, celery, chocolate, grapes, nuts, rhubarb, and spinach.

Salt. Too much salt in your diet increases your risk for kidney stones because it makes the calcium in your urine more concentrated.

Vitamin C. In high doses, vitamin C (an oxalate) can cause problems if you're prone to kidney stones. If you're like many people who take a vitamin C supplement to boost your immune system, be aware of this. However, some research suggests that vitamin C–rich foods don't have the same effect.

flaxseed, hempseed, inca peanuts, and walnut oil. This substance could be particularly helpful if you're at high risk, so you might want to eat more fish.

★**Nuts** Some naturopathic doctors say that low levels of lecithin may be linked to gallstones. Lecithin is a nutritional substance that helps water and fat mix more easily, and it's believed that it helps cholesterol move within your system. The more cholesterol moves, the less likely it is to settle and form stones. Foods rich in lecithin include peanuts, soybeans, and wheat germ. On a dry weight basis, soybeans may contain 1.5 to 2.5 percent lecithin, but Brazil nuts and velvet beans may contain as much as 10 percent.

Healing Foods for Kidney Stones

You might want to try these food remedies and nutrients to help prevent painful kidney stones from forming:

★★★**Cranberry** Dr. Murray suggests that cranberry reduces the volume of ionized calcium in the urine by more than half in patients with recurrent kidney stones. He cautions, however, that it would take 16 ounces of cranberry juice a day to prevent stone formation under such high-risk conditions.

★★★**Fiber** Foods rich in fiber have proven to reduce the amount of calcium in urine, making kidney stones less likely, so include lots of fruits, vegetables, and whole grains in your diet. Fiber may be one reason that vegetarians are at lower risk for developing these stones, but studies show that even meat eaters can lower their risk for kidney stones by beefing up on fiber.

★★**Cranberry juice** Dr. Murray, also the author of *The Complete Book of Juicing*, says that cranberry juice is a good choice if you're prone to kidney stones. Too much calcium causes them, and cranberry juice contains quinic acid, which reduces cal-

Gallstone Remedy Rumor

There's one old-time remedy I probably *wouldn't* try if I had gallstones. Rumor has it that fasting for 3 days and then dosing yourself heavily with olive oil and fruit juice will give your gallbladder such a boost that it spews out any stones. Some people have reported seeing their stones pass as "greenish blobs" when they follow this remedy, but experts are skeptical. Andrew Weil, MD, professor at the University of Arizona College of Medicine in Tucson, isn't convinced this works. He says it's possible that the greenish blobs are residues of the olive oil, not gallstones.

cium in your urine. Dr. Murray suggests drinking two 8-ounce glasses a day to help prevent stone formation.

★★**Dandelion** Eric Yarnell, naturopath; Kathy Abascal, an herbalist; and Carol Hooper, an MD—all good friends of mine—suggest large volumes of dandelion leaf tea for kidney stones. Animal studies confirm that it is useful in preventing kidney stone formation. If you can't find it in your supermarket, weed it from your lawn, but don't pick plants that are too close to a road or driveway. The roots are very good at soaking up chemical pollutants from passing cars.

★★**Magnesium** Eat foods rich in magnesium. Magnesium regulates calcium by binding with calcium salts in your urine, which keeps them dissolved so that they can't form stones. Foods rich in magnesium include green vegetables, whole grains, beans, and nuts.

★★**Potassium** People with low potassium levels are at higher risk for kidney stones because of potassium's role in maintaining healthy urine. Eating a diet full of vegetables and fruits, especially citrus fruits and juices, is often recommended. My friend Alan Tillotson, PhD, notes that lemon juice is an inexpensive form of citrate; 4 ounces per day provide sufficient concentration to increase urinary citrate levels and reduce urinary calcium excretion.

From the Herbal Medicine Chest

When it comes to herbal remedies for gallstones and kidney stones, it basically boils down to tea. Try steeping a preventive, healing tea with any of these:

For gallstones:

Celandine	Milk thistle
Peppermint	

For kidney stones:

Beggar-lice	Java tea
Couchgrass	Lovage
Ginger	Parsley
Goldenrod	Stinging nettle
Horsetail	

Gingivitis

BE FRUITFUL AND MULTIPLY—that sound advice takes on menacing overtones when you're talking about bacteria in the mouth, bacteria that build up between the teeth and near the gums. Over time—and particularly in those who don't floss, brush, or get regular dental care—that bacteria can cause swelling, redness, and even bleeding in your gums. If left untreated, gingivitis can develop into more serious gum diseases, such as periodontitis, or the loss of teeth.

Where do the bacteria come from? I hate to tell you this, but they're already in your mouth. They've been there the whole time. Normally they're kept in check with flossing and brushing, but when you avoid regular dental care, the sugars and starches in your food form a plaque—a sticky film—on your teeth. After a couple of days, the plaque hardens into tartar, the bacteria set up permanent residence, and your gingiva—the part of the gum closest to the teeth—starts getting irritated.

During pregnancy, women are at greater risk of developing gingivitis because of hormonal changes that make their gums more sensitive to the negative effects of plaque.

Poor nutrition is another possible cause of gingivitis, which means that getting the wrong nutrients or not enough of the right ones is the second way that food can gum up your health, in addition to creating plaque. But while food can get you into this mess, food can also get you out.

Healing Foods for Gingivitis

★**Citrus fruits and more** In some cases, a deficiency in vitamin C can lead to inflamed or bleeding gums, but with a recommended Daily Value of only 60 milligrams, as determined by the FDA, that total isn't too hard to reach if you add a few fruits to your diet. Nutritionists, working with as-purchased values, suggest oranges (84 milligrams), strawberries (84 milligrams in a cup), kiwi (70 milligrams), grapefruit (45 milligrams in one-half), and cantaloupe (25 milligrams in one-eighth). Black currants pack in even more vitamin C, with 180 milligrams in 100 grams, while a single guava boasts 125 milligrams.

For best results, don't sprinkle sugar on the strawberries or otherwise adorn the fruit because then you're defeating the purpose of eating the fruit in the first place. The goal is to keep your teeth clean of sugar and starches. Note that having lots of vitamin C in your diet doesn't seem to affect your risk of developing gingivitis; just make sure that you're at least getting the minimum amount recommended.

★**Cranberries** Cranberry juice is widely known to prevent urinary tract infections, but a study in the *Journal of the American Dental Association* found that cranberry juice can also reverse and inhibit the growth of dental plaque bacteria—and taking out the bacteria should lessen the risk of gingivitis. One catch, though, is that cranberry juice typically includes a lot of sugar, and dumping sugar in your mouth will undo the positive effects of the juice, so try to keep the cranberries plain.

★**Red and green peppers, Brussels sprouts, and broccoli** If you prefer savory foods over sweet ones, no worries—plenty of vegetables have decent amounts of vitamin C. The best choices are sweet red and green peppers, as one medium red pepper contains 152 milligrams of vitamin C, while a green pepper of the same size has 95 milligrams. One cup of broccoli features 81 milligrams of vitamin C, while a cup of Brussels sprouts has nearly the same amount at 75 milligrams.

★**Sardines and salmon** When you think about building strong bones, you'll probably think of calcium, and even though teeth aren't bones—because they don't contain marrow, among other reasons—calcium intake is a good indicator of dental health. A study in *Journal of Periodontology*, for example, showed that those with a lower calcium intake had a higher risk of periodontal disease: a 54 percent higher risk for women who took in only 2 to 499 milligrams of calcium and a 27 percent risk for women who had moderate calcium intake levels of 500 to 799 milligrams.

You can turn to the coastlines for calcium in the form of sardines—325 milligrams in 3 ounces of Atlantic sardines in oil—and canned pink salmon—181 milligrams in a 3-ounce serving. Note that while canned salmon has some calcium clout, fresh salmon has much less, roughly 10 milligrams for that same 3-ounce serving. What's the difference between canned and fresh? When salmon is canned, the calcium-rich bones are canned as well, and these bones soften during the canning process, which makes them digestible.

★**Soy and tofu** Not everyone can take dairy products, but thanks to the diversity of our food supply, you don't have to. Many calcium-enhanced soy beverages are available, and they typically include about 300 milligrams of calcium per cup. Even more amazing, raw firm tofu prepared with calcium sulfate contains 861 milligrams of calcium in just a half cup. (Hard tofu prepared with nigari contains 345 milligrams of calcium in a 100-gram serving, just under half the amount of calcium in the same amount of tofu prepared with calcium sulfate.)

★**Yogurt, milk, and cheese** The FDA recommends that you take in 1 gram of calcium daily, and if you want more calcium in your diet, your first thought might be to turn to various dairy products. Good choice! An 8-ounce container of plain nonfat yogurt contains almost half the calcium you need, a total of 452 milligrams. A 1.5-ounce chunk of Romano cheese contains the same amount of calcium, and 2 ounces of pasteurized processed Swiss cheese has 438 milligrams. Many cheeses have more than

300 milligrams of calcium in 1- to 2-ounce servings, including ricotta, provolone, mozzarella, cheddar, muenster, and even individually wrapped slices of American cheese.

Milk fits into the calcium package as well, with a cup of milk—whether skim, 1 percent, or whole—providing between 276 and 300 milligrams of calcium.

Glaucoma

GLAUCOMA, A BLANKET TERM FOR A GROUP OF DISEASES, is a leading cause of blindness, both in the United States and around the world. The most common cause of glaucoma is an increase in fluid pressure within the eye (intraocular pressure) caused by a failure in the normal drainage mechanism, but some versions of the disease have no increase in fluid pressure.

In all cases of glaucoma, damage is done to the optic nerve—the bundle of nerves that transmit visual information from the retina to the brain—and you start to develop blind spots in your peripheral vision (your vision directly to the side). Closed-angle glaucoma, one of the less common forms, might be accompanied by severe eye pain, blurred vision, and headaches, while other forms of glaucoma cause almost no pain as they develop.

An estimated three million Americans have glaucoma, but only about half of them are aware of it. This is a shame since the condition can be treated and controlled, although not completely cured. It's only when glaucoma is left untreated that blindness might result, and any damage that has already occurred cannot be undone by treatment.

If you fall into one of the two risk groups—those with a family history of glaucoma and African Americans over age 40 (who are 15 times more likely than white persons of the same age to go blind as a result of glaucoma)—then you should be checked every 2 years. If you find yourself turning your head to see objects at the side of your vision that once were clear and visible, then hasten to an ophthalmologist for a battery of tests. Once you're over age 60, you also need to be checked biennially, no matter what your background.

Ideally, you'll never need to resort to daily medication or turn to surgery to create a new drainage system for fluid in the eye simply to keep spots at bay and your peripheral vision clear.

Healing Foods for Glaucoma

★★**Almonds** A 2001 study in the *Archives of Ophthalmology* of more than 4,500 participants found that vitamin E intake had an inverse relationship with intraocular pressure. The relationship wasn't incredibly strong, but it's there.

Adding sources of vitamin E to your diet is easy to do. Almonds, for example, have 40 percent of the Daily Value of vitamin E in a 1-ounce serving. You can eat dry roasted almonds plain or mix them into salads, rice, or other meals.

★★**Wheat germ oil** Another good source of vitamin E is wheat germ oil. One tablespoon of the stuff contains 20 milligrams of the alpha-tocopherol form of vitamin E, which equals 30 International Units (IU) or 100 percent of the Daily Value.

Wheat itself contains only a tiny bit of vitamin E in the germ inside the kernel. When wheat germ oil is made, however, all of that vitamin E is extracted; this makes the oil a medicinal wonder. Use wheat germ oil as the base ingredient in salad dressings or mix it with freshly cooked pasta to get your daily dose.

★**Black currants and guava** Some studies have shown that vitamin C can lower intraocular pressure, which would most likely alleviate future damage to the optic nerve, but (1) the studies have involved intravenous or oral delivery of vitamin C supplements and (2) the doses of vitamin C are incredibly high, on the order of 500 milligrams per kilogram of body weight. The US National Library of Medicine notes that taking more than 2,000 milligrams of vitamin C per day can lead to diarrhea and upset stomachs, and nearly all of the study participants did experience these problems.

In your quest for more C, you can turn to oranges and orange juice, the standard bearers of the vitamin, or you can try a couple of fruits that contain way more C than Florida's best-known product. Black currants, for example, contain 180 milligrams of C in 100 grams, while a single guava boasts 125 milligrams.

★**Green peppers** Another way to boost your vitamin C naturally is to turn to green peppers—a medium-sized pepper contains 95 milligrams of vitamin C, 150 percent of the Daily Value. Before you start popping peppers at breakfast, lunch, and dinner to megadose on vitamin C, however, consult your physician so that he or she can monitor your progress.

★**Liver** Only 6 micrograms of vitamin B_{12} are needed daily according to the FDA— but a Japanese study on the long-term treatment of glaucoma with B_{12} found that glaucoma patients taking a daily dose of 1.5 milligrams (or 1,500 micrograms) suffered no further loss in their visual field.

While 5 milligrams is a big step up from 6 micrograms and probably would require a supplement to reach that level, you can take in a lot of vitamin B_{12} by eating liver. This food has been the butt of many jokes over the decades, but it does include almost 60 micrograms of B_{12} in a 100-gram serving, making it one of your best choices for this vitamin.

★**Oysters and clams** Another option for increasing your vitamin B$_{12}$ intake is to eat clams, which contain 42 micrograms in 3 ounces, or oysters, which have 14 micrograms in the same amount.

★**Sunflower seed kernels and hazelnuts** Other sources of vitamin E include these snack-appropriate items; dry roasted sunflower seed kernels boast 30 percent of the Daily Value in 1 ounce, and hazelnuts have 20 percent in 1 ounce.

Gout

I KNOW FROM PERSONAL EXPERIENCE HOW PAINFUL GOUT CAN BE. I had my first attack shortly before I turned 50. A day after working in my herb garden—one of the great passions of my life—I woke up with telltale symptoms: pain and swelling in my big toe. It was so intense that the weight from my bed sheet felt like a ton of bricks. When I got up, I was barely able to walk.

Gout results from a buildup of uric acid in the blood. If levels become too high, uric acid crystals form in the joints—usually but not always in the big toe—which causes excruciating and incapacitating pain. Once considered a disease of royalty and royal excess—England's King Henry VIII, a notorious overindulger in food and drink, is the prime example—gout actually afflicts rich and poor alike. Although 95 percent of its victims are older men—more often African Americans rather than Caucasians or Hispanics—an increasing number of women are developing the disease.

In my case, after some initial hesitation, I finally agreed to my doctor's recommendation that I take allopurinol (Lopurin, Zyloprim), a drug that flushes pain-causing uric acid crystals from the body. That helped me regain my footing, so to speak, and effectively prevented the gout attacks that kept me from puttering in my beloved herb garden or walking in the nearby forests.

With all due respect to conventional medicine, however, I eventually found a natural alternative to allopurinol in celery seed extract and whole celery stalks. I also think there are many other possible dietary interventions that can help.

Healing Foods for Gout

A number of food remedies may be effective at helping to prevent gout or reduce its symptoms. Here are some to try.

★★★**Celery** Two of the better sources of natural COX-2 inhibitors are celery and celery seed, which contain high amounts of painkilling apigenin. When I was diagnosed with gout and was looking for alternatives to allopurinol as a way to reduce my uric acid levels, I found that either eating four celery stalks or taking two to four tablets of celery seed extract daily all but eliminated my gout attacks. Alternatively, you might try preparing a tea by pouring boiling water over 1 teaspoon of freshly crushed celery seeds and letting it steep for 10 to 20 minutes before drinking it.

★★★**Cherries** Although the Arthritis Foundation insists that there's no conclusive evidence that cherries can prevent or reduce the pain of gout or any other form of arthritis, this longstanding folkloric remedy has strong anecdotal support. When *Prevention* magazine conducted a reader survey, some 67 percent of respondents said that cherries were effective for gout pain. Some alternative medicine practitioners recommend drinking two to three glasses of black cherry juice diluted with an equal amount of water daily until the pain subsides. According to some reports, this regimen can help relieve an acute attack of gout within 48 to 72 hours.

An increasing body of evidence suggests that these anecdotal reports may be accurate. Cherries contain many antioxidants and other compounds that may help reduce the painful inflammation of gout. In one study, researchers at the University of California, Davis, measured blood levels of uric acid—a marker for gout—in 10 healthy women before and after they ate 45 fresh Bing cherries for breakfast. Following the meal, they showed significantly lower levels of uric acid. In a follow-up study, 18 women and two men consumed 45 fresh Bing cherries throughout the day every day for a month. The researchers found that levels of three inflammatory indicators—nitric oxide, C-reactive protein, and a marker for T-cell activation—decreased by 18 to 25 percent.

That's no guarantee that cherries will work for everyone with gout. They didn't do much for me, although they did help my younger brother and many other people who have consulted with me. But there's no question that cherries contain dozens of analgesic and anti-inflammatory compounds, including natural COX-2 inhibitors such as apigenin, caffeic acid, and quercetin. Some of these same compounds are found in green tea, so it seems to me that the easiest herbal way to control uric acid production may be to eat cherries, drink green tea, and watch your diet.

★★**Coffee** If you're a java lover, here's some of the best news you could possibly imagine: The more coffee you drink, the lower your risk of developing gout. If you already have gout, it's possible that an extra cup or two of coffee a day could help you manage your symptoms. In 2007, researchers from the University of British Columbia in Canada and Harvard University in the United States published fascinating findings in the journal *Arthritis and Rheumatism*. The results, based on two large-scale studies, suggest that coffee—caffeinated and, to a lesser extent, decaffeinated—contains substances that reduce blood concentrations of uric acid, the vile substance that causes gout.

In the first study, researchers assessed data from the landmark Health Professionals Follow-up Study of 45,868 male health professionals, who were gout free when the study began in 1986. Of these, 757 subsequently developed gout.

When the researchers looked at participants' coffee consumption, they found that drinking four to five cups a day lowered the risk of developing gout by 40 percent. The reduction was even greater among men who drank six or more cups a day: 59 percent. But apparently caffeine wasn't the most important factor. Men who

FOODS TO WATCH

Yes, it's true: Alcohol is associated with a higher risk of gout. In a 2004 study published in the *Lancet*, researchers crunched data from the Health Professionals Follow-up Study and found that men who consumed more than four or five alcoholic drinks a day were 2½ times more likely to develop gout than teetotalers were. Interestingly, beer consumption (two drinks a day or more) was associated with the highest risk, while equivalent hard liquor consumption had a slightly lower risk and equivalent wine consumption had none.

Using data from the same study, a 2008 study reported in the *British Medical Journal* identified an additional risk factor for gout: sweetened sodas. The researchers found that men who drank five or six sodas per week were 29 percent more likely to develop gout than men who drank no soda.

At one time, it was thought that consumption of all foods rich in purines, which form uric acid when they break down, was associated with gout. Doctors often advised patients to minimize or eliminate consumption of purine-rich meat, seafood, and vegetables. Then a 2004 study published in the *New England Journal of Medicine* showed that men with high intakes of meat and seafood—particularly beef, pork, and lamb—had a significantly increased risk of gout. But the study also found no increased risk from consumption of purine-rich vegetables such as peas, beans, mushrooms, and spinach. The researchers actually found a protective effect from vegetable as well as dairy proteins.

drank four or more cups a day of decaffeinated coffee also had a 27 percent reduced risk, while tea consumption had no effect.

So what's in coffee that makes it so special? According to the study's lead investigator, it could be the high content of chlorogenic acid, a strong antioxidant that also may improve insulin sensitivity. People with gout often have impaired insulin sensitivity—a precursor of diabetes.

In the second study, the researchers looked at another large group—the more than 14,000 men and women who were enrolled in the landmark US Third National Health and Nutrition Examination Survey study between 1988 and 1994—and found that levels of uric acid decreased with increasing coffee intake.

Although these studies aren't conclusive, they do seem to suggest that drinking at least four cups of coffee a day could be of enormous help in preventing as well as managing this painful condition. And to be realistic, most of my Starbucks buddies would rather have four cups of coffee a day than four stalks of celery.

★★**Mint** Peppermint, spearmint, Chinese mint, and other mint oils contain high amounts of menthol, which when applied topically can help relieve the pain associated with gout. Although you can buy commercial products containing menthol, it might be a better (and cheaper) bet to apply mint oils directly to your gouty joints. Be aware, though, that such oils are toxic when consumed internally. Another option is to drink peppermint tea two or three times a day. Although many commercial mint teas are available, I'd recommend making your own by pouring 1 cup of boiling water over 1 heaping teaspoon (5 grams) of dried peppermint leaves, steeping it for 5 to 10 minutes, and drinking three to four cups daily. For extra benefits, consider using a licorice stick to stir a delicious peppermint/chamomile tea, which will give you a host of analgesic and anti-inflammatory compounds. Another option is taking 3 to 6 grams a day of peppermint leaf tablets or capsules.

In Japan, a weedy, aromatic mint called chiso is often used to relieve gout. You'll find it in a few Asian specialty markets here but certainly not in many American supermarkets. The leaves are often consumed with sushi. It's rich in xanthine oxidase inhibitors, which can prevent the production of uric acid. I often add a little chiso to my mint teas and find that it's good for what ails me.

★★**Turmeric** Human studies of curcumin have found that it can reduce the pain and stiffness associated with rheumatoid arthritis as well as help relieve postsurgical inflammation, which suggests it may also be effective for gout.

I prefer a whole-foods approach whenever possible because I believe you get more healing power from whole foods than from the individual components found in supplements, so I often add liberal amounts of curry to rice and other dishes. I would also consider adding other anti-inflammatory foods such as pineapple and papaya. You can also make tea with turmeric.

Unfortunately, it's difficult to get medicinal doses of curcumin from just diet. According to naturopaths, that dose is 250 to 500 milligrams of pure curcumin a day between meals, which translates into 5 to 25 teaspoons of dried turmeric a day. That's a good deal more than even a curry fan like me would want in my food. I would recommend adding as much turmeric as possible to your diet to help prevent pain and taking turmeric supplements—standardized to 90 to 95 percent curcumin—to help relieve acute pain. Take it with freshly ground black pepper to enhance absorption.

★★**Vitamin C–rich foods** According to a study published in *Arthritis and Rheumatism*, uric acid levels are considerably lower in people who have high blood levels of vitamin C. The researchers randomly assigned 184 participants to take either 500 milligrams a day of vitamin C or placebo. Uric acid levels were significantly lower in the vitamin C group, suggesting that vitamin C–rich fruits such as strawberries, kiwifruit, oranges, and other citrus fruits, as well as vegetables such as bell peppers, broccoli, and Brussels spouts, may help prevent or alleviate gout symptoms. The richest source of vitamin C that I know of is Amazonian camu-camu. You won't find it in your local supermarket, but you can buy capsules or powder made from the fruit from Internet sources.

★**Chamomile** Although best known as a calming herb, chamomile also contains potent anti-inflammatory compounds such as apigenin, luteolin, and quercetin. Naturopaths recommend drinking three or four cups of chamomile tea daily to treat painful joint conditions. You might also try taking 2 to 3 grams of the herb in tablet or capsule form, taking 4 to 6 milliliters of tincture three times a day between meals. or applying a topical chamomile cream or ointment to the affected area three or four times daily.

★**Chile peppers** Hot peppers contain a pungent substance known as capsaicin, which is number one among my painkillers. When applied topically, capsaicin temporarily depletes substance P, a chemical in nerves that transmits pain sensations. Without substance P, pain signals can no longer be sent. Dozens of studies show that capsaicin can temporarily relieve many painful conditions, including gout. After a lot of digging, I've found that capsaicin is more potent (almost 20 times more) as an anti-inflammatory than the now-banned drug rofecoxib (Vioxx).

You can buy a commercial topical cream containing 0.025 to 0.075 percent capsaicin and apply it to your gouty joints three or four times a day. Or perhaps do what people outside the United States often do: buy a chile pepper, mash it, and apply it directly. You can also mix mashed hot pepper with a skin cream such as cold cream. Either way, you'll save money. A fresh pepper costs a few pennies, whereas a commercial capsaicin product such as Zostrix can cost up to $16.

No matter which route you choose, you may experience a burning sensation the first few times you use capsaicin, but it usually subsides with repeated use. Just be sure to thoroughly wash your hands after using it. If you get any in your eyes, nose, or mouth, it may be even more painful than your gouty joints.

Although capsaicin is best used topically, it may be helpful to add more peppers and pepper-derived hot sauces to your diet. Another option is taking a cayenne tincture (0.3 to 1 milliliter) three times a day. You also can make an infusion by stirring ½ to 1 teaspoon (2.5 to 5 grams) of cayenne powder into 1 cup of boiling water, letting it steep for 10 minutes, and taking 1 teaspoon mixed with water three or four times daily.

★**Ginger** This spice contains high amounts of zingibain, a powerful anti-inflammatory enzyme. Ginger contains 180 times more proteolytic enzymes than does the papaya plant and may be even more effective at relieving inflammation-related conditions, including gout. It also contains at least four natural COX-2 inhibitors.

It's easy to get enough ginger in your diet to help reduce pain. You can take it as an herb in tea by steeping three or four slices of fresh ginger in a cup of boiling water. If you prefer, you can get clinically significant doses in tinctures or capsules. However, I love the taste of ginger, so I use it often in foods. Try sprinkling ½ teaspoon of powdered ginger into foods or eating an ounce (6 teaspoons) of fresh ginger every day.

Recently, I have been enjoying New Chapter's commercial ginger salve in honey. It reminds me pleasantly of an exotic pain remedy I encountered during my travels down the Amazon River. I dubbed it Soccorro's Secret, after Soccorro Guerrero, who brewed it in her kitchen. Her salve is made of ginger, honey, rum, and other ingredients, including the herb dragon's blood. But if I were to improve on it, I'd add pineapple. In your own kitchen, you could make a tea with a tablespoon of dried ginger and sweeten it to taste with honey; if you're feeling adventurous, add a splash of rum.

★**Pineapple** This exotic fruit is rich in a number of substances that can help people with conditions such as gout. Foremost among them is bromelain, an enzyme that helps reduce swelling and inflammation in many painful inflammatory conditions.

Its anti-inflammatory effects are so profound that the German government has approved its use for healing after injuries and surgical procedures. Pineapple also contains high amounts of manganese, which is essential for the formation of collagen, the tough, fibrous protein that builds connective tissues such as bone, skin, and cartilage. You can get 100 percent of the daily value for manganese (2 milligrams) from just a cup of fresh pineapple chunks or pineapple juice. Pineapple is also a rich source of vitamin C, also necessary for collagen formation, and it contains more of this important vitamin than apples, cranberries, or tomato juice. A cup of fresh pineapple chunks contains 40 percent (24 milligrams) of the Daily Value for vitamin C. To get the maximum antioxidant punch, try "Gold" pineapple, which is imported from Costa Rica and contains four times as much vitamin C as other varieties.

Unfortunately, recent research suggests that levels of bromelain in fresh pineapple and a related enzyme—papain in fresh papaya—may be too low to have much of an effect. While I would encourage enjoying these fruits—either whole or as juice—you'll probably need to use supplements to achieve effective doses. Naturopaths suggest taking anywhere between 250 and 500 milligrams three times a day. In human studies, a daily dosage of up to 2,000 milligrams has not proven harmful.

From the Herbal Medicine Chest

Ermiao wan is a traditional Chinese herbal medicine made up of phellodendri cortex and atractylodis rhizome. For thousands of years, it has been used to reduce inflammatory swelling. In a study published in a 2004 issue of the *Journal of Ethnopharmacology,* researchers studied the effects of ermiao wan in mice with elevated levels of uric acid and found that it reduced the levels as effectively as the prescription medication allopurinol, the drug I've sometimes used to control my gout. If you decide to try this remedy, which you can purchase on the Internet, be sure to consult a certified herbalist who can advise you about appropriate dosages and possible side effects.

Alternatively, you might try a pain remedy that's a favorite of Andrew Weil, MD, professor at the University of Arizona College of Medicine in Tucson. Zyflamend (available at health food stores), is a blend of ginger, turmeric, oregano, rosemary, holy basil, green tea, and other herbs with anti-inflammatory properties. It's safe to take indefinitely if you follow the label directions.

Hangover

IN GERMANY, THEY CALL IT THE WAILING OF THE CATS. In Norway, it's known as carpenters in the head. The Spanish refer to it as backlash. But a hangover by any name is just as painful in every land and culture. A lucky few don't experience the horrible morning-after effects of alcohol, but most of us do—and you don't have to be a two-fisted drinker to suffer the boozy consequences. The severity of your headache, dry mouth, nausea, and muscle aches is determined by what you drink, when you drink, and your body's metabolism.

Sadly, hangovers are all too common because alcohol abuse is on the rise. More than 14 million Americans meet the diagnostic criteria for alcoholism. However, there are many responsible ways to enjoy the occasional libation without sacrificing your health—or your dignity.

Why Hangovers Hurt

The nausea and skull-splitting headache many people feel after a night of partying is the body's way of reacting to low blood sugar, dehydration, and inflammation.

Alcohol hampers the production of glucose, the sugar that fuels every cell in your body, particularly the brain. A glucose-deprived brain can cause irritability, weakness, and dizziness. Alcohol also acts as a diuretic, so the kidneys are continually flushing out vital nutrients such as magnesium and potassium. If you ended your "happy hour" with an episode of vomiting, your hydration stores are taxed even more. As if that weren't enough, alcohol causes inflammation of the stomach lining and blood vessels in the brain. To add insult to injury, it also prevents a good night's rest by disturbing rapid eye-movement sleep. The result? A ghastly kabob of aches and pains from head to toe.

Obviously, the best way to circumvent a hangover is to avoid alcohol altogether. However, if you do drink, there are several ways to minimize or even prevent morning-after misery.

One of the simplest defenses against hangover is to replace the liquids that alcohol has leached out of you. The National Institutes of Health recommends drinking a glass of water after each alcoholic drink. This will not only hydrate your parched insides but may also curb your drinking. You should also abstain from darker-colored drinks such as whiskey, bourbon, and red wine. They contain by-products called congeners that fuel inflammation and can turn a headache into a headquake. Finally, before you propose a toast, be sure to break some bread. Having even a few morsels of food in your stomach will slow the absorption of alcohol, and your body will metabolize it more efficiently.

Healing Foods for Hangover

So what do you do if a hangover already has you in its talons? Fortunately, there are several steps you can take to loosen the grip.

★★★**Teaberry and wintergreen** I don't know if you still can buy teaberry gum. Teaberry and wintergreen are one and the same—flavorful sources of the analgesic methyl-salicylate, along with a dozen or so anti-inflammatories. Here at home, I like to brew myself a cup of wintergreen tea and spike it with hot-pepper sauce.

★★**Cinnamon** One of Mrs. Duke's favorite remedies for an upset stomach is cinnamon toast. Cinnamon contains several stomach-settling compounds, along with almost a dozen pain relievers. No wonder people will drink cinnamon tea after a night out.

★★**Hot pepper** Whenever I overindulge—which isn't frequently—my favorite hangover remedy is a freshly squeezed vegetable juice cocktail or commercial V8 juice seasoned with hot pepper sauce. The vegetables contain antioxidants to repair cell damage, and the hot pepper sauce is rich in capsaicin, a chemical that triggers the body to release natural opiates called endorphins. Hot peppers also contain aspirin-like compounds called salicylates. You can buy hangover pills and sprays that contain capsaicin, but my hot pepper cocktail offers more complete sustenance for a nutritionally deprived body.

★★**Prickly pear** When you think of popular fruits, the prickly pear probably doesn't come to mind. However, these sweet cactus fruits, called tunas, are commercially produced at twice the rate of strawberries or apricots! Prickly pears are a common dessert ingredient, particularly in Mexico and Central America. It's not the pulp, however, but rather the spine-studded skin that could hold a hangover cure. A group of doctors from Tulane Health Sciences Center in New Orleans gave two groups of graduate students either prickly pear extract or a placebo 5 hours

FOODS TO WATCH

You've heard of that oft-recommended remedy for a barking hangover—order up another glass of whatever "bit you" the night before. This notion is based on the belief that hangovers are caused by alcohol withdrawal, so giving your body the alcohol it's craving will temporarily calm those beastly symptoms. But drinking to squelch a throbbing headache will only delay, and possibly compound, the inevitable repercussions of tying one on. Even more important, this practice can encourage alcohol abuse, so give your body a much-needed reprieve from the booze and let sleeping dogs lie.

before drinking alcohol. The prickly pear group reported less severe symptoms of nausea and dry mouth than the students who were given a placebo. The extract appeared to reduce the inflammation caused by alcohol consumption.

★**Bananas** Knocking back a few sends your kidneys into overtime. They keep pace by flushing out toxins, but vital fluids and nutrients, such as electrolytes, are also excreted. A banana can help replenish these important minerals. Bananas are a very good source of electrolytes, such as potassium, which you lose when you become dehydrated. Once electrolytes are restored, you shouldn't have that weak or shaky feeling. To take that remedy one step further, make a banana smoothie with a dollop of honey; the honey will bring those glucose levels back up.

★**Fruit juice** Alcohol disrupts your body's manufacture of glucose, the very fuel that drives your cells. Your brain is especially dependent on this fuel, so a glucose drought can cause headaches and dizziness. Booze also signals your liver to accumulate fat compounds and produce lactic acid, both of which can create mild hypoglycemia. Dousing the flames of a hideous hangover with fruit juice will restore your reservoir of glucose. There's some evidence that fructose, the natural sugar in fruit juice, may have the added benefit of burning up alcohol in your body faster. Other good sources of fructose include dates, chicory, and onion bulb.

★**Leafy greens** These are another good source of potassium, one of the all-important electrolytes that we discussed earlier. You could make a soothing sald of lettuce, endive, radish, Chinese cabbage, and/or spinach.

From the Herbal Medicine Chest

Since 600 AD, the Chinese have believed that the herb kudzu snuffs out hangover headaches by turning off alcohol cravings. In fact, the name *kudzu* loosely translates into "drunkenness dispeller."

Researchers at McLean Psychiatric Hospital, affiliated with Harvard Medical School, were intrigued by kudzu's mystique and put its teetotaler's effects to the test. Much to their surprise, this invasive vine caused some pretty dramatic results. Students who were given kudzu extract before drinking as many beers as they wanted (up to six) drank significantly less than students who were given a placebo. In fact, the kudzu group drank about half the amount of beer compared to the non-kudzu group. It's not clear exactly how the herb hampers the desire to drink alcohol, but it appears to make the drinker feel more satisfied with less beer. The researchers caution that this isn't a magic bullet and that more research is needed, but it could certainly be a tool for cutting back on alcohol intake.

Hay Fever

MOST OF US GET A RUSH OF ENERGY AT THE FIRST SIGN OF SPRING, when we wake up to the sound of birds chirping and crocuses begin poking out of the ground. And yet, just as we're ready to shed our winter coats and breathe in the fresh spring air, hay fever symptoms send some of us back inside, sniffling and miserable.

Hay fever is one of the most common allergies, with one in five Americans experiencing a runny nose, congestion, sneezing, itchy eyes and ears, sinus pressure, sleeplessness, and fatigue during the spring, summer, or fall. Most people with hay fever react to pollen, which is light enough to be carried by the wind anywhere—even through the front door of your home. But other outdoor allergens, such as grass, weeds, and mold, can also bring on the symptoms. Likewise, some people are sensitive to indoor allergens, such as dust mites, cockroaches, and pet dander. And some irritants, such as cigarette smoke, perfume, and room deodorizers, can make hay fever feel even worse.

It's easy to mistake hay fever for a cold because the symptoms are similar, but they're actually quite different conditions. Colds are caused by viruses and clear up in 5 to 7 days. Hay fever is caused by your body's reaction to common substances in the air. Your immune system characterizes pollen and dust as invaders, and in response to them, it releases histamine, a chemical that makes you alert but unfortunately also causes allergy symptoms.

In addition to making you generally miserable, hay fever makes you more likely to have asthma, eczema, and sinusitis.

What's the best way to control hay fever, according to experts? Avoid the offending allergens. Of course, that's easier said than done. Even if your allergies are so bad you decide to pack up and move to another part of the country, you may develop new sensitivities in the new locale.

Antihistamines, decongestants, and nasal sprays will help relieve symptoms, but they don't work on what's causing the allergies: the inappropriate response from your immune system. In severe cases, allergy shots may help, but results sometimes don't occur until after years of treatment.

Leigh Broadhurst, PhD, a biochemically trained nutritionist whom I invited to help structure this chapter, has an excellent protocol for allergies. For milder allergies, she leans toward a nutritional approach to boost the immune system and reduce symptoms without medication. Minimize or eliminate alcohol, artificial colors and flavors, food preservatives, caffeine, dairy products, egg yolks, formaldehyde, MSG, meat, refined sugar, soda, sulfites, and trans fats—then go ahead, and feel the exhilaration of breathing in the sweet spring air without fear of allergies.

Healing Foods for Hay Fever

In addition to Dr. Broadhurst's suggestions, adding the following foods to your daily diet may help keep hay fever at bay.

★★★**Broccoli** Broccoli is high in vitamin C, which acts as an antihistamine, blocking the inflammation that causes allergy symptoms. Studies have found that consuming up to 500 milligrams of vitamin C a day, from either diet or a supplement, can relieve allergies, asthma, respiratory infections, nasal congestion, and watery eyes. It's also a member of the crucifer family, a family of vegetables with properties that may help unclog your sinuses.

★★★**Citrus fruits** Oranges, grapefruits, lemons, and limes also contain vitamin C to help relieve allergy symptoms. I advise getting as much C as you can not only from broccoli and citrus fruits but also from other foods, such as guavas, strawberries, cantaloupe, tomato juice, mangoes, potatoes, cabbage greens, and raw spinach. If you'd like to boost your vitamin C intake after you've gotten all you can at meals, you may want to take a supplement.

★★★**Collard greens and kale** These leafy greens have two things going for them when it comes to relieving hay fever: They're crucifers, a type of vegetable that opens up the sinuses, and they're packed with carotenoids, which are associated with fewer allergy problems.

Allergy Soup, Coming Right Up!

Because Andrew Weil, MD, professor at the University of Arizona College of Medicine in Tucson, recommends stinging nettle as one of the best allergy relievers, and my database lists onions and evening primrose as major sources of the antihistamine quercetin, I've created a concoction that I call AllerGreens or AllergEase. Boil a whole onion (with the skin) and a clove of garlic. Add ½ cup chopped leaves and diced taproots of evening primrose. After boiling the concoction for 3 to 5 minutes, add a cup of nettle leaves and a cup of diced celery stalks (with leaves) and boil gently for another 3 to 10 minutes. Before eating, remove the onion skins from the soup and enjoy it while it's still warm, seasoning to taste with wine vinegar, black pepper, diced raw onions, hot pepper, turmeric, curry powder, or celery seed.

★★★**Elderberries** Immunity-boosting elderberries have a long folk history for treating allergies, along with colds, coughs, fever, and flu. They contain flavonoids and anythocyanins, which stimulate the immune system and reduce inflammation. Studies have found Sambucol, an elderberry extract sold in drugstores, to be an effective remedy, but I advise enjoying elderberry wine, juice, and jam. I'd wager that elderberry wine would prove quite competitive with Sambucol, but there haven't been studies to prove it. I always trust the food first and the extract second.

★★★**Onions and garlic** Onions and garlic contain quercetin, another antihistamine that acts like vitamin C to lower inflammation and give you relief from allergies. They're major ingredients in my SinuSoup, which also includes hot spices such as curry, horseradish, hot pepper, mustard seed, and black pepper.

★★★**Tea** According to my database search, onions have the highest amount of quercetin, but tea comes in second. Citrus fruits, apples, parsley, olive oil, grapes, dark cherries, blueberries, blackberries, and bilberries also contain significant concentrations of this antihistamine.

★★**Parsley** According to Michael Castleman, who has written several books on herbs, this culinary herb inhibits the secretion of histamine, which triggers allergy symptoms. If you have hives from hay fever, try adding parsley to your diet.

★★**Pumpkin** Whether you roast it or puree it for a soup, pumpkin has high amounts of three specific carotenoids, a type of vitamin A found in colorful fruits and vegetables, which can help relieve your allergies. One study of 547 adults showed that having high blood levels of carotenoids was associated with fewer allergy symptoms. Carrots are also high on the list for carotenoid content.

★**Celery** When I searched for foods that could be possible treatments for hay fever, celery came out on top as having the most evidence for alleviating allergy symptoms. Also on the list were carrots, ginger, peppermint, parsley, turmeric, chamomile, and cabbage.

★**Chile peppers, ginger, cayenne, horseradish, and mustard** Chronic congestion is an unfortunate side effect of allergies, but you can get relief from spicy foods. Hot peppers dilate blood vessels to clear out congestion. They also cause your nose and throat to produce a watery secretion that helps remove mucus when you cough or blow your nose. The Mayans traditionally used hot pepper for these purposes and even added it to their hot chocolate. Irwin Ziment, MD, of the UCLA School of Medicine, recommends eating a chile pepper a day with meals. I suggest adding one

FOODS TO WATCH

If you have hay fever, you may have what doctors call cross-sensitivity, meaning that certain foods can bring on hay fever symptoms.

Milk and meat. Richard Firshein, DO, director of the Firshein Center for Comprehensive Medicine in New York City, recommends a vegetarian-style diet that focuses more on fish and vegetables than on meat and dairy. That's because cows consume grass, which contains hay fever allergens, and drinking milk or eating meat can cause your hay fever to act up. Milk and beef also contain saturated fat, which can lead to inflammation.

Wheat and tree fruits. Because of cross-sensitivity, someone with hay fever may be allergic to wheat or fruits that come from trees, such as pears and apples. By eating those foods, especially in the spring, when allergen levels are highest, they may experience hay fever symptoms.

Foods that cause acid reflux. People with allergies and asthma often have digestive problems that can increase acid reflux, which in turn can make allergies worse, Dr. Firshein says. To avoid reflux, it's a good idea to stay away from acidic foods and heavy, high-fat sauces and dishes.

to chicken soup as a decongestant. Horseradish and wasabi (Japanese horseradish) are also good options.

★**Mint** The Eclectics, a group of late 19th- and early 20th-century American medical doctors who employed botanical remedies with their patients, used menthol vapors from inhalants and chest rubs to relieve hay fever, asthma, and morning sickness, according to Castleman. Cornmint has the highest amount of menthol, followed by muticous mountain mint, peppermint, European pennyroyal, watermint, Virginia mountain mint, and scented geranium. I wouldn't recommend using these herbs during pregnancy, however.

★**Pineapple** This sweet fruit contains a compound called bromelain, which fights inflammation caused by hay fever. The German Commission E, a government agency that evaluates the safety and efficacy of medicinal herbs, has approved bromelain for sinus and nasal swelling after ear, nose, and throat surgery.

From the Herbal Medicine Chest

More and more people with hay fever are turning to alternative therapies, including herbs, to relieve their symptoms, and studies show that the herbs are working. In one study, 52 patients with seasonal allergies were given either a combination of acupuncture and Chinese herbal medicine or a sham acupuncture treatment (acupuncture applied to nonacupuncture points) and a nonspecific Chinese herbal formula. Those receiving both acupuncture and Chinese herbal medicine reported significant improvement in their symptoms and quality of life.

Here are the herbs I recommend if you have hay fever.

Butterbur *(Petasites hybridus)* In a study of 580 people with seasonal allergies, taking butterbur leaf extract Ze339 for 2 weeks helped nearly all of them—90 percent saw an improvement in their symptoms. Another study found the extract to be as effective as an antihistamine.

Because butterbur is related to the ragweed family, it can make your symptoms worse if you're allergic to ragweed. The Mayo Clinic advises avoiding butterbur if you're allergic to ragweed, marigolds, daisies, or chrysanthemums.

If you try butterbur, be sure to choose a preparation that's PA-free— that is, toxic chemicals called pyrrolizidine alkaloids have been removed from the herb during processing. These chemicals can damage your liver and kidneys and may cause cancer.

German chamomile *(Matricaria recutita)* This herb can be taken for a wide variety of ailments, from gout to insomnia. It works by reducing inflammation.

Licorice *(Glycyrrhiza glabra)* Licorice has a high synergy score for hay fever, which means it can help relieve allergy symptoms. You can use it as a sweetener in teas when you buy it as a standardized herb, but don't use it regularly for more than 6 weeks. Long-term use can cause head-aches, lethargy, sodium and water retention, loss of potassium, and high blood pressure. Women who are pregnant or nursing and anyone with severe liver, kidney, or heart disease or high blood pressure or who is taking a prescription diuretic should not take licorice.

Stinging nettle *(Urtica dioica)* Taking nettle as capsules or liquid extract may get rid of an itchy throat and help soothe irritated, watery eyes. Freeze-dried nettle, which you can find in capsules, is the most potent for giving you allergy relief. I have frozen nettle in my downstairs freezer. In the spring when I weed the garden and hay fever makes my nose run, I pour boiling water over the nettle and add fresh and powdered onion and garlic, along with salt, for a great-tasting anti-allergy pot liquor. Then I cook the nettle and eat it. (The leaves lose their sting when cooked.)

Andrew Weil, MD, professor at the University of Arizona College of Medicine in Tucson, suggests taking nettle and quercetin instead of prednisone and other steroids. He advises taking 400 milligrams of quercetin twice a day between meals a week or two before pollen season. Also take one or two capsules of freeze-dried nettle leaf extract every 2 to 4 hours as needed.

Headaches

HEADACHES ARE AMONG HUMANKIND'S MOST COMMON AFFLICTIONS. In the United States, about 15 percent of us—some 45 million Americans—are stricken with at least one a week.

The vast majority of these attacks—about 90 percent—are tension headaches, which start with knotted muscles in the neck and scalp and spread dull pain through the skull. The other 10 percent are the real bangers: migraines and cluster headaches caused by the nerve-jangling opening and closing (dilation and constriction) of blood vessels in the brain.

Moderate to severe migraines affect about 28 million Americans and are about three times more common in women than in men. The pain usually starts on one side of the head—often preceded by visual disturbances known as auras (or scintillating scotoma)—and develops into a severe and throbbing headache that can last for hours or even days. It can also come with nausea and vomiting. In women, migraines frequently develop before menstrual periods and disappear after menopause.

Cluster headaches—which are shorter but can be even more painful—are seven times more common in men than in women. They're sometimes known as suicide headaches because they're so intense. They affect about one million Americans.

For about 1 in 10 of us, headaches are the worst source of pain, according to a 2005 survey of 1,200 adults conducted by Stanford University School of Medicine. Although respondents relied most on prescription drugs and prayer to treat their pain, only 50 percent of them said that these methods were effective. About 1 in 10 of respondents took daily over-the-counter painkillers, while 2 in 10 relied on daily prescription painkillers. That means a sizable number of Americans are gobbling mounds of drugs each day but realizing little benefit.

If you frequently take over-the-counter or prescription medications for headaches, you may be at especially high risk of developing a difficult-to-treat and debilitating condition called chronic daily headache (CHD), which affects 3 to 5 percent of Americans, according to a 2004 review article published in the journal *Headache Currents*.

Healing Foods for Headaches

To help prevent or manage headaches, a number of food remedies can prove useful.

★★★**Spinach and other magnesium-rich foods** People who get migraines often have low levels of magnesium. In one study, researchers gave intravenous magnesium to magnesium-deficient patients in the midst of migraine attacks and found that 85 percent of them obtained relief within minutes. In another study, researchers randomly assigned migraine patients to take either 600 milligrams of magnesium a day or a placebo. After 12 weeks, the magnesium group had a dramatic 42 percent reduction in migraine symptoms compared with only a 15.8 percent reduction in the placebo group.

Good dietary sources of magnesium include spinach, fish, buckwheat, avocados, barley, quinoa, amaranth, almonds, Brazil nuts, sunflower seeds, pumpkin seeds, and oysters. Although nuts are good sources of magnesium, many anecdotal reports suggest that they are migraine trigger foods, so be wary of them.

You could easily get the daily value of 400 milligrams of magnesium by eating 1 cup of cooked spinach (which contains almost 40 percent of the recommended amount), a 3-ounce fillet of baked or broiled halibut (23 percent), and any dish made with 1 cup of buckwheat flour (a whopping 75 percent).

You may also want to try my Magnesium Medley of greens (see page 91), which is especially rich not only in magnesium but also in many anti-inflammatory compounds.

★★**Garlic** This "bodacious bulb," as I've sometimes heard it described, plays a key role in inhibiting the activity of platelets, the blood cells involved in triggering migraines. Naturopaths often suggest consuming more garlic to help thin the blood and possibly reduce the risk of heart attack. This thinning effect may also have benefits in terms of reducing the severity of headaches.

If you can handle the odor, I'd recommend eating one or two whole cloves of raw garlic each day. If you can't, you may prefer enteric-coated tablets or capsules with approximately 1.3 percent allicin, garlic's active ingredient. Most clinical trials with garlic involve taking 600 to 900 milligrams a day in two or three doses.

Probably the most troublesome headache-inducing foods are those rich in tyramine, a substance produced by the natural breakdown of the amino acid tyrosine. These foods include chocolate, beer and other alcoholic beverages, ripened cheeses, bananas, nuts, and beans. Other problematic foods contain high levels of nitrates, such as cured meats, hot dogs, and bologna.

Until recently, Chinese restaurant food often contained high levels of monosodium glutamate (MSG), which was used to enhance flavor but inadvertently also triggered migraines. Fortunately, many restaurants have now eliminated this ingredient. Still, if you're dining out on Chinese cuisine, ask if the menu item has been verified to be MSG free. If your server simply asks the chef about MSG content or looks at the recipe, it's not the same as verifying that the dish is MSG free.

You may also want to watch your carbohydrate intake. In a 2006 study, researchers from the Albert Einstein College of Medicine in New York City found that 50 percent of headache sufferers obtained as much relief from a low-carbohydrate diet as from a standard migraine medication. They suggested that the reason may be that people prone to headaches are more sensitive to allergens in carbohydrates, such as gluten and wheat protein.

If I were prone to migraines or other types of headaches, I'd keep a daily food diary so I could keep track of the foods that seemed to hurt--or help--my head.

★★**Ginger** Since ancient times, ginger has been used to treat a variety of ailments, including headaches. It helps prevent blood vessels in the brain from dilating, a process that often precedes headaches. It also helps inhibit the formation of prostaglandins, a group of complex fatty acids that cause inflammation, pain, and swelling.

Preliminary research from Denmark suggests that ginger can prevent a migraine as effectively as standard migraine drugs but without any of the adverse side effects. I'd follow the same regimen used by the Danish researchers at Odense University: ⅓ teaspoon of fresh or powdered ginger a day.

Add ginger to your diet whenever you can. Try drinking a few cups of ginger tea, grating fresh ginger into juice, noshing on Japanese pickled ginger, using fresh or powdered ginger when you cook, or nibbling on a piece or two of crystallized ginger.

You can make a tasty ginger tea by steeping three or four slices of fresh ginger in a cup of boiling water. Or add ½ teaspoon of powdered ginger or about 6 teaspoons of fresh ginger to your daily diet.

Ginger and the herb feverfew may work together to fight headaches even more effectively. Researchers from the Headache Care Center in Springfield, Missouri, recruited 30 people with a history of migraines to test a product, Gel-Stat, that contained both herbs. Participants took GelStat at the onset of a migraine, when symptoms were still mild. After 2 hours, the pain had disappeared in 48 percent of the participants, and the intensity had lessened in another 34 percent.

★★**Mint** Drink peppermint tea two or three times a day. Although many commercial mint teas are available, I'd recommend making your own by pouring 1 cup of boiling water over 1 heaping teaspoon (5 grams) of dried peppermint leaves and steeping them for 5 to 10 minutes; drink three to four cups daily.

★★**Walnuts** The regal nut of King Solomon's garden might help with a royal headache. I'm not a devout believer in "brain foods," but the kernels of walnuts—corrugated and folded like the brain—contain high levels of serotonin, one of the brain chemicals sometimes implicated in migraine. Further, walnut contains a dozen different pain-relieving compounds.

★**Turmeric** This yellow curry spice is a rich source of curcumin, a strong antioxidant that protects against free radical damage. Curcumin contains natural pain-relieving COX-2 inhibitors, which makes it an attractive, side effect–free alternative to prescription COX-2 inhibitors such as celecoxib (Celebrex). It also reduces inflammation by reducing histamine levels and possibly by stimulating the adrenal glands to produce more cortisone, the body's natural painkiller.

I prefer whole foods over supplements whenever possible because I believe you get more healing power from whole foods than from individual components, so I often add liberal amounts of curry to rice and other dishes and would consider adding other anti-inflammatory foods such as pineapple and papaya. You also can make tea with turmeric.

Unfortunately, it's difficult to get medicinal doses of curcumin from your diet alone. According to naturopaths, that dose is 250 to 500 milligrams of pure curcumin a day between meals, which translates into 5 to 25 teaspoons of dried turmeric a day. That's a good deal more than even a curry fan like me would want to add to my food. I'd recommend adding as much turmeric as possible to your diet to help prevent pain and taking turmeric supplements—standardized to 90 to 95 percent curcumin—to help relieve acute pain.

From the Herbal Medicine Chest

Feverfew and butterbur are the only two herbal headache remedies that have been evaluated by the gold standard of medical research: randomized, placebo-controlled, double-blind trials. Some studies have shown that feverfew—in dried leaf preparations but not alcohol extracts—can lessen the severity, duration, and frequency of migraines and may also reduce nausea and vomiting. Other studies have shown that butterbur can help reduce the frequency of migraine attacks but not shorten their duration.

Feverfew contains a compound called parthenolide, which reportedly prevents excessive clumping of blood cells known as platelets. More important, it prevents platelets from releasing the neurotransmitter serotonin, which appears to play a causative role in migraine.

If I were prone to migraines, I'd start eating one to four leaves a day of fresh feverfew or making a tea with two to eight fresh leaves steeped in boiled water for prevention. As is the case with many herbal remedies, you may need to take feverfew for 4 to 6 weeks before you notice any benefits.

Butterbur contains a compound called petasine, which helps relax blood vessels and smooth muscles such as those in the lungs and uterus. This compound also helps reduce inflammation—all of which shows why butterbur has proven more effective in treating migraine than placebos. If I were prone to migraines, I'd take one or two capsules three times a day of an extract of butterbur rhizome standardized to contain 7.5 milligrams of petasine per capsule. This type of extract does not contain components of butterbur—pyrrolizidine alkaloids—that can cause liver damage.

Heartburn

HEARTBURN HAS NOTHING TO DO WITH YOUR HEART. That burning sensation in your chest occurs when digestive acids back up into your esophagus because the muscle that separates it from the stomach, the lower esophageal sphincter (LES), relaxes and remains partially open.

Chronic heartburn is sometimes called nonulcer dyspepsia or gastroesophageal reflux disease (GERD), a condition that causes frequent or constant acid backflow.

Heartburn is very common, and it's more likely to develop when you eat too quickly, wolfing down your food without chewing it well—so in this case, an ounce of prevention, as they say, is worth a pound of cure. Don't eat on the run. Try to have meals and snacks when you're relaxed and can take the time to chew. Also, eat lots of fruits, vegetables, and whole grains instead of heartburn-producing foods such as like high-fat dishes, fried foods, chocolate, coffee, and alcohol.

Healing Foods for Heartburn

Along with avoiding foods and eating habits that aggravate heartburn, here are some food remedies that can help put out the fire.

★★**Bananas and plantains** These fruits are an old folk remedy for many gastrointestinal problems because they soothe the digestive tract. In particular, plantains—close cousins of the banana—contain an enzyme that stimulates mucus production in the lining of the stomach, helping to relieve upset and heartburn. Plantains that are green and a bit unripe are best because they contain leucocyanidin, an anti-ulcer flavonoid that can even protect the lining of the stomach from damage caused by aspirin. In addition, current research is under way at the University of Liverpool in England to confirm initial findings that the soluble fiber in plantains can soothe the painful inflammation of Crohn's disease and ulcerative colitis.

★★**Carob** Many Americans might become nauseated at the very thought of sitting down with John the Baptist for a meal of locusts and honey, but some scholars believe the "locusts" were in fact the carob, a Mediterranean relative of our honey "locust." Carob, which grows well in the Mediterranean climate of California, contains a honey-like substance that surrounds the seeds. Some naturopaths suggest consuming 20 grams of carob powder for GERD. That's about what doctors gave me daily in Panama when I contracted salmonella poisoning.

★★**Chamomile** Widely used as a digestive aid in Europe, chamomile is well suited to treating digestive ailments such as heartburn. This is because it has a unique combination of anti-inflammatory, antiseptic, antispasmodic, and stomach-soothing properties. If I had heartburn, I'd drink chamomile tea with licorice.

★★**Ginger** Ginger contains certain chemicals (gingerols and shogaols) that soothe the entire gastrointestinal tract, making it helpful for all kinds of digestive troubles. It relaxes the walls of the esophagus, aiding digestion and making

FOODS TO WATCH

Certain foods tend to bring on heartburn more than others. Here are a few to avoid.

Chocolate. Chocolate may contain compounds that relax the lower esophageal sphincter (LES), allowing stomach acid to bubble up and cause heartburn. Researchers at Bowman Gray School of Medicine at Wake Forest University in North Carolina found that when study participants ate chocolate, they experienced acid reflux for up to an hour afterward.

Coffee. Caffeine can make heartburn worse, so if you have it, avoid coffee and other caffeinated drinks.

High-fat foods. Studies show that foods high in fat, especially fried foods, can weaken the LES. Researchers at Bowman Gray found that for people who ate high-fat meals, the risk of acid reflux was four times higher than for people who ate less fat.

Onions. Scientists aren't exactly sure why, but it's been found that onions can bring on heartburn—and for some people, it took as little as one slice. Stephen Brunton, MD, director of family medicine at Long Beach Memorial Medical Center in California, says that there are three kinds of onions that don't cause heartburn—the Maui, Texas sweet, and Walla Walla varieties.

Salt. Researchers in Sweden suggest that adding salt to your food increases your risk of heartburn. The study found that people who regularly salted their food were 70 percent more likely to develop gastroesophageal reflux disease, a common cause of heartburn.

heartburn less likely. It also helps tighten the LES, which keeps stomach acid down and out.

Ginger has been used for centuries for its digestive healing powers. The ancient Greeks ate ginger wrapped in bread after large meals to prevent all kinds of digestive repercussions. Eventually, they added it to dough to give us gingerbread. In 16th-century Europe, ginger became such a popular digestive herb that it was put on every table right along with salt and pepper.

For instant relief of heartburn, make a cup of ginger tea by adding ½ teaspoon of ground or freshly grated ginger to 1 cup of hot water. For added protection, sip it 20 minutes before you eat. Pickled ginger is tastefully effective, too.

★★**Peppermint** Peppermint is an age-old indigestion remedy, and a good deal of research validates the folklore. Many traditional cultures—from the ancient Hebrews to the Pilgrims, who brought mint to the United States on the *Mayflower*—used peppermint for all sorts of digestive problems, including heartburn.

Some controversy surrounds this use of peppermint, however: A few herb advocates believe that it can actually aggravate heartburn. If this happens to you, then obviously, don't use the herb. But I doubt you'll have any trouble. My experience has been that most mints ease digestion and help prevent heartburn.

You can use peppermint along with other carminative herbs from the mint family, such as spearmint and lemon balm (also known as melissa), to make a soothing tea.

★**Cinnamon** Cinnamon is a carminative, an herb that soothes the digestive tract and minimizes gas. When Mrs. Duke experiences occasional heartburn or acid indigestion, you'll find her drinking cinnamon tea, sprinkling cinnamon on her toast, or both. She's also using cinnamon almost daily now to keep her blood sugar down.

★**Dill and fennel** During medieval times, the emperor Charlemagne provided dill on his banquet tables to calm the stomachs of guests who overindulged. Like cinnamon, dill is a carminative and has been used for thousands of years to treat heartburn and soothe the digestive tract. If I had heartburn, I'd try crushing a few teaspoons of dill seed and steeping them hot water for a tea.

A Biblical GERD-Guard Salad

Several plants mentioned in the Bible have folkloric reputations as being helpful for heartburn. These include almonds, chicory, dandelion, watercress, lettuce, mustard, olives, and walnuts. If I had frequent heartburn, I'd try making a salad with several of these anti-heartburn ingredients, and I might add a vinegar/garlic/olive oil/mustard/onion dressing. Lazier folk might just take a dash of bitters a half hour or so before eating. In either case, eat slowly and chew your food well. And follow your meal with ginger/peppermint tea.

Fennel is a similar herb that's been used for as long as dill, and you can use the seeds in the same way.

★**Papaya** This tropical fruit contains papain, an enzyme that soothes the stomach. Naturopaths believe that papaya juice is good for relieving indigestion and heartburn. If they're right, you should also get benefits from eating other fruits that contain proteolytics, such as kiwifruit and figs, after meals. If I had heartburn, I'd eat more of these fruits for dessert, and maybe follow up with my chamomile and licorice heartburn tea.

★**Pineapple** Pineapple is also loaded with digestive enzymes and proteolytics. It has been widely used to relieve heartburn and indigestion. In particular, pineapple contains glutamine, a compound that helps protect the lining of the stomach. Bite-size chunks of pineapple drizzled with a bit of honey as an appetizer or between courses just may help prevent heartburn.

From the Herbal Medicine Chest

If you're troubled by heartburn, you can give the following herbs a try.

Angelica (Angelica archangelica) and its relatives Angelica is a carminative and a relative of the carrot. Many members of this plant family seem to produce a soothing effect on the digestive tract. If you have heartburn, you might want to mix up a batch of my AngelAde, which contains six relatives of angelica. In a juicer, combine angelica stalks, carrots, celery, fennel, garlic, parsley, and parsnips. Feel free to add some water and spices to make it more drinkable. If you can't get fresh angelica, just use any of the other ingredients, all of which have heartburn-soothing benefits. Mix and match to create a juice you like.

Licorice (Glycyrrhiza glabra) Licorice contains several compounds that help protect the lining of the stomach and intestine. Deglycyrrhizinated licorice (DGL), a processed form of the herb, is your best choice for heartburn and indigestion and may reduce the risk of some unwanted side effects that licorice can sometimes cause.

The flavonoids in licorice are especially helpful in preventing ulcers. DGL has been shown to promote the release of certain compounds in saliva that may stimulate the healing of stomach and intestinal cells. If you have heartburn, add ½ teaspoon of DGL powder to your favorite herbal tea or use a bit of DGL by itself to make a sweet, pleasant-tasting infusion.

Heart Disease

IF WE COULD GET RID OF ALL MAJOR FORMS of cardiovascular disease, we could increase life expectancy in the United States by 7 years. Compare that to cancer: Getting rid of all forms of cancer would increase life expectancy by only 3 years. Yet despite our best medical efforts, cardiovascular disease, which includes atherosclerosis, heart attacks, congestive heart failure, and arrhythmias, still kills about 2,400 American every day. That's an average of one death every 37 seconds. It's responsible for as many deaths each year as all cancers, chronic lower respiratory diseases, accidents, and diabetes *combined!*

The good news is that we're doing much better at identifying the underlying causes of heart disease and trying to address them early through diet, lifestyle changes, and medication. Two factors I want to focus on here are inflammation and oxidative damage. Inflammation is like the unintended consequences that sometimes happen when you're trying to be a Good Samaritan. It occurs when elements of your immune system rush in to "fix" something gone awry or banish an invader. The very act of protecting you unleashes a chemical cascade that can inadvertently damage tissues.

You've seen inflammation if you've ever cut yourself. The cut healed, but only after becoming red and warm and perhaps swollen. Imagine that effect on your blood vessels. Not very pretty, is it?

When injuries occur to blood vessels, immune cells rush in to repair the damage, but they do so as part of an inflammatory process that actually damages blood vessels further, thickens blood, and contributes to the formation of blood clots. That's why many of the healing foods you'll read about here are intended to reduce inflammation.

One reason immune cells often feel compelled to rush to the walls of blood vessels is because that's where plaque builds up. This occurs when low-density lipoprotein (LDL) cholesterol becomes oxidized or damaged by molecules called free radicals, which are like the exhaust from your car—an unavoidable but dangerous by-product resulting from the creation of energy. Ideally, other compounds in your cells, called antioxidants, neutralize these free radicals before they can do much damage, just as the catalytic converter in your car is designed to prevent most of the gasoline combustion exhaust from reaching the air. If the LDL is oxidized, however, it becomes much easier for it to stick to and burrow into artery walls. This in turn attracts immune cells, leading to inflammation, which increases the buildup of gunk on artery walls, raises the risk of blood clots, and spurs more free radicals.

It's all a nasty, circular process. Your goal is to short-circuit that process through a diet filled with foods and herbs that reduce inflammation and oxidation and provide other benefits that support heart health.

Healing Foods for Heart Disease

★★★**Beans** Some nutrient-rich breads contain not only whole grains but beans as well. I've preached for decades that replacing 90 percent of the red meat in your diet with a wide variety of beans—and the darker the color, the better—could reduce your risk of dying from cancer as well as of developing cataracts, heart failure, and diabetes. How? Beans are high in folate, a B vitamin that works to reduce levels of homocysteine, an inflammatory risk factor for heart disease, by converting it back to methionine, which doesn't damage arteries. While naturopaths suggest taking 5 milligrams of folic acid (the synthetic form of folate) a day under medical supervision, the Daily Value is 400 micrograms. It's easy to get this much because so many of our foods these days, including cereal, bread, and grains, are enriched with folic acid. I focus on beans not only because of their high folate content (180 micrograms in ½ cup of black-eyed peas or lentils, 140 micrograms in ½ cup of chickpeas, and 136 micrograms in ½ cup of lima beans) but also because they're such good sources of fiber. Fiber helps to reduce blood levels of cholesterol and contributes to maintaining a healthful weight, each of which is important when it comes to reducing your risk of heart disease or managing an existing heart condition.

★★★**Olive oil** I keep a bottle of olive oil on my kitchen counter, in plain view and within easy reach, because I use it so much. I use it to make scrambled eggs, to dip bread into, to whip up a quick salad dressing, and to sauté chicken breasts. My garden crew and I daily douse our bread with a mixture of olive oil, vinegar, diced garlic, and hot pepper. In fact, it's about the only oil or fat I use in cooking. Why? Because olive oil is to heart disease what a sudden downpour is to a forest fire. It soothes inflammation, reduces oxidation, and lowers cholesterol levels.

Olive oil forms the basis for the so-called Mediterranean diet, which is high in vegetables, whole grains, legumes, and fruits and which studies find can substantially reduce the risk of heart disease. This way of eating uses olive oil, a monounsaturated fat, as a more healthful alternative to cholesterol-raising saturated fats like butter. Consuming monounsaturated fat doesn't increase cholesterol levels. In fact, replacing saturated fat with olive oil can reduce total cholesterol half as much as saturated fat raises it!

Recent studies find that olive oil's ability to reduce LDL oxidation may play an even greater role in keeping your circulatory system in good shape. In a major Spanish study involving 372 people at high risk for cardiovascular disease, one-third ate a low-fat diet, while the others followed a traditional Mediterranean diet with either virgin olive oil or nuts as the primary source of fat (nuts, like olive oil, are high in healthful monounsaturated fat). After 3 months, LDL oxidation levels dropped significantly in those on the Mediterranean diets with olive oil and nuts but not in those on the low-fat diet.

Olive oil also reduces inflammation in several ways. For one, the fatty acids in olive oil are less likely to be oxidized by free radicals. For another, compounds in olive oil have their own antioxidant effects.

I could go on and on, but this isn't supposed to be a chapter about olive oil. Suffice it to say that the benefits of this monounsaturated fat are so significant that the FDA allows olive oil manufacturers to put a label on their bottles noting the benefits of the oil in reducing cardiovascular disease risk.

★★★**Onions and garlic** Important elements of the Mediterranean diet, onions and garlic are used to prevent and/or treat coronary heart disease, obesity, high cholesterol, and hypertension, among other conditions. These activities are partially related to pungent volatile sulfur compounds called thiosulfinates. While eating these bulbs raw is super for the heart, cooked onions and garlic can also add these cardioprotective compounds to your arsenal. If you're after the quercetin glycosides in onions (the outer husk is perhaps the best source), it's better absorbed with oils (fish oil, soy oil, tallow, and, best of all, lecithin)—all the more reason to add garlic and onions to your olive oil salad dressing.

★★★**Pomegranate** With a long folk history as being heart-friendly, pomegranate recently was proven cardioprotective in clinical trials in Israel. It lowered blood pressure, helped prevent atherosclerosis, and demonstrated properties similar to pharmaceutical ACE inhibitors. (ACE is short for angiotensin-converting enzyme.)

★★★**Sardines** Sardines are a great source of coenzyme Q10, or CoQ10. This vitamin-like substance exists in every cell of your body but is particularly important in heart cells. It not only helps cells produce energy but also provides important antioxidant protection against free radical damage. If you take drugs called statins to reduce your cholesterol levels, you may be inadvertently reducing your CoQ10 levels.

Studies examining the use of CoQ10 in heart disease primarily focus on its benefits for congestive heart failure, in which the heart weakens and can't pump blood very well. But studies have found low levels of CoQ10 in people with all forms of heart disease, not just congestive heart failure. For instance, one study of patients who underwent cardiac surgery found that three-fourths had CoQ10 deficiencies in their cardiac tissue. Studies have also found that supplementing with CoQ10 reduces cholesterol oxidation.

FOODS TO WATCH

Fatty red meat, butter, and whole-fat dairy products all contain high amounts of saturated fat. You know something has saturated fat if the fat is solid at room temperature (just think about what happens to the fat left in the pan after sautéing ground meat). This fat stimulates the production of LDL cholesterol, which underlies atherosclerosis. Study after study after study has found that reducing the amount of saturated fat in your diet can protect you against heart disease.

Other food sources of CoQ10 include organ meats like kidneys, liver, and sweetbreads as well as beef, soy oil, mackerel, and peanuts. If you're going to eat beef, I recommend that it come from grass-fed, free-range cattle. Grass-fed beef contains less fat and more healthful nutrients than beef from cattle fed with cereal grains.

Sardines and other fish are also a good source of L-carnitine, another essential nutrient required to help cells make energy. L-carnitine has been evaluated in people with a variety of cardiovascular problems, including angina (chest pain caused when blood can't get through blocked arteries), erratic heart rhythms, peripheral vascular disease (a kind of angina in the legs, also called intermittent claudication), congestive heart failure, and heart attacks. In a study of 81 people who had had recent heart attacks, those who received 4 grams of L-carnitine a day for 4 months afterward had a 12-fold improvement in survival compared with those who received a placebo. The supplement improved participants' heart rate, blood pressure, angina, and cholesterol levels.

★★★**Walnuts** Clinically proven to be cardioprotective, walnuts have much more than omega-3's and COX-2 inhibitors going for them. They also offer a collection of ACE-inhibiting, blood-thinning, and diuretic compounds. A handful a day should help keep the cardiologist away.

★★★**Wine** A persuasive body of evidence suggests that one 5-ounce glass of wine a day for women and two glasses for men may keep the cardiologist away. And while I'm not suggesting you start drinking if you're a teetotaler, the fact is that studies find you're more likely to die from heart disease if you don't drink at all than if you drink moderately. In addition, more than 30 long-term studies suggest that moderate drinking reduces heart attack risk by 25 to 40 percent, while Finnish researchers found that men who imbibed up to 12 drinks a week (still a moderate amount) had only half the risk of clot-related strokes compared with those who didn't drink. Once you go past the moderate level, however, the risk of death due to alcohol-related causes starts increasing.

By the way, you won't get as great a health effect from beer or liquor. Studies suggest that some compound in red wine greatly improves the heart benefit you may get from alcohol. When it comes to heart disease, wine's benefits probably stem from high levels of flavanols and bioflavonoids found in grapes and grape skins. These plant-based chemicals have numerous heart-healthy effects. For instance, they increase nitric oxide production in artery cells, which helps blood vessels dilate. The chemicals also block production of other chemicals that can lead to the buildup of plaque on artery walls. Flavonoids in red wine appear to be even more effective than vitamin E for preventing LDL cholesterol oxidation, and they also work effectively at preventing blood clots.

★★**Almonds** I think vitamin E is an important antioxidant, particularly when it comes to preventing heart disease. But recent large clinical trials found that supplementing with large doses of E actually *increased* the risk of heart disease over time. I firmly believe the reason we keep finding negative results in trials of antioxidant supplements is that these compounds were not meant to be pulled out of food and taken singly but instead to work in synergy with other nutrients, so I don't recommend swallowing lots of vitamin E pills. Instead I recommend a handful of almonds a day. Almonds provide a whopping 7.4 milligrams of vitamin E per 1-ounce serving. And while supplementing with vitamin E isn't great for reducing heart disease, a study of 5,133 Finnish men and women ages 30 to 69 found that the richer their diets were in vitamin E, the lower their risk of death from heart disease. Try almonds as a midmorning or pre-dinner snack or toast them and add to salads and pasta.

★★**Dark green leafy vegetables** I'm talking about spinach, kale, mustard, and turnip greens. They're chock-full of magnesium, a mineral that relaxes the heart muscle and improves heart function. I'd aim for at least one serving (about ½ cup) a day; two, of course, is better! Consider making spinach salads, tossing a handful of greens into a soup, and using these greens instead of lettuce on sandwiches.

★★**Rosemary** I just love this herb. It's so easy to grow in your garden, and it winters beautifully in many warmer parts of the country. Its fragrance enhances nearly any poultry, game, or fish, so getting it into your daily diet shouldn't be too difficult. And believe me, you want to start adding it to soups, stews, and potato dishes or sprinkling it on vegetables. Rosemary is a rich source of antioxidants. In days of yore, it was used to preserve meat, preventing the fat from turning rancid. That rancidness occurs through the same oxidative process that leads to atherosclerosis, so if rosemary can prevent oxidation in meat, imagine what it could do for your heart!

★★**Tea** I'm not talking about fancy herbal teas here, although there are several that could be recommended for heart disease. I'm just talking about plain old teabags— black or green. Tea contains compounds called polyphenols and flavonoids, which work to reduce oxidative damage from free radicals. Flavonoids also improve the ability of blood vessels to dilate and contract and may have some anti-clotting benefits. A Dutch study of nearly 5,000 people found that those who drank a cup and a half a day had about half the risk of heart attack compared with people who drank none. If the tea drinkers *did* have a heart attack, they were only one-third as likely to die from it as non–tea drinkers.

Meanwhile, a study of 1,900 people who had already had heart attacks found that heavy tea drinkers (14 or more cups a week) were 44 percent less likely to die in the 3½ years following their attacks than non–tea drinkers.

If this convinces you to take up tea drinking, I urge you to dunk the teabag in the water several times. When researchers compared dunking teabags to soaking them, they found dunking for 3 minutes released up to five times more polyphenols than simply letting the bag sit in the hot water.

★★**Tomatoes** I'm used to thinking of tomatoes as beneficial for preventing prostate cancer thanks to an antioxidant called lycopene (though recent research has cast doubt on this benefit). But it turns out that lycopene also works pretty well to prevent heart disease. When researchers for the Harvard Women's Health Study tested lycopene levels in the blood of 485 women who developed heart disease and 485 who didn't, they found that those with the highest levels were about one-third less likely to develop heart disease than were those with the lowest levels. The protection extends to us men, too. In fact, men with the lowest amounts of lycopene in their diets had more than triple the risk of a heart attack or stroke compared with men who ate higher amounts. Another reason to reach for tomatoes? They contain a compound called gamma-amino butyric acid (GABA), which can help lower blood pressure and strengthen the heart muscle. Other good sources of lycopene include guavas, pink grapefruit, and watermelon, all available at your supermarket. And I recommend you try them all since each has its own special group of nutrients.

★★**Wheat germ** I suggest adding a tablespoon or so of wheat germ to your morning cereal, yogurt, and salads, and even sprinkle it over ice cream. Wheat germ is rich in vitamins, minerals, and other nutrients required for a healthy heart. One of these is the amino acid L-arginine, which helps reduce inflammation and improve blood vessel function. Even more important is the fact that your body uses it to create nitric oxide, an enzyme that helps blood vessels dilate, inhibits blood clotting, improves production of smooth muscle in blood vessels, reduces oxidation, and prevents white blood cells from sticking to and burrowing into blood vessels. In one review, 12 of 16 studies of people supplementing with L-arginine showed positive cardiovascular benefits. I'd like to have a head-on analytic comparison of wheat germ oil and palm germ oil. The latter has more carotenoids and tocotrienols, I'll wager, but I recommend both.

★**Purslane** A high-risk situation for heart attack develops when blood thickens and becomes more susceptible to clotting. Numerous natural remedies and foods can reduce the risk of blood clots, including omega-3 fatty acids. You know fatty fish as a great source of omega-3's, but few people know that purslane, a delicious vegetable that can be found in many supermarkets and farmer's markets, is the best vegetable source of green omega-3 fatty acid. In this plant, the fat exists primarily as alpha-linolenic acid. As mentioned often in this book, other good sources include certain seeds and/or their oils, such as chia, chiso, flax, Inca peanut, and walnut.

Purslane is easy to grow; it's even considered a weed in many places. It's also high in vitamin C and glutathione, both great antioxidants that can help stem heart disease. Want another reason to add purslane to your garden? It's also a great source of calcium and magnesium, which together in a 1:1 ratio can significantly reduce heart attack risk.

Hemorrhoids

IN MEDIEVAL TIMES, HEMORRHOIDS WERE KNOWN AS "St. Fiacre's curse." The story goes that St. Fiacre, the patron saint of gardeners, was given the chance to farm all the land he could farm in one day and was handed a very small shovel by a merciless bishop to do it. After many, many hours of intense spading, St. Fiacre developed a terrible case of hemorrhoids. Seeking relief, he sat on a stone and prayed for a cure, which miraculously occurred, and according to legend, the imprint of St. Fiacre's hemorrhoids remains on the stone today. Folklore has it that hemorrhoid sufferers from around the world still sit on the stone in hopes of relief.

It's estimated that some 75 million Americans have St. Fiacre's curse, with about half of all adults experiencing its typical pain, itching, and bleeding by age 50. Hemorrhoids are actually varicose veins that form inside your rectum or around the opening of your anus. They're caused by increased pressure on the veins from sitting, being constipated, or straining too hard to "go." Hemorrhoids can rupture and bleed when they're irritated, most often by dry, hard stools.

The best way to deal with hemorrhoids is to prevent them, and the best way to do that is to prevent constipation—which is all about eating right.

Healing Foods for Hemorrhoids

The great thing about healing foods for hemorrhoids is that there's a lot of overlap. You'll notice that many of them serve more than one purpose, with some foods giving a hemorrhoid sufferer plenty of collateral reasons to eat them.

Go High-Fiber

When it comes to preventing hemorrhoids, fiber is king because it's the secret to avoiding constipation, the number one cause of hemorrhoids.

Unlike vitamins and minerals, fiber isn't absorbed during digestion. It stays in your intestine and absorbs large amounts of fluid. When fiber absorbs water, your stools get bigger, wetter, and heavier—better for moving down and out more quickly and easily. Fiber also softens your stools, requiring less of the pushing and straining that causes hemorrhoids. A high-fiber diet can help ward off a host of other digestive disorders, too, including diarrhea, irritable bowel syndrome, diverticulitis, and maybe even colon cancer.

If you need to add more fiber to your diet, do so gradually. Eating lots of fiber-rich foods when your body isn't used to it can bring on cramping and gas. Start slowly by eating more fiber over the course of several weeks or months.

Here are some top high-fiber picks:

★★★**Apples** Apples are an excellent choice because they contain both kinds of fiber—soluble fiber to keep your stools soft and easy to pass, and insoluble fiber to give your intestines a slippery, gel-like coating. Most of the fiber in apples is in the skin, so eat your apples unpeeled. If you're constipated, try eating three or four small apples a day to clear things up.

★★★**Beans** Beans are another super-fiber food. They're also high in both soluble and insoluble fiber, which makes them great ammo against constipation and hemorrhoids. Black beans, for example, have 6 grams of fiber per serving. Chickpeas, kidney beans, and lima beans contain about 7 grams of fiber, with black-eyed peas beating them all at 8 grams of fiber in a ½ cup serving. Beans can be incorporated into your diet many different ways, making them extremely versatile. Add them to soups, salads, casseroles, and dips.

However, beans are well-known gas producers, so try this trick: Flavor your beans with fresh or ground ginger (yet another natural laxative and hemorrhoid-helper), which reduces the gas beans can create. In fact, any herb that soothes your digestive tract (carminative) can help, including allspice, basil, caraway, cinnamon, cloves, coriander, dill, fennel, garlic, nutmeg, onion, oregano, rosemary, sage, tarragon, and thyme—to name just a few.

★★★**Berries** Berries are tiny powerhouses in the fight against constipation and hemorrhoids. Packed with fiber, berries help your stools absorb lots of water so they can travel faster and easier. Elderberries top the list for fiber, packing a powerful 5 grams in a half-cup serving. Raspberries are next, which have 4 grams per serving, with blackberries coming in third with more than 3 grams. Blueberries and strawberries are good, too. When it comes to berry juice, mulberries and boysenberries make for gentle laxatives.

★★★**Flaxseed** Also known as linseed, flaxseed is very high in fiber and rich in omega-3 fatty acids (a "good" kind of fat that helps keep your bowels moving), both of which are helpful for constipation and hemorrhoids. Three tablespoons of flaxseed has about 3 grams of fiber. Flaxseed has a sweet, nutty taste and can be added to almost anything. It's great in salads, cereals, casseroles, and breads.

However, whole flaxseed provides little benefit because your digestive tract is unable to crack open the hard shell that surrounds the seed (which is where all the benefits are). Go for ground or crushed flaxseed because it's easier to digest. Ground flaxseed has a pleasing flavor and crunch.

Also, don't fall for common claims that flaxseed oil is just as good for you. While flaxseed oil has some nutritional benefits, it doesn't retain the fiber and omega-3's needed to help with constipation and hemorrhoids.

★★★**Prunes** Prunes are the oldest and most effective food remedy for constipation, and therefore a top choice for preventing hemorrhoids. Prunes contain three ingredients to help keep you regular. First, they're very high in fiber, with 3 grams in just three prunes. Second, they contain a compound called dihydroxyphenyl isatin, which stimulates the contractions in your intestines that give you regular bowel movements. Third, prunes contain a natural sugar called sorbitol, which, like fiber, soaks up large amounts of water in your digestive tract to help things move on through without trouble.

Most fruits are less than 1 percent sorbitol. Prunes, however, are about 15 percent, which is why they're such a potent natural remedy for constipation and hemorrhoids. Prunes are a sweeter option than laxatives from the drugstore.

Like prunes, other dried fruits—such as raisins and figs—are wonders at relieving constipation and preventing hemorrhoids, too. Raisins contain a compound called tartaric acid, which acts as a natural laxative. Figs are also an excellent source of fiber, providing about 5 grams of fiber in just three dried or fresh figs.

★★**Dark leafy greens** A salad tossed with various dark leafy greens is a good choice to combat constipation and hemorrhoids. Throw in a few handfuls of apple slices, raisins, blackberries, red cabbage, and toasted flaxseed, and you have the makings of a digestive dream. Dark leafy greens are also a great source of omega-3's.

FOODS TO WATCH

Certain foods can worsen constipation and aggravate hemorrhoids. Try to avoid these:

Alcohol. Don't drink alcohol while hemorrhoids are flaring. Alcohol is a diuretic, which means it causes your body to lose water. You need more, not less, water when you have hemorrhoids.

Coffee. Although the caffeine in coffee signals your large intestine to contract and keep your bowels awake and working, drinking too much coffee removes more fluids from your body than it puts in. When used addictively, caffeine prevents your bowels from maintaining their natural rhythm. If you drink coffee, try to limit yourself to fewer than five cups a day to avoid constipation and hemorrhoids.

Dairy foods. Foods such as cheese, milk, and ice cream have little or no fiber and contain an insoluble protein called casein, which slows digestion and worsens constipation. Steer clear of the dairy case if you have hemorrhoids.

Separated oils. If I had hemorrhoids, I'd try not to eat oils that have been removed from their sources, such as corn, olive, and soy oil. (For example, flaxseed is an excellent source of fiber, but flaxseed oil has almost none.) These oils actually form a film in your stomach that makes it difficult to digest certain foods, and this can back you up—and set you up for hemorrhoids. Go for oils from actual food sources, like those you get from eating avocados, olives, nuts, and fish.

Spicy foods. Hot, spicy foods can cause the tender nerves around hemorrhoids to burn when you "go." Pass on foods such as hot peppers, and opt for blander items until after the flare.

Tea. Tea is rich in tannins, which bind stools and hold back bowel movements. If you have hemorrhoids, avoid drinking tea.

Berry Power

Besides being high in hemorrhoid-fighting fiber and flavonoids, dark-colored berries such as blueberries and blackberries, as well as cherries, contain anthocyanins, pigments that tone and strengthen the walls of hemorrhoidal veins, which can reduce pain and swelling. According to John Neustadt, ND, medical director of Montana Integrative Medicine in Bozeman, when the walls of the capillaries and veins in the anus are strengthened, they're less likely to stretch under pressure and lead to hemorrhoids. You can get the benefits of anthocyanins from eating whole berries, but they're more concentrated in berry juice.

Good greens to choose include kale, Swiss chard, endive, dandelion greens, beet greens, turnip greens, chicory, and spinach. When it comes to color, dark greens offer the biggest benefit.

Dandelion, in particular, has long been considered an effective natural laxative. More than just a backyard weed, dandelion increases bile flow into your large intestine, which helps prevent constipation. Dandelion greens can be found in popular "spring mix" salad combinations in many restaurants and produce sections. And you'll probably find it flowering near your supermarket, if not in it.

★★**Pineapple** High in soluble fiber, pineapple is a tasty way to promote healthy bowels and avoid hemorrhoids. Pineapple also has lots of bromelain, a natural anti-inflammatory that helps reduce the swelling and inflammation of the varicose veins that make up hemorrhoids.

★★**Rhubarb** Eating the stalks of rhubarb has long been used in folk medicine to relieve constipation. Rhubarb is a member of the buckwheat family, which makes it a good source of fiber. A ½ cup of rhubarb stalks contains large amounts of insoluble fiber. However, you should eat only rhubarb stalks. Rhubarb leaves contain very high levels of toxins, called oxalates, that can cause stomach irritation and kidney problems.

★★**Whole grains** Foods made with whole grains—grains that haven't had their bran and germ removed by milling—are great sources of fiber. Some of the best include barley, buckwheat, bulgur, cracked wheat, millet, oat, and rye.

Oats, for example, are high in both soluble and insoluble fiber. Bulgur, which is wheat in its whole form, is one of the most healthful foods you can eat. Besides being extremely high in fiber, studies show that bulgur might also help prevent colon and breast cancer as well as heart disease and diabetes.

Many food companies are making whole-wheat versions of bread, cereal, pasta, crackers, tortillas, and even cookies. And for those of you who prefer white bread, you're in luck. Many bakeries now offer whole-grain versions of white bread, which traditionally contains very little fiber. Look for the word "whole" on food packages, which should be listed in one of the first three ingredients.

By the way, don't forget that water goes hand-in-hand with fiber. Aim for eight full glasses a day to keep things moving through easily. If you don't like drinking that much water, substitute soups and juices—or eat lots of watermelon and cucumbers, which are nearly 100 percent water by weight.

★★The Flavonoid Family

To take the benefits of vitamin C one step further, flavonoids are powerful antioxidants that enhance vitamin C's ability to protect and improve blood vessel function. Without getting too technical, the most beneficial flavonoids for hemorrhoids include diosmin, hesperidin, naringin, rutin, and quercetin, which can be found in these flavonoid-rich foods (among many others):

Apples	Citrus fruits	Grapes
Beans	(grapefruit,	Green beans
Berries	lemons, limes,	Green tea
Black tea	oranges,	Kale
Broccoli	tangerines)	Onions
Buckwheat	Cherries	Red pepper
Celery	Cranberries	Tomatoes

★★Think Zinc

Zinc is an infection-fighting mineral that's important for the healing process and can help reduce irritation while hemorrhoid tissue mends. Foods high in zinc include:

Avocados	Bulgur	Shellfish
Beans	Lentils	Wheat germ
Buckwheat	Oysters	

★★Vital Vitamin C

Vitamin C can help reduce swollen varicose veins and protect against free radicals (molecules that contribute to aging and the onset of many diseases) that can weaken blood vessels. If you have hemorrhoids, here's just a few of the many foods rich in vitamin C to try:

Artichokes
Asparagus
Berries
Broccoli
Brussels sprouts
Cabbage

Cranberries
Citrus fruits
  (grapefruit,
  lemons, limes,
  oranges,
  tangerines)
Kiwifruit

Pineapple
Peppers
Rhubarb
Strawberries
Sweet potatoes
Tomatoes

Other Hemorrhoid Helpers

Because preventing constipation means avoiding hemorrhoids, here are a couple other food remedies to try as natural laxatives:

★★**Chamomile** Externally applied, chamomile can be used as a liniment for bruises, hemorrhoids, inflammation, and sores. It contains dozens of helpful compounds, many of which may be synergic. Apply a spent or moist chamomile tea bag to external hemorrhoids to help soothe irritation.

★★**Ginger** Long known for its many healing properties, ginger is a great way to deal with constipation and ward off hemorrhoids. Ginger contains certain chemicals that stimulate your digestive system by increasing the wavelike muscle contractions (peristalsis) that move food through your intestines.

There are many ways to get the health benefits of ginger, which comes in a variety of different forms, including fresh, dried, crystallized, candied, pickled, and powdered. However, fresh ginger is best. Pickled ginger, often found in Asian restaurants and served alongside sushi, is thought to be as beneficial as fresh ginger. Candied ginger can be sweet to nibble on and handy for baking. Seasoning meats and vegetable stir-fry with fresh ginger is a good option, too.

Tea, Topically Speaking

Although you shouldn't drink tea if you have hemorrhoids, try it topically instead. The tannins in tea have been found to ease the pain of hemorrhoids, third-degree burns, and open wounds. Moisten a tea bag of conventional tea (without any fancy herbs or spices added) with cold water and tuck it into place as a compress whenever you feel the need for a little soothing.

And then there's ginger ale. Although most varieties aren't made with real ginger and often contain unhealthy additives, soda made with real ginger is available and makes for a refreshing option. One brand, Reed's Ginger Brew, is made with real ginger (up to 25 grams of fresh ginger in one variety) and other natural ingredients—such as apple, raspberry, pineapple, and honey—which are also constipation and hemorrhoid fighters.

Much of the ginger available in the United States comes from Jamaica, but the varieties grown in Africa and India are more potent. You can't see the difference, so ask the produce manager at your local supermarket or health food store where the ginger was grown. When buying fresh ginger, look for firm roots that have smooth skin with a spicy smell.

★★**Honey** Honey contains large amounts of fructose, a sugar that can act as a natural laxative by helping draw water into your bowels and soften your stools. Honey is higher in fructose than almost any other foods. If I had hard stools and problems with hemorrhoids, I'd substitute honey in place of regular sugar or artificial sweeteners. Drizzle honey over fresh berries to get double the benefits.

From the Herbal Medicine Chest

Therapeutic herbs can also go a long way toward bringing the discomfort of hemorrhoids under control. Here are a few to try.

Aloe (Aloe vera) Aloe juice is a natural laxative. Ayurvedic doctors suggest drinking a ½ cup three times a day until hemorrhoid flare-ups have cleared. You can buy aloe juice at most health foods stores. Don't try to prepare your own because the inner part of the aloe leaf itself is an extremely powerful laxative and, when juiced, could cause serious gastro-intestinal problems.

Butcher's broom (Ruscus aculeatus) This woody herb has a long history as a treatment for venous problems, such as hemorrhoids and varicose veins. Butcher's broom contains chemicals called ruscogenins, which have anti-inflammatory and vasoconstricting properties. I'd try 5 rounded teaspoons of powdered root in a cup of boiling water and sweeten it with honey.

Psyllium (Plantago ovata) Psyllium seeds are high in fiber and constitute the main ingredient in many over-the-counter laxatives. They contain mucilage, a fiber that adds bulk to your stools, which makes them softer and easier to pass. Psyllium needs lots of water to work, so be sure to drink plenty if you decide to try it. Because of its allantoin content, you can apply the leaves of the psyllium plant topically. If you have allergies or asthma, don't ingest this herb. Some people have had allergic reactions to psyllium, including serious asthma attacks from inhaled psyllium seed dust. This warning does not apply to the leaves.

Rooibos (pronounced *roh'-ih-bus*) (*Aspalathus linearis*) This herb is rich in flavonoids (antioxidants that give plants their color) and can help with hemorrhoids. You can find a variety of rooibos teas in health food stores. They are caffeine-free and have less than half the tannins of regular tea, so they're less likely to cause the constipation problems that regular coffee and tea can.

High Blood Pressure

A FEW YEARS AGO, 50 MILLION PEOPLE went to sleep one night certain that one thing they *didn't* have to worry about was their blood pressure, only to wake the next day and learn they were wrong. That's because the Joint National Committee on Prevention, Detection, Evaluation, and Treatment of High Blood Pressure had identified a condition called prehypertension, defined as a systolic blood pressure reading (the top number) of 120 to 139 or a diastolic reading (the bottom number) of 80 to 90. One result? More people now visit doctors for hypertension (the fancy word for high blood pressure) than for any other condition except the common cold.

I'm one of those people. Yes, I have high blood pressure. And I can tell you that although it is often described as a "silent" disease with no symptoms, I nearly always know when my pressure rises. It's that uptight feeling I get when I'm filling out bureaucratic forms or wrestling with typos in preparing a book manuscript. But I avoid pharmacologic management of my blood pressure, always preferring to take the natural rather than the chemical route. For instance, when I feel that my pressure is up, I can bring it down with 15 to 20 meditative deep breaths. There are also numerous foods that can do the same thing.

Healing Foods for High Blood Pressure

★★★**Celery** I'm puzzled by the fact that after more than 30 years of prescribing beta-blockers for high blood pressure, the medical establishment has produced no study showing that using them alone reduces the complications of high blood pressure or of cardiovascular deaths when compared to a placebo. In all the studies showing their effectiveness, beta-blockers were combined with a diuretic, a drug that helps you get rid of excess fluid—so I suggest you munch on some celery instead.

Celery and its seeds have long been used for their diuretic properties. Laboratory studies also find that the active ingredient in celery can relax the smooth muscles that line blood vessels, enabling the vessels to open wider for blood flow. In one key study on this vegetable, researchers found that the equivalent of about four stalks of celery a day lowered blood pressure by 2 to 14 percent in rats and about 7 percent in humans.

Not into eating the stringy veggie? Try making a celery tea. Just pour 1 cup of boiling water over a teaspoon of celery seeds. I'd also heartily recommend that you puree four sticks of celery with two cloves of garlic, half an onion, and half a tomato for a daily anti-hypertensive drink.

★★★**Garlic** You can buy garlic capsules in health food stores, but the best way to use this aromatic herb is in its natural form. Slice it, mash it, mince it—then walk away for 10 minutes to let its powerful chemical allicin form. Allicin is a potent antioxidant that animal studies find can reduce blood pressure in rats as effectively as the ACE inhibitor enalapril (Vasotec) does. It can make blood vessels more elastic so they can dilate more easily.

Garlic also contains other components helpful in lowering blood pressure, such as potassium, vitamin C, calcium, and magnesium. Human studies evaluating garlic's benefits for blood pressure, whether using aged garlic extract, garlic powder, or fresh garlic, found average reductions in systolic blood pressure of 7.7 mmHg and in diastolic pressure of 5 mmHg. You don't need much; just one to two cloves of raw garlic a day should do it.

Low Blood Pressure Soup

Too often, we think we can take a pill to get the same benefits we would from a healthful diet. What we don't understand is that the various nutrients and chemicals in foods often work in synergy with each other to produce specific benefits. That's where my Low Blood Pressure Soup comes in. You've seen my top-ranking food for high blood pressure, celery; some others are broccoli, carrots, garlic, onions, saffron, and tomatoes. But why eat them separately when you can use them all to make a wonderful soup? Not only are the various ingredients known for their blood pressure–reducing effects, but the way you eat soup—sipping it slowly as it cools—is very calming and should help further lower your blood pressure. And don't forget to add seasoning. Obviously, you shouldn't use salt if you have high blood pressure, but pepper, basil, and tarragon contain six anti-hypertensive compounds each, while oregano has seven, and all can do a great job of spicing up the soup.

★★★**Green tea** Despite its caffeine, tea has more ACE-inhibiting compounds than most of the other herbs mentioned in this chapter, plus at least 10 beta-blockers, 7 calcium channel blockers, and 16 diuretics. So instead of an agitating coffee break, I recommend taking a reflective green tea break. That plus some deep breathing can lower my blood pressure significantly.

★★★**Fish** When it comes to heart health, you probably know fish best for its high levels of omega-3 fatty acids. But fish also contains high levels of the antioxidant coenzyme Q10, or CoQ10. This nutrient helps cells create energy. While it's available in all cells, the greatest supply resides in heart cells. Supplementing with it can make a big difference in blood pressure, which is what makes me think that getting enough of it through your diet may also help. In one study of 109 patients with serious high blood pressure (serious enough that they had been taking medication for at least a year), half were able to completely stop taking one to three antihypertensive medications an average of 4 months after they started on CoQ10 supplements.

★★★**Onions** Like its tough cousin garlic, onion has many attributes that prove useful in managing high blood pressure. For one, it's a great source of quercetin, found mostly in the husk. This powerful antioxidant flavonol is linked to a reduced risk of heart disease and stroke. When people with hypertension took 730 milligrams of quercetin a day for 28 days, their blood pressure dropped between 2 and 7 points systolic and 2 and 5 points diastolic compared with no change with a placebo. Other studies find just 2 or 3 tablespoons a day of onion essential oil can drop blood pressure by an average of 25 points systolic and 15 points diastolic. That would, however, translate to a lot of onions—more than anyone who has to be around other people would want to eat in a single day. I'm sure you can still get good benefits from just an onion or two a day, particularly if you can eat it raw or lightly cooked. (Onions that are barely cooked seem to reduce blood pressure much more than fully cooked onions.)

FOODS TO WATCH

Canned and processed foods are full of sodium; even breakfast cereal has added salt. And as you probably know, a diet high in sodium is a no-no for hypertension. High-salt diets draw water into your bloodstream, increasing the volume of blood and thus increasing blood pressure. That's how diuretics work: by pulling the water *out* of the bloodstream. Avoid the drugs. Instead, eat fresh, natural foods, and you'll cut your sodium intake significantly and painlessly.

★★**Banana** An average-sized banana contains more than 400 milligrams of potassium and only 1 milligram of sodium. Potassium is one of the most important electrolytes in the body, helping to regulate heart function and fluid balance, a key factor in controlling blood pressure. Potassium-rich foods like bananas are known to lower blood pressure and protect against heart disease and stroke.

★★**Chamomile** I view this floral food as the herbal answer to the beta-blocker atenolol (Tenormin), which slows your heartbeat and relaxes blood vessels. Chamomile is the best food source of apigenin, a powerful antioxidant that studies find works really well to relax blood vessels and reduce blood pressure. Sip a cup of chamomile tea when you feel your stress or anxiety levels rising.

★★**Spinach and other bitter greens** These foods, which include beetroot greens and the biblical "bitter weeds," a.k.a. chicory, dandelion, endive, fenugreek, horseradish, lettuce, and nettle, spur the production of nitric oxide, a molecule that helps relax blood vessels. Other edible greens such as amaranth, chard, lamb's-quarters, purslane, and sorrel can also work. You can use them in a salad, sauté them with diced onion and garlic, or toss them into my Low Blood Pressure Soup (see page 233) just before you're ready to eat it.

They all have different benefits for treating high blood pressure. For instance, dandelion roots and leaves are highly diuretic, with high levels of potassium, and are sometimes used by naturopathic physicians in place of the common prescription diuretic furosemide (Lasix). Meanwhile, fenugreek, which is served as part of the Indian dish *alu methi,* is a fabulous source of choline and beta-carotene, both of which help reduce high blood pressure. Overall, fenugreek contains eight different diuretic agents.

★★**Tomatoes** I recommend tomatoes for my blood pressure–reducing soup because cooked tomatoes are a fabulous source of lycopene. Tomatoes also contain beta-carotene and vitamin E, which help protect cells from oxidative damage. In a study of 31 people with hypertension who didn't require medication, researchers gave them a tomato-like placebo for 4 weeks, followed by 8 weeks of a tomato extract and then another 4 weeks of the placebo. During the tomato extract period, their systolic readings dropped by 10 mmHg and their diastolic readings by 4 mmHg; no changes were seen during the placebo phases. One of my favorite ways to fix tomatoes is to drizzle them with olive oil (which helps your body absorb the lycopene and other antioxidants), then roast them slowly in a 250°F oven for a few hours. Serve over pasta, on toasted bread rubbed with a bit of garlic, or as a side dish for fish or chicken. Delicious!

★**Fava beans** Years ago, frustrated by my recalcitrant high blood pressure, I tried a daily serving of fava bean soup with seven dandelion leaves and lots of blood pressure–reducing onions and garlic. Fava beans are among the richest natural sources of L-dopa, a precursor of the chemical dopamine, which acts as a diuretic. In one study, eating 40 grams of freshly chopped fava beans significantly increased the amount of sodium and dopamine in the urine—a good thing when it comes to reducing blood pressure.

★**Saffron** At prices upwards of $60 an ounce, saffron is the world's most expensive spice. Its cost is due to the intensive work required to get that ounce. The bright golden powder comes from the stigmata of hand-picked saffron plants, and it takes 75,000 flowers to make up 1 pound of the spice. However, since you use only a pinch at a time, that ounce can last a long time. It's probably also cheaper than blood pressure medication, which is why I recommend it. The herb contains a chemical called crocetin, which my database shows reduces blood pressure.

From the Herbal Medicine Chest

The next time you think about a PB&J sandwich, consider using hawthorn jelly (found in health food stores and online) instead of grape. Hawthorn, a close relative of the apple, shares many compounds with grapes. It appears to have some vasodilating effects, a fancy way of saying it helps your blood vessels relax and open wider. In particular, it dilates the coronary artery, increasing blood flow to the heart and reducing blood pressure.

In one study of hawthorn, 79 people with type 2 diabetes, most of whom were taking drugs for high blood pressure, were randomly assigned to take either 1,200 milligrams a day of hawthorn extract or a placebo for 4 months. Those taking hawthorn saw an average drop in their diastolic blood pressure (the bottom number) of 2.6 mmHg compared to the placebo group, whose blood pressure actually increased slightly. One of the best studies of hawthorn and high blood pressure found a drop in systolic blood pressure (the top number) from 160 mmHg to 150 mmHg and in diastolic readings from 89 to 85. One reason for the herb's benefits may be its high flavonoid content. Flavonoids are powerful antioxidants, some of which are linked to lower blood pressure.

If you can't find hawthorn jelly, make a tea with 1 teaspoon of dried herb per cup of boiling water and drink up to two cups a day.

High Cholesterol

EVERYONE WORRIES ABOUT THEIR CHOLESTEROL LEVELS, but the reality is that high cholesterol levels won't kill you. Heart disease will. The problem is that heart disease and cholesterol are inextricably linked, with one contributing to the other. If you have high levels of low-density lipoprotein (LDL) cholesterol—the so-called bad cholesterol—you have more of those fatty compounds in your blood available for oxidation by free radicals, molecules produced as a by-product of energy production. Once oxidized, those little blood fats get sticky and are more likely to glom onto artery walls, beginning the gradual narrowing of your coronary arteries known as atherosclerosis. The key is to halt the process before it begins keeping LDL cholesterol levels low. One way to do that is by *increasing* levels of another form of cholesterol—high-density lipoprotein (HDL) cholesterol. This form of cholesterol acts like a garbage truck in your blood system, picking up LDL and escorting it to the liver, where it can be processed for disposal.

These days, if you have high cholesterol, most doctors will immediately start you on a statin medication such as atorvastatin (Lipitor). These drugs, which are among the 10 most used medications *in the world,* work well when it comes to lowering blood cholesterol and possibly the risk of heart disease. But they are not benign. They carry their own risks, including memory problems, muscle aches and pains, and loss of a very important antioxidant in the heart called coenzyme Q10. That's why I prefer to start with cholesterol-lowering foods; it's amazing what they can do when it comes to reducing the numbers. And it doesn't take much of a drop to get a big heart-healthy benefit. Each 1 percent drop in cholesterol levels may reduce your heart attack risk by 2 percent.

Healing Foods for High Cholesterol

Here are some foods that can give you a real boost in your fight against unhealthy cholesterol levels.

★★★**Almonds** Nuts may be high in fat, but they're a great source of beneficial monounsaturated fat. That's probably why people who eat a handful of nuts a day are less likely to be severely overweight than those who don't. The high fat content helps fill you up—without filling you out. One study found that replacing half of your normal fats with fat from almond oil reduced total cholesterol levels by about 4 percent and LDL levels by about 6 percent in people with normal cholesterol levels.

★★★**Barley** If you're feeling smug because you down a bowl of "heart-healthy" oatmeal every morning, I've got news for you: You may like barley even better. I suggest you cook up a pot of barley once a week, then have some as a side dish at dinner or sprinkle some nuts and cinnamon on top for a unique breakfast. Barley is one of the richest sources of beta-glucans, the plant components that also give oatmeal its cholesterol-reducing power. But a cup of barley can offer three times more beta-glucans than a cup of oatmeal. In fact, it's so rich in cholesterol-lowering fiber that I don't even mind if you mix a soft-boiled egg with it, especially if you use eggs from free-range chickens.

★★★**Beans** Most if not all edible bean varieties pack a double whammy in terms of cholesterol control, with their fiber and lecithin, a plant-based fat that—believe it or not—is used in milk chocolate to keep the milk and chocolate from separating. It turns out that lecithin can also help lower cholesterol. The two together—fiber and lecithin—are probably behind beans' amazing benefits when it comes to blood fats. One study found that just 1½ cups of dried lentils or kidney beans a day could slash cholesterol levels by a whopping 19 percent!

★★★**Edamame** Of the many types of soy I have tried, these green soybeans are the most palatable. You just steam or boil them for about 5 minutes, sprinkle them with salt, and pop them out of the pod into your mouth. But let me warn you—they can be addictive, though that's not such a bad thing given the huge declines in cholesterol levels studies find when soy protein is substituted for high-fat protein sources like most red meats. One study found that 25 grams a day of soy protein could lower LDL levels by about 5 percent. You can also try soy milk. One study found that about two cups a day reduced LDL levels by an average of 8 mg/dl and increased HDL levels by about 4 mg/dl on average.

★★★**Oatmeal** Don't nix oatmeal altogether. The protein in oats (yes, oats have protein!) is a good source of the amino acid L-arginine, from which your body eventually produces nitric oxide. Nitric oxide has many jobs to do in keeping your heart healthy, including reducing oxidation and inflammation. Although arginine may help treat high blood pressure and other markers of heart disease, some research finds it also helps reduce cholesterol. In one study, 45 healthy elderly volunteers took either an arginine supplement or a placebo for 2 weeks. Those taking

Cholesterol-Dropping Hummus

Drain and rinse a couple of cans of cannellini beans, then put them in a blender with a couple of garlic cloves, a tablespoon of lemon juice, and salt and pepper to taste. Voilà! Cholesterol medicine in a dip. The beans are a fantastic source of fiber, which binds to cholesterol in the gut and helps escort it out of your body, while garlic has long been known for its cholesterol-reducing benefits. Studies find garlic can drop cholesterol levels by 4 to 12 percent.

the supplement showed significant drops in their total and LDL cholesterol levels, but those taking a placebo experienced no change.

By the way, peanuts are another rich source of arginine, as are seeds such as pine nuts, black cumin, butternut, watermelon, pumpkin, sesame, and soy.

★★★**Olive oil** This oil is another of the richest sources of monounsaturated fatty acids. It's also one main reason for the healthy hearts of those who follow a Mediterranean diet. I think it's a must if you're trying to keep your cholesterol levels within a healthy range, and studies support my thinking. Just use it in place of butter or other oils for everything from sautéing to dipping bread.

★★**Avocados** I hope you don't limit these fruits to just the Super Bowl and guacamole. Avocados are packed with healthy monounsaturated fats like those found in olive oil. When researchers had 45 people, 30 of whom had high cholesterol, add an avocado a day to their diets for one week, the healthy volunteers' total cholesterol levels dropped by 16 percent, while those with high cholesterol saw their levels drop by 17 percent. LDL and triglyceride readings fell by 22 percent each, and HDL cholesterol levels jumped by 11 percent. A control group that didn't eat avocados had no change in their cholesterol levels.

★★**Carrots** Carrots (along with apples and the rind of oranges and grapefruits) are high in a form of fiber called calcium pectate, or pectin. You may know it as the powder you add to homemade jams and jellies. Mixed with liquid, it turns into a gel that's high in a soluble fiber that studies find can help reduce cholesterol. It seems that pectin binds to bile acids in the gut, which helps transport cholesterol out of your body. As for the carrots—well, I like to cite a favorite Scottish study in which participants snacked on two carrots a day for 3 weeks and saw their cholesterol levels plummet by 10 to 20 percent! A study we did at the USDA found similar results. These are drops you'd be lucky to get with statins. So you decide: Carrots or a pill?

★★**Chocolate** Chocolate isn't going to lower your cholesterol per se, but it will help prevent the oxidation of those cholesterol molecules that turn an otherwise innocuous compound into a biological dirty bomb. That's because dark chocolate (and it must be dark to be healthfully helpful) packs a powerful wallop of antioxidants, which neutralizes nasty free radicals. One study found that supplementing a typical American diet with 0.5 ounce of dark chocolate and about 0.75 ounce of cocoa powder was all it took to reduce LDL oxidation.

★★**Cinnamon** The cinnamon that I often suggest folks sprinkle on their barley or oatmeal breakfast has its own cholesterol-reducing benefits. About ½ tablespoon a day slashed LDL cholesterol levels by nearly a third in one study, cutting total cholesterol by 26 percent. Try putting a sprinkling of cinnamon in your coffee before brewing. It also makes a pretty good tea, either on its own or with fenugreek.

> It's not the cholesterol in eggs and shellfish you should worry about if you have high cholesterol but rather the saturated fat in red meat and full-fat dairy products. That's what turns into LDL cholesterol in your bloodstream, and that's why diets low in this type of fat are so important if you have high cholesterol.

★★**Cranberries** This fruit is good for more than just holiday meals and preventing urinary tract infections. Not only are cranberries (and cranberry juice) one of the best sources of antioxidants around but they also yield extracted chemicals that can increase the amount of cholesterol your liver takes out of your bloodstream. Once in the liver, that cholesterol can be processed for removal from your body.

★★**Orange juice** In addition to eating an orange (including the white part so you get that valuable pectin), swig a glass of orange juice. In one study, drinking three glasses a day for a month helped increase levels of HDL by an average of 21 percent and reduce the LDL/HDL ratio by an average of 16 percent—a good thing when it comes to cholesterol. The benefits are probably linked to high levels of antioxidant flavonoids in the juice. The best part is that the benefits lasted 5 weeks after people stopped drinking the juice.

If you're not an orange juice person, you can try apples. A study found that either eating two apples or drinking 12 ounces of apple juice daily significantly reduced LDL oxidation.

★★**Peanuts** Just an ounce of peanuts a day will provide a good amount of the coenzyme Q10 I mentioned earlier. Studies find that supplementing daily with about 120 milligrams of the enzyme can increase HDL cholesterol and reduce a form of dangerous cholesterol called lipoprotein(a), which significantly contributes to heart disease.

★★**Tea** Black or green—it doesn't seem to matter. Either can lower your cholesterol. Aim for about five cups a day; a government study found that after 3 weeks of drinking this amount, total cholesterol dropped by 6.5 percent and LDL cholesterol by 11.1 percent.

From the Herbal Medicine Chest

You may be getting this herb in food if you eat a lot of Indian cuisine; otherwise, it probably doesn't hold a prominent place in your spice rack. But I recommend you pick up a bottle of fenugreek seeds or supplements. Studies find that chewing an ounce of seeds three times a day can reduce total and

LDL cholesterol levels without negatively affecting HDL levels. Fenugreek stimulates the formation of bile in your liver, which binds to cholesterol and escorts it out of your body so it can't be released into the bloodstream. The seeds can be bitter, however, so try soaking them overnight or just rinsing them with running water to reduce the bitterness.

Hives

HIVES, ALSO KNOWN AS URTICARIA, are pale pink swellings that can itch, burn, or sting. They can be as small as a pencil eraser or as large as a dinner plate. Hives are as mysterious as they are annoying; often, people never figure out exactly what triggered the itchy bumps. We know they signal an allergic reaction, but just about anything can be the culprit—medications, food, infections, insect bites, stress, or even sunlight or cold air. The good news is that they usually disappear within a few hours; the bad news is that they *can* hang around as long as a few weeks.

If you have hives in or around your eyes or mouth, or if you're having trouble breathing, go directly to an emergency room. You may need a shot of a chemical called epinephrine, a form of adrenaline that's used to treat allergic reactions. It can help prevent the hives from causing your throat to swell shut.

Still with me? If you haven't set this book down to run to the ER, and you're just plagued by an irritating case of garden-variety hives, here are some food remedies to dull the itch.

Healing Foods for Hives

★★**Chamomile** The sedative chamomile is one of the best sources of apigenin, a natural anxiolytic (anti-anxiety) compound, which would seem to make it an ideal remedy for stress-induced hives. It also scores well in my database for antihistaminic compounds. Of course, you shouldn't try chamomile if you're sensitive to it, as some people are.

★★**Oregano** In their *Condensed Encyclopedia of Healing Foods*, my colleagues Michael Murray, ND, and Joseph Pizzorno, ND, recommend oregano specifically for hives. My database shows that the herb contains 10 anti-allergic and 10 antihistaminic compounds. Knowing this, I'd certainly try it if I came down with hives.

★**Baking soda** Pour half a box of baking soda into a warm bath and step in. Soaking in the solution may bring some relief. Or you could make a paste of baking soda and water and pat it right onto your hives.

Ironically, because this is a book about healing with food, I have to warn you that foods often actually trigger hives, which can appear any time from minutes to several hours after eating. The most common culprits are nuts, chocolate, shellfish, tomatoes, eggs, berries, and milk. Although fresh foods cause hives more often than cooked foods, food additives and preservatives–such as yellow dye #5–can also cause hives.

This being said, true allergies to foods are actually relative rare. Only about 2 percent of the population has them, according to the American Academy of Allergy, Asthma, and Immunology. But if you have a food allergy, you'll become quite the detective, scrutinizing labels for your trigger foods. Peanuts and soy can be especially challenging to avoid because they're inexpensive and used in lots of recipes and processed foods. For example, peanuts can be found in foods as diverse as baked goods and pasta sauces.

★**Cornstarch** Toss a few tablespoons of cornstarch into a cool bath and soak.

★**Cream of tartar** Make a paste of water and cream of tartar and apply the mixture liberally to your hives. When the paste crumbles off, reapply it.

★**Milk** To soothe inflamed skin, wet a clean cloth with cool milk and place it on your hives for 10 to 15 minutes.

★**Oatmeal** Oatmeal baths are a classic anti-itch remedy. Add 1 cup of oatmeal to a warm bath and soak in it for 10 to 15 minutes to soothe irritated skin. Don't use hot water, though; it can make hives worse. I think applying applesauce topically might work as well since apples can contain at least 10 antihistaminic compounds. Whether they're present in antihistaminic levels remains to be determined.

From the Herbal Medicine Chest

Although it isn't widely available, stinging nettle *(Urtica dioica)* would be my top choice of any remedy for hives, with a half-dozen anti-allergic compounds and as many as eight antihistaminic compounds. The Paiute Indians, native to the American West, make a nettle root decoction to treat hives. I take my Allergreens, which consists of cooked stinging nettle mixed with garlic and onion.

Indigestion

HERBALISTS WORLDWIDE HAVE USED HUNDREDS OF NATURAL REMEDIES for indigestion (dyspepsia) throughout recorded history. Asian Indians use the seeds of coriander to treat gas and colic. The Chinese use cinnamon for stomachaches. Even the Bible makes reference to the healing herbs: "Woe to you, teachers of the law and Pharisees, you hypocrites! You give a tenth of your spices—mint, dill, and cumin" (Matthew 23:23).

Indigestion plagues all of us from time to time, quite often because of what we eat. However, the great thing about foods is that right ones can fix a sour stomach just as easily.

Healing Foods for Indigestion

There are many foods and herbs that can help soothe a troubled tummy. Here are several that I recommend.

★★★**Basil** Like most members of the mint family, basil and holy basil are traditional remedies for settling an upset tummy, and for good reason. They're loaded with carminatives (gas-dispelling phytochemicals). Today, on a nerve-wracking stressful day, I'll have pesto, which is made with basil, on celery with a dash of powdered rosemary, thus incorporating three of my top anti-dyspeptic herbs. And yes, I believe that three herbs are better than one. Each brings some unique phytochemicals to the dyspepsia, and many of them work additively or synergistically.

★★★**Celery** Hungarians have long used celery to calm indigestion, and Germany's Commission E, a government agency that evaluates the safety and efficacy of medicinal herbs, has approved its use for dyspepsia. It can contain two dozen painkillers, more than two dozen anti-inflammatories, 11 anti-ulcer compounds, and more than two dozen sedatives to complement the activities of its three carminative compounds.

★★★**Peppermint** Herbalists have a special regard for peppermint's ability to soothe the lining of the stomach. This mint has been used for centuries to treat a wide range of digestive ailments. It's an age-old remedy for gas and abdominal cramps, so it's easy to see how the after-dinner mint came to be.

Commission E endorses peppermint tea for treating indigestion. However, being a native of Alabama, I'm partial to mint juleps, which, it turns out, work better than peppermint tea. Varro Tyler, PhD, late dean and professor emeritus of pharmacognosy (natural product pharmacy) at Purdue University in West Lafayette,

Indiana, noted that most of the carminative oils in peppermint and other mints are relatively insoluble in water. As a result, peppermint tea doesn't contain much of the plant's stomach-soothing constituents. It does contain enough to make it effective, but a peppermint tincture, which is made with alcohol, contains more.

★★★**Rosemary** As with celery, Europeans have long used rosemary for indigestion, and Commission E has approved it for that use. To strengthen the case for this herb even further, scientific evidence is now accumulating showing that rosemary contains more than a dozen analgesics, 11 anesthetics, and more than a dozen each of anti-inflammatories, anti-ulcer compounds, and sedative phytochemicals, all of which support its seven carminatives.

★★**Chamomile** Commission E considers chamomile an effective herb for relieving many gastrointestinal problems, including indigestion. According to Michael Berry, PhD, a pharmacognosist in Liverpool, England, chamomile is safe, effective, and particularly useful for small children with colic and teething pain.

When I'm at risk for stress-induced indigestion, I chew on a chamomile flower as I take a stress-busting walk through my Green Farmacy Garden. Both actions can help calm my stomach.

Andrew Weil, MD, professor at the University of Arizona College of Medicine in Tucson, suggests sipping chamomile and peppermint tea to soothe your digestive tract. These two herbs together are particularly effective for relieving indigestion, so I mix them often.

★★**Cinnamon** Mrs. Duke swears by cinnamon toast and cinnamon tea when she gets an upset stomach. Cinnamon has been used medicinally for thousands of years, and modern science has shown it can prevent and soothe indigestion. It's also a rich carminative, helping to minimize gas. Chinese scientists use cinnamon to treat a wide variety of gastrointestinal disorders, including indigestion, gastritis, and even gastric cancer. Cinnamon is approved for such ailments by Commission E.

★★**Ginger** Ginger contains certain chemicals (gingerols and shogaols) that not only soothe the gut but also aid digestion by increasing the wavelike muscle contractions (peristalsis) that move food through the intestines. In fact, ginger contains 180 times the protein-digesting power of papaya and stimulates fat-digesting bile, which helps restore proper digestive balance.

The medicinal part of ginger is the rhizome, an underground stem of the plant that's often mistaken for the root. This stem is ground up and used in many Chinese herbal prescriptions. Ayurvedic doctors call ginger the universal medicine.

The ancient Greeks used ginger wrapped in bread after large meals to prevent

Assorted Anti-Indigestion Herbs

If anything, there are too many herbal carminatives. I have more than 500 carminative entries in my database, most supported by research. Along with those I've already highlighted, here are some other notable indigestion fighters.

Coriander. This herb is loaded with indigestion-fighting elements. Its oil is carminative, antiseptic, antibacterial, antifungal, and a muscle relaxant. No wonder coriander helps soothe indigestion. People in Amazonia add wild coriander to beans to reduce the gas that beans often produce.

Marjoram. The British like marjoram sandwiches to treat indigestion. They also use diluted marjoram tea to relieve colic in infants. Marjoram is a fragrant mint with digestion-soothing benefits similar to those of peppermint.

As I've said, there are many others. Feel free to try any of the following to relieve indigestion: agrimony, allspice, anise, basil, bay, bee balm, buckwheat, burdock, caraway, cardamom, catnip, celery, chervil, chives, cloves, cumin, dill, fennel, hyssop, lemon balm (also known as melissa), lemongrass, lovage, oregano, parsnips, pennyroyal, sage, savory, tarragon, vanilla, and yarrow.

all kinds of digestive repercussions. Eventually, they simply added ginger to bread dough to give us gingerbread. In the 19th century, barkeepers in English pubs put ground ginger in small containers so patrons could sprinkle the herb into their beer, creating ginger ale.

Ginger is particularly helpful for relieving gas, bloating, and cramps. It settles the intestines and removes gas from the digestive tract. Try spicing your favorite dishes (especially beans) and drinks with ginger. Dr. Weil recommends fresh (not dried or ground) ginger as being best for indigestion, but never on an empty stomach.

★★**Radishes** Radishes contain a variety of chemicals that help improve digestion (in addition to keeping your gallbladder healthy and protecting against cancer). Many cultures have used radishes for gastrointestinal disorders, especially stomachache and gas. Both the root and juice of the plant have medicinal benefits. Michael Murray, ND, a natural medicine expert and author of *The Encyclopedia of Healing Foods*, suggests eating fresh radishes if you're constipated.

★**Chile pepper** Despite popular American beliefs, hot spices don't upset the stomach. In fact, some, such as chile pepper (cayenne), actually help soothe it. Additionally, recent studies have reported that carotenoids, the natural pigments that give the pepper its bright color, seem to protect the lining of the stomach, and capsaicin, the compound that gives it heat, may help prevent ulcers. Chile pepper also stimulates digestion.

★**Garlic, onions, and leeks** Eating foods known as prebiotics—indigestible food elements that stimulate the growth of "good" bacteria in the digestive tract—can be helpful in preventing many gastrointestinal problems. Natural sources of prebiotics include garlic, onions, and leeks, important elements of the Mediterranean diet. According to studies in India, garlic's link to good bacteria in the intestine improves digestion and enhances absorption of minerals. It also combats diarrhea and ulcers.

★**Papaya** This fruit contains digestive enzymes called proteolytic enzymes that break down proteins and aid in digestion. Naturopaths and people who advocate juicing for health maintain that papaya juice is good for relieving indigestion. If they're right, you should also get benefits from eating other fruits that contain proteolytics, such as kiwifruit and figs, after meals here in temperate America, but papaya and pineapple and ginger in tropical America. If I had chronic indigestion, I might have these fruits for dessert more often.

★**Pineapple** High in fiber, pineapple is a sweet way to promote healthy bowels and avoid indigestion. Pineapple contains glutamine, a compound that helps protect the lining of the stomach. It also has proteolytic enzyme bromelain, a natural anti-inflammatory that can help reduce the painful inflammation of ulcers.

★**Turmeric** This culinary herb, the main ingredient in Asian and Indian curry dishes, has been used as a natural medicine for thousands of years and is believed to have a number of gastrointestinal benefits. India's traditional Ayurvedic doctors used turmeric for all kinds of ailments. In addition, researchers have found that curcumin, the most active ingredient in turmeric, stays in the gastrointestinal tract, where it appears to fight colon polyps and possibly colon cancer. Scientists are also studying the effects of curcumin against other abdominal diseases such as colitis and inflammatory bowel disease.

From the Herbal Medicine Chest

South African physicians recommend rooibos (pronounced *roh'-ih-bus*) as an effective stomach soother that's gentle enough to treat babies with colic, according to the late economic botanist Julia Morton, DSc, author of *The Atlas of Medicinal Plants of Middle America*. Rooibos leaves are fermented and sun dried for use in teas; health food stores carry a variety of them. Rooibos is caffeine free and has less than half the tannins of regular tea, so it's less likely to cause the constipation problems that regular coffee and tea can.

Insect Bites and Stings

MY GOOD FRIEND JOHN DUVALL never joined me in the Amazon, but he was there with me in spirit. John once gave me his special formula to repel Amazonian bugs, but the bugs there didn't bother me—except once, at a place where my Shaman, Antonio Montero Pisco, made his spiritual offerings. Antonio had chosen the place because of its wild animals—the boa, deer, big cats, and, unfortunately, the deerflies and sweat bees.

On one particular occasion, Antonio wore a bright red baseball cap that was completely covered with these flying critters. I put a drop of John's special recipe on Antonio's hat, and a moment later, there was a red bull's-eye where the formulation had instantly repelled the insects—even more effectively than the well-known DEET. What was in this magical brew? Almond from the Mediterranean, citronella from the Orient, pennyroyal from America, and catnip from Europe—an international smorgasbord of insect repellents.

No matter where they are, in the Amazon or your backyard, insects bite and sting. Some, including mosquitoes, ticks, chiggers, and fleas, see you as food. Others, such as yellow jackets, bees, wasps, fire ants, and spiders, bite or sting to defend themselves.

Regardless of the insects' motivation, once you realize one has bitten or stung you, the faster you use a remedy, the more effective it will be. First, if you were stung by a bee, remove the stinger. If you leave it in place, it will continue to pump venom into your skin. The best way to remove it is with a flicking motion, using a dull knife blade or your thumbnail. If you pinch the stinger, you risk squeezing the venom sac and releasing even more toxins.

Next, assess the severity of the bite or sting. If the perpetrator was a poisonous spider, or if it was a bee and you know you are allergic, no food I know of is going to help you, so seek medical attention immediately. You should also seek emergency care if you feel faint, have swelling in your mouth or throat, have trouble breathing, or experience a rapid pulse after a bite or sting. And if you have muscle aches, a fever, headaches, and/or a bull's-eye rash within a few weeks of a tick bite, see your doctor; you could have Lyme disease.

Healing Foods for Insect Bites and Stings

There's not much new among insect repellents and bug bite remedies since I wrote *The Green Pharmacy*. In fact, they've been around so long and work so well that science's role is generally just to figure out how they work. Ironically, the scents that repel insects are often the ones humans and other animals find most attractive. After all, John's concoction included citronella, almond, and catnip, ingredients that appeal to humans (and felines, in the case of the catnip). Below are some you might try.

★★**Basil** This herb, especially the so-called holy basil or *tulsi* in India, is used extensively by traditional healers. Indians rub their skin with fresh basil leaves to repel insects, and people in Africa do the same. If I were bothered by insects in my garden and some of my culinary basil was within reach, I might rub some on my skin as an impromptu repellent.

★★**Garlic** When it comes to insect bites and stings, garlic can play two roles: as a repellent and as a treatment. It also helps when used either topically or ingested. In an Italian study, volunteers who received a topical application of garlic oil were well protected against insect bites. As a treatment, you can use the oil or make a poultice with crushed garlic and apply it directly to the bite or sting. If you prefer to ingest the garlic but don't want to smell it—and thus repel people in addition to insects— Jim LaValle, ND, a pharmacist, naturopathic physician, and founder of the LaValle Metabolic Institute in Cincinnati, suggests you take aged garlic extract instead of eating the raw cloves. He says the extract contains enough of the compounds to give your skin a slight sulfur scent that's detected by insects, but it isn't strong enough that your fellow humans will smell it. I agree with him, but I think that the more garlic stinks to my friends, the more it stinks to the bugs, and the more potent its physiological activities.

★★**Lemongrass** One of the ingredients in my friend John's magical Amazonian insect deterrent was citronella, a common scent used in insect-repelling candles and a staple of Thai and Vietnamese cooking. A close relative of citronella, lemongrass

FOODS TO WATCH

> Janet Maccaro, ND, PhD, a holistic nutritionist in Ormond Beach, Florida and author of *Natural Health Remedies A-Z*, reminds us that insects are attracted to excess sugar and alcohol. If you don't want to attract bugs, avoid eating or drinking anything sugar- or alcohol-laden before you go outdoors.

contains many of the same bug-repellent compounds. If you have some of this fresh herb available, crush it and rub it directly on your skin before you head outside. It has an appealing lemony smell, and I'd certainly rather smell like lemonade than like plastic- and body-dissolving DEET.

★★**Meat tenderizer** This is a tried-and-true remedy for the pain of insect bites and stings, and there's actually some good science behind its use. Dr. LaValle says meat tenderizer contains an enzyme (papain) that breaks down insect venom and proteins that cause inflammation, which decreases swelling and pain. Dr. LaValle recommends mixing a few tablespoons of meat tenderizer with enough water to form a paste, spreading the paste over the sting site, and leaving it on for about an hour.

★★**Onions** Although they may burn your eyes when you slice them, raw onions, when rubbed directly onto an insect bite or sting, can reduce inflammation. I'm not sure how it works, but it may be because the herb contains enzymes that can break down biochemical substances called prostaglandins, which actually increase your perception of pain. You can also get some relief from a bite or sting by eating foods containing onions. Onion skin is particularly good at relieving inflammation because it has a good supply of an anti-allergy chemical called quercetin. You can get a nice dose of quercetin by leaving the skin on onions when you add them to soups or stews. In addition, the skins will give the broth a rich brown color. Just be sure to fish them out before serving.

★★**Peppermint** Mint causes a cool, refreshing sensation in your mouth, and it will do the same for an insect bite or sting. Just a drop of peppermint essential oil increases blood flow to the sting, helping to flush out the venom. Peppermint also has a cooling effect, which will decrease pain and itching and take away the urge to scratch. Also, instead of peppermint oil, you can try a salve or ointment made from crushed peppermint leaves and lard, oil, or beeswax to help relieve the itching. Or you can dab a little toothpaste that contains peppermint oil on the irritated area. Peppermint and many other members of the mint family also contain piperitone, which is a potent repellent. Other essential oils that have insect-repelling powers come from eucalyptus, basil, and laurel.

★**Apple cider vinegar** Immediately after you've removed an insect stinger, give the irritated area a cool application of apple cider vinegar to decrease the inevitable redness and swelling. Depending on where you were stung, you can either soak the spot in the vinegar or dip a cotton ball in it and tape it to the site of the sting.

★**Baking soda** Although baking soda is more of an ingredient in baked goods than a food, baking soda paste can work well to relieve the inflammation associated with an insect bite or sting. Natural healers suggest dissolving 1 teaspoon of baking soda in 1 cup of water, applying the liquid to a cotton ball or washcloth, and using it as a compress for about 20 minutes.

★**Cinnamon** When it comes to preventing insect stings, cinnamon appears to pack a double whammy. Pure cinnamon appears to help kill mosquito larvae and act as an insect repellent at the same time. To make your own natural repellent, add a few drops of cinnamon oil to your lotion or sunscreen before you head outdoors. Use just a few drops—enough so you can just begin to smell the cinnamon over the other ingredients.

★**Ice** It may sound simple, but applying an ice cube to an insect bite or sting will decrease the pain and swelling. Place the ice on the sore spot for 10 minutes, remove it for a few minutes, and repeat. You can leave the cube on for up to 20 minutes if you wrap it in a washcloth or small towel. If ice feels too cold, use a washcloth soaked in cool water instead.

★**Oatmeal** A tried-and-true remedy for soothing chickenpox, oatmeal also makes a nice poultice for relieving the itch of insect bites and stings. Cook the oatmeal, let it cool, and put some in a soft cotton cloth. Place the filled cloth over the bite, cover with a dry cloth, and apply a heating pad.

★**Papaya** Like meat tenderizer, the papaya fruit contains papain, the enzyme that helps neutralize insect venom, so if you're planning to be outside for a few hours, you may want to pack some papaya as a snack. That way, if you're stung, you can place a slice of the fruit on the sting for an hour or so. On the Amazon, there are often wild papaya seedlings that ooze milk when broken. That milk is probably more effective than a slice of fruit.

★**Parsley** To freshen your breath after you've eaten garlic, munch on some parsley. And be sure to leave a few leaves to rub on your skin should you be unfortunate enough to be bitten or stung, since fresh parsley is a folk remedy for insect bites.

From the Herbal Medicine Chest

Some herbal treatments are just as effective as food remedies for insect bites and stings. Here are a few that may help ease the pain after an insect attack.

Beautyberry (*Callicarpa americana*) The leaves of the plant, which bears distinctive pinkish-purple—and occasionally white—berries, are as effective as any commercial product for repelling ticks and mosquitoes. Try rubbing some beautyberry leaves on your skin or clothing before heading out into a field or other tick- or mosquito-infested area, or perhaps plant beautyberry shrubs where your pets can rub against them for natural tick control.

Calendula *(Calendula officinalis)* For decades, the Shakers planted calendula as a pot herb for cooking and as a medicinal herb to treat insect stings. Nowadays, many herbal bug bite products contain calendula extract. Some experts suggest applying calendula ointment every 4 to 6 hours, hinting that a few dabs of the ointment may keep insects away.

Clove *(Syzygium aromaticum)* When applied to the skin, clove oil is one of the most effective natural insect repellents available. Here are some ways you can dilute and mix clove oil to use it to repel mosquitoes, fleas, and other pests.

- Dilute the oil with rubbing alcohol, witch hazel, vodka, or olive oil. Mix 1 part clove oil with 10 parts diluting liquid in a container with a lid, shake well, and apply directly to your skin. Reapply every 1 to 2 hours when you're outside, and more often if you're sweating. Wash off the solution when you go in.

- Using the same 1:10 ratio, dilute the oil with distilled water, put it in a spray bottle, and spray the solution onto outdoor areas such as planters and fences.

Plantain *(Plantago major)* Herbalists often recommend this versatile plant as an effective remedy for numerous conditions, including insect bites and stings. It's the first thing I apply when I'm at home, since it's a common weed in my lawn. Rub fresh plantain leaves on a bite or sting three or four times a day.

Insomnia

MRS. DUKE READS WOMEN'S MAGAZINES and follows many of their recommendations. In particular, she has enforced the often-cited rule, "Make sure your bedroom is quiet and dark." Why? The darker your bedroom is at night, the more melatonin you secrete. This natural chemical helps regulate your wake-sleep cycle, and supplements of the stuff have been linked to better sleep in some people.

Other tips that may help you sleep better include retiring and rising at the same time during the week and on weekends and avoiding extended naps during the day (although for me, a post-lunch nap is part of my daily routine).

In addition, a strategy utilizing foods that encourage sleep may help you doze off more easily and keep you slumbering through the night.

Healing Foods for Insomnia

★★★**Cherries** Some tart cherries contain significant quantities of melatonin, a hormone produced in the pineal gland (at the base of the brain) that influences the sleep process. According to studies at the University of Texas, Montmorency cherries contain 0.1 to 0.3 milligram of melatonin per serving. At this amount, melatonin has been shown to be an effective sleep inducer.

★★★**Grains** Many other foods contain small doses of melatonin. Particularly rich plant-based sources include corn, rice, and barley, as well as ginger and bananas. My Mela-Tryp Sleep Aid Soup, which provides melatonin and tryptophan (which I discuss on the next page) may be a helpful snack to try before bed. Simmer corn, rice, barley, and perhaps some oats and wheat in turkey broth and milk. Sprinkle in some walnuts for their serotonin and add some chickpeas for their tryptophan. Enjoy a cupful in a dark room a half hour before bedtime.

★★**Dill** My database shows me that dill contains multiple plant chemicals that act as sedatives, stress fighters, central nervous system depressants, muscle relaxants, and tranquilizers. And dill smells nice. Pickles are obviously a traditional source of dill, and many people use the herb as the main flavoring in dips made with sour cream and mayonnaise. You can also make a fresh-tasting tea by pouring hot water over dill seed.

★★**Soybeans** People with restless legs syndrome develop strange sensations in their lower extremities while they're lying at rest, which gives them a strong urge to move their legs. This, of course, doesn't bode well for falling sleep.

FOODS TO WATCH

If you drink caffeinated or alcoholic beverages, cut back on them during the day and definitely avoid them during the evenings. Consuming either too close to bedtime can keep you from getting a good night's sleep.

One common cause of restless legs syndrome is iron deficiency. If you've recently developed the condition, it's a good idea to have your doctor check your iron level. In addition, some people find that folate, vitamin E, and magnesium are helpful. Near the top of the list of food sources of iron are cooked green soybeans, which modern diners call edamame. Good folate sources include fortified breakfast cereals, black-eyed peas, cooked spinach, and asparagus. For vitamin E, try wheat germ oil, almonds, sunflower seeds, and peanut butter.

★★**Squash seeds and pumpkin seeds** One reason people nod off after Thanksgiving dinner, aside from trying to escape doing the dishes, is because of the tryptophan in the turkey. Your body turns this amino acid into serotonin and then converts serotonin into melatonin.

In a 2005 study, one group of participants consumed a food high in tryptophan (butternut squash seed meal, in this case) combined with the carbohydrate glucose; a second group took a supplement of pharmaceutical-grade tryptophan along with a carbohydrate; and a third group ate only a carbohydrate. The food source of tryptophan turned out to be similar to the pharmaceutical-grade tryptophan for treating insomnia. Here's why having some carbohydrate along with the tryptophan is helpful, according to the authors: Tryptophan, which is relatively rare, competes with other amino acids, which are plentiful, to get into your brain, and it often loses. But when you eat a carbohydrate, your body responds with a burst of insulin that lowers levels of the other amino acids, giving tryptophan an advantage.

If you don't happen to have a stash of butternut squash seeds in your kitchen, try pumpkin seeds—they're also a good source of tryptophan.

★**Halibut and other magnesium-rich foods** If your magnesium stores run low, the deficiency may stimulate your brain, which could interfere with your sleep. The recommended intake of magnesium for adult men is 400 milligrams up to age 30 and 420 milligrams thereafter. For adult women, it's 310 and 320 milligrams for those respective age groups. Halibut is one good source, with 90 milligrams in 3 ounces. Others, with magnesium content in milligrams, include:

1 ounce almonds—80

½ cup cooked spinach—75

1 cup oatmeal—55

1 baked potato—50

Other good sources of magnesium include purslane (an edible plant with juicy leaves and stems that many consider a weed), green beans, poppy seeds, cowpeas, and lettuce.

Several herbal teas are commonly recommended for insomnia, such as lemon balm (also called melissa) and chamomile. Lemon balm contains chemicals called terpenes that are sedating, and chamomile—often used as a relaxing after-dinner beverage in Latin America—contains an effective sedative called apigenin.

Intermittent Claudication

HAVING SEVERE CRAMPS AND TINGLING in your buttocks, thighs, and/or calves when you walk is called intermittent claudication (IC) and is a symptom of a condition called peripheral artery disease (PAD). In PAD, clogged blood vessels prevent adequate blood flow in your legs, starving them of oxygen and nutrients and sometimes leading to pain when you walk, stand, or move. People with the condition find it difficult to walk even short distances, say, from bed to the bathroom, without severe pain. It's important to note that about half of all people with PAD do not experience this leg pain and go undiagnosed. If you have been diagnosed, however, you're probably taking prescription medication. Don't stop taking it without talking to your physician, but consider the following healing foods. All contain nutrients and phytochemicals shown to benefit IC.

Healing Foods for Intermittent Claudication

★★★**Bilberries, blueberries, and other dark berries** In their great book, *Principles and Practice of Phytotherapy,* my friends Simon Mills and Kerry Bone give top billing to bilberries under the heading "Peripheral Vascular Disorders and Venous Disorders." The bilberry is just a strain of blueberry that's royal blue all the way thru, while blueberries are green at the center. But any dark blue or purple berries loaded with anthocyanins should help.

★★★**Garlic and onions** I still bet on garlic for IC because of the many biologically active compounds it contains that should help relieve the condition. My Multiple Activities Menu for garlic lists nearly two dozen activities related to this condition among the 147 phytochemicals so far listed in my database for garlic. As always, onions come in a close second, with the same activities and almost as many phytochemicals as garlic. These compounds can reduce oxidation as well as make blood less sticky and less likely to clot. In one 12-week study of garlic, people with IC who were given 800 milligrams of garlic a day were able to walk with much less pain after 5 weeks. Not only that, but they had lower cholesterol levels and blood pressure.

★★★**Ginger** Ginger contains 241 different plant chemicals (at last count), many of which have various activities that can help with overall heart health. For IC, I focus on ginger's ability to prevent blood clots. It slows the production of thromboxane, a compound that causes blood platelets to clump together and clot, which is beneficial because too much clotting increases the risk of heart attack and stroke. Studies find these benefits almost as powerful as those from aspirin. Since clotting in the leg can be one cause of PAD pain, I recommend using ginger throughout the day. Sprinkle dried ginger on your cereal or over yogurt, mince it with garlic and onions to form the base for sauces and meat dishes, and grate it over steamed vegetables as a spicy additive.

★★**Anti-PAD spices** Spices that help alleviate PAD include allspice, cardamom, and cloves. I suggest adding a dash of each to herbal teas and oatmeal. These spices are part of an amazing Tibetan formula called Padma 28 (even though it contains only 20 herbs). In one study of people with PAD, those who used Padma 28 for 6 months had greatly improved blood flow to their feet, with more than half saying they could walk farther without pain.

★★**Carob and other arginine sources** Although exercise therapy is the most effective conservative treatment for IC, early trials indicate that L-arginine, an amino acid that helps cells create energy, may yield significant benefit in lessening symptoms. Some writers suggest that this condition is rather like angina (chest pain due to an oxygen shortage in the heart) and believe that natural treatments for angina may also help relieve IC.

It certainly wouldn't hurt to eat more foods containing high levels of L-arginine. Not only does it help with energy production, it also converts into nitric oxide, an enzyme that helps blood vessels dilate. The wider your blood vessels, even if they are thick with plaque, the easier time your blood has getting through.

In one study, 41 people with angina ate two energy bars supplemented with L-arginine, one supplemented energy bar and one placebo bar, or two placebo bars every day for 2 weeks. At the end of the trial, the group getting two supplement bars increased their pain-free walking distance by 66 percent and their overall walking distance by 23 percent. The benefits lasted for 10 weeks after participants stopped eating the bars. There was no improvement in either of the other groups.

★★**Codfish** This sweet, white, flaky fish is one of the best food sources of the amino acid L-carnitine, which is vital for energy production, particularly in the heart muscle. Studies evaluating its use in people with IC find that the worse their disease, the greater the benefit they derived when supplementing with L-carnitine. In one study, 485 people received either a placebo or 1 gram of propionyl-l-carnitine twice a day for 12 months. Those getting the supplement were able to nearly double their walking distance compared with those in the placebo group. The overall quality of life for people in the supplement group also increased significantly, compared with no improvement in those taking placebos.

★★**Salmon** As I've said elsewhere, salmon is rich in omega-3 fatty acids, healthful fats that benefit the heart and arteries in numerous ways. A Spanish study of people with IC found that supplementing with a liquid form of fish oil made from salmon combined with olive oil for 3 months reduced the risk of oxidation of low-density lipoprotein (LDL) ("bad") cholesterol. What does this mean? Simply that the LDL is less likely to undergo chemical changes that make it stick to artery walls—possibly improving blood flow in people with IC. In fact, a review of several studies of omega-3 supplementation in people with IC found that blood did become less thick and sticky. In another study, when participants drank a milk-like liquid fortified with omega-3's, folic acid, and vitamins B_6 and E for 3 months, their pain-free walking distance increased significantly. Researchers also found that the supplementation reduced artery wall inflammation.

From the Herbal Medicine Chest

Ginkgo biloba is among my favorite herbs for intermittent claudication. It prevents blood clotting and stickiness, improves blood flow, and helps dilate blood vessels. It also has potent antioxidant benefits. The herb was evaluated in an analysis of nine clinical studies in which people with IC were treated with a ginkgo supplement called EGb 761. Most studies found a significant increase in the distance people taking the supplement could walk without pain. Overall, when results from six studies were pooled, people walked an average of 23 percent farther after taking the supplement for several months.

Irritable Bowel Syndrome

IRRITABLE BOWEL SYNDROME (IBS) is a rather elusive disease that affects between 25 and 45 million people in the United States. Doctors aren't exactly sure what causes it, but they do have some good ideas about what makes it worse and how to control it.

Basically, IBS consists of waves of intestinal distress. A person with IBS can experience intermittent bouts of constipation, diarrhea, cramping, and gas on and off for weeks at a time. These flare-ups have been found to be closely linked to trigger foods, which vary from person to person. The key to controlling IBS and preventing its flare-ups, doctors believe, is a healthy, closely managed diet.

Fat vs. Fiber

IBS flare-ups are commonly caused by your bowel working overtime to digest fat, something Americans eat plenty of. When you eat high-fat foods, your bowel contracts, and for people with IBS this means lots of pain and discomfort. Eating less fat can help you prevent a flare-up. Additionally, high-fat foods tend to have very little fiber, and when it comes to controlling IBS, fiber is the key.

Here's why fiber is so great for people with IBS. There are two kinds of fiber: soluble and insoluble. Soluble fiber forms a sticky gel that acts like a protective coating inside your digestive tract, preventing irritants from causing problems such as cramping and gas in your already upset intestine. Insoluble fiber soaks up water as it passes through your intestines, helping to bulk up, weigh down, and soften your stools. Both kinds of fiber are important because together they help sweep things along, from your stomach to your intestines to your stools—on out.

However, if you have IBS and want to start eating more fiber, do so gradually. Eating more fiber when your body isn't used to it can bring on even more digestive problems. You need to ease your system into it. Start slowly by adding more fiber-rich foods to your diet a few at a time over the course of several weeks or months. And be sure to drink lots of water, which fiber needs to work well.

Healing Foods for IBS

Because IBS is famous for causing a host of miserable intestinal problems, let's look at foods that can help to calm and soothe the most common symptoms of IBS—constipation, diarrhea, cramping, and gas. From these suggestions, you can pick and choose which healing foods you might like to try based on what tends to trouble you the most. Because everyone with IBS reacts to foods differently, finding natural remedies that work for you can take a bit of trial and error.

Constipation: Keeping Things Moving

★★★**Apples** Apples are an amphoteric food, which means they can work in either direction, plugging you up if your bowels are loose or loosening you up if you're constipated. Because they contain lots of both soluble and insoluble fiber, apples are an excellent choice if you're constipated.

★★★**Berries** Berries contain large amounts of fiber, helping your stools absorb lots of water to become heavier and travel through your intestines faster. Elderberries top the list with 5 grams of fiber in a ½ cup serving. Raspberries are next at 4 grams of fiber per serving, with blackberries coming in third with 3 grams. Blueberries and strawberries are good, too. When it comes to berry juice, mulberries and boysenberries make for gentle laxatives.

★★**Dark leafy greens** A salad tossed with various dark leafy greens is a good choice to combat constipation. These greens provide some omega-3 fatty acids, a "good" kind of fat, that help keep your bowels moving. Deep-colored greens offer the best benefit. Dandelion greens, in particular, are an effective natural laxative. Dandelion increases bile flow into your large intestine, which helps prevent constipation. Dandelion greens can be found in popular "spring mix" salad combinations in many restaurants and produce sections. And while not recently sold in my local Bloom, I know they grow outside it. Dandelions are pushing through my new $12,000 asphalt hard top. They shall inherit the earth. But tough plants make good sources of fiber.

★★**Flaxseed** Also known as linseed, flaxseed is very high in fiber and rich in omega-3's, both helpful for constipation. Three tablespoons of flaxseed has about 3 grams of fiber. Flaxseed has a sweet, nutty taste and can be added to almost anything. It's great in salads, cereals, casseroles, and breads. However, whole flaxseed provides little benefit because your digestive tract cannot crack open the hard shell that surrounds the seed (which is where all the benefits are). Go for ground or crushed flaxseed because it's easier to digest. Also, don't fall for common claims that flaxseed oil is just as good for you. While flaxseed oil has some nutritional benefits, it doesn't retain the fiber that helps with constipation. If you try flaxseed, be sure to drink plenty of water to keep all that bulk moving through. And, as I've pointed out in other chapters, there's also the seed of chia, chiso, hemp, inca peanut, and walnut as sources of alpha-linolenic acid, one "vegetarian" omega-3.

★★**Ginger** Long known for its many healing properties, ginger is a tasty way to deal with constipation. Ginger contains certain chemicals that stimulate your digestive system by increasing the wavelike muscle contractions (peristalsis) that move food through your intestines, which is especially helpful for IBS. Fresh ginger offers the most medicinal benefit. Pickled ginger, often found in Asian restaurants and served alongside sushi, is thought to be as beneficial as fresh ginger.

FOODS TO WATCH

Although people with IBS react to foods differently, there are some common food triggers that IBS sufferers seem to share:

Beans. It's no surprise that beans often don't agree with people who have IBS—they're quite the gas producers. You might find that certain beans are more tolerable than others, or that you need to avoid them altogether. To help reduce gas, flavor your beans with fresh or ground ginger (a natural laxative). In fact, any herb that soothes your digestive tract (a carminative) might help.

Coffee. Both regular and decaf coffee can make your bowels more sensitive. If coffee seems to aggravate your IBS but you can't give it up entirely, you might try cutting back to only a cup or two a day.

Corn. Corn and foods that contain corn, such as corn cereals, can cause problems. Corn tends to irritate 20 percent of people with IBS.

Milk and dairy products. Although these foods have a reputation for binding you up, dairy products can also cause diarrhea because they contain a natural sugar called lactose, which some people with IBS can't digest (lactose intolerance). However, yogurt is lower in lactose than other dairy foods, so you might find it easier to digest. It's also a probiotic, a food that contains "good" living bacteria to fight "bad" bacteria in your intestines that can cause gastrointestinal distress.

Sweets. Foods high in natural sugar (fructose) often aren't the best choice if you have IBS. Fruit juices and honey, for example, can move into the large intestine undigested, causing gas and diarrhea. Artificial sweeteners found in sugarless gums and candies can also be hard to digest.

★★**Prunes, raisins, and figs** Well known as effective food remedies for constipation, prunes contain three active ingredients. First, they're very high in fiber, with 3 grams in just three prunes. Second, they have a compound called dihydroxyphenyl isatin, which stimulates the contractions in your intestines that are needed for regular bowel movements. Third, prunes contain a natural sugar called sorbitol, which, like fiber, soaks up large amounts of water in your digestive tract to keep things moving on through. Most fruits generally contain less than 1 percent sorbitol. Prunes, however, have about 15 percent sorbitol, which is why they're one of the best natural remedies for constipation.

Like prunes, other dried fruits—such as raisins and figs—are wonders at relieving constipation. Raisins contain a compound called tartaric acid, which acts as a natural laxative. Figs are also an excellent source of fiber, providing about 5 grams of fiber in just three dried or fresh figs.

★★**Rhubarb** Eating the stalks of rhubarb (not the leaves) has long been used in folk medicine to relieve constipation. Rhubarb is a member of the buckwheat family, which makes it a good source of fiber. It's important to know that you should eat only rhubarb stalks because rhubarb leaves contain very high levels of toxins called oxalates that can irritate your stomach.

★★**Squash** The fiber found in dark yellow and orange winter squash, such as acorn, butternut, and Hubbard squash, can be particularly helpful with constipation. Pale summer squash, on the other hand, is lower in fiber and not as beneficial.

Diarrhea: Slowing Things Down

★★★**Apples** Handy for treating diarrhea, apples contain both pectin and tannins. These two substances work together to bind up your stools and soothe your digestive tract. Both the skin and the pulp of apples are beneficial, which is why whole apples as well as applesauce (good for babies) are common food remedies for diarrhea.

★★★**Tea** One of the most astringent natural remedies for diarrhea is conventional tea in traditional tea bags—just plain, without any other herbs or spices added. Tea is rich in tannins, which help bind stools and hold back bowel movements.

★★**Bilberries and blueberries** These berries are particularly effective against diarrhea because they, too, are rich in both pectin and tannins. Dried, not fresh, bilberries and blueberries are best.

★★**Carrots** Cooked carrots seem to soothe the digestive tract and control diarrhea. They also provide nutrients that are lost during an attack. Interestingly, the Appalachians cook their beans with a small, whole carrot to reduce their gas-producing ability.

★★**Garlic, onion, and leek** Eating foods known as prebiotics—nondigestible food elements that stimulate the growth of "good" bacteria in the digestive tract—can be helpful in preventing diarrhea. Natural sources of prebiotics include garlic, onion, and leek. Eating lots of these flavorful foods can boost your immune system and ward off diarrhea-causing bacteria. According to studies in India, garlic's link to good bacteria in the intestine also improves digestion and enhances absorption of minerals, a helpful bonus during and after a bout of diarrhea.

★★**Pomegranate** This biblical fruit is often used to treat diarrhea. Pomegranate's seeds can be astringent, helping to bind and dry up your bowels. Sipping pomegranate juice is a good option. Some of the rind of the fruit, even richer in binding tannins, is often incorporated in commercial pomegranate juice

Gas and Cramps: Calming the Storm

Any herb that soothes the digestive tract and minimizes gas is called a carminative. Dozens of herbs fall into this category, and naming them all would be exhausting. Here are a few of the best:

★★★**Ginger** Ginger is a particularly helpful digestive aid because it helps to relieve gas, bloating, and cramps. It settles the intestine and removes gas from the digestive tract. Try a nice cup of ginger tea by adding ½ teaspoon of ground or freshly grated ginger to 1 cup of hot water.

★★★**Peppermint** Peppermint has been used for centuries to treat a wide range of digestive ailments. Its gas-relieving chemicals make it an age-old remedy for flatulence and abdominal cramps. It's also quite helpful in relieving heartburn.

★★**Other assorted herbs** Here are just a few more carminative herbs that can help tame the effects of IBS:

Allspice	Cloves	Nutmeg
Caraway	Coriander	Peppermint
Cardamom	Dill	Sage
Cinnamon	Fennel	Thyme

Licorice (Glycyrrhiza glabra) Licorice contains several compounds that help protect the lining of the stomach and intestine. Deglycyrrhizinated licorice (DGL) is a processed form of the herb and the preferred type to treat a handful of digestive ailments. DGL has been shown to promote the release of certain compounds in saliva that may stimulate the healing of stomach and intestinal cells. To soothe your digestive tract, try adding ½ teaspoon of DGL powder to your favorite herbal tea.

Psyllium (Plantago ovata) Tiny psyllium seeds are very high in fiber and are a common ingredient in many over-the-counter laxatives. They contain a specific fiber called mucilage, which absorbs a great deal of fluid in your gut. This makes the seeds swell, adding bulk to your stools to help with the constipation of IBS. Psyllium seeds need lots of water to work well, so be sure to drink plenty if you try them. If you have allergies or asthma, don't use this herb. Some people have had allergic reactions to psyllium, including a few reports of serious asthma attacks from inhaled psyllium seed dust.

Macular Degeneration

THE NAME OF THIS DISEASE TELLS YOU PRECISELY WHAT IT IS: the degeneration of the macula, the central and most sensitive part of the retina, the nerve-rich area at the back of the eye that's needed for sight. If you develop macular degeneration, then you'll have blurred areas right in the center of your vision—and without clear central vision, tasks such as driving a car or reading become extremely difficult because you can't look where you want to see!

Macular degeneration, also known as age-related macular degeneration (AMD), is the leading cause of vision loss for Americans over the age of 60, according to the Institute of Medicine. There's no pain associated with AMD, and once you develop the condition, treatment can slow the loss of vision but not restore vision already lost. Sometimes people developing AMD experience hallucinations of patterns or geometric shapes, a phenomenon called Charles Bonnet syndrome.

The causes of macular degeneration are varied, and contributing factors include age, gender (women develop AMD more frequently than men), race (AMD is more common among whites, especially after age 75), family history, smoking, obesity, exposure to sunlight, and low levels of nutrients. While you can't do much about your age, race, gender, and family history, you can stop smoking, bring your weight down to healthy levels, and get more of the right nutrients.

Healing Foods for Macular Degeneration

★★**Broccoli (and other cabbage relatives) and spinach (and other beet relatives)** Multiple studies have shown that consumption of carotenoids—natural pigments that color vegetables yellow, orange, and red—are associated with a lower risk of developing AMD, and two carotenoids in particular stand out from the pack: lutein and zeaxanthin. These two carotenoids accumulate in the retina and other ocular tissues and are thought to prevent oxidative damage caused by free radicals. They might also aid in protecting the retina by filtering out blue light, which isn't stopped by the cornea and may damage the retina over time.

The FDA hasn't established Daily Values for lutein and zeaxanthin, but Macular Degeneration Support, a nonprofit organization that provides information about the condition, recommends taking 20 milligrams of lutein and 6 to 10 milligrams of zeaxanthin daily. These carotenoids are listed together in the US Department of Agriculture database of nutrient data. Broccoli and spinach are both decent suppliers, with 1.3 milligrams of lutein and zeaxanthin in a cup of broccoli and 3.6 milligrams in a cup of spinach. (The only risk from an overdose of lutein is carotenoderma, yellow-orange discoloration of the skin. If you cut down on the foods that contain lutein, this unnatural coloring will vanish over time.)

★★**Kale, collard greens, and turnip greens (all cabbage relatives)** What's better than broccoli and spinach when you want to add more lutein and zeaxanthin to your diet? Kale, collard greens, and turnip greens, all leafy, dark-green vegetables that don't get nearly enough press compared with the spinach loved by Popeye and the broccoli disliked by President Bush. A cup of kale has more than 26 milligrams of lutein and zeaxanthin, a cup of collard greens has 3.2 milligrams, and a cup of turnip greens (not the turnips themselves) has 7 milligrams.

★★**Salmon, mackerel, sardines, and tuna** This fishy line-up contains an oceanful of vitamin D, something that a 2007 study in the *Archives of Ophthalmology* showed had an inverse relationship with AMD—participants who had the highest levels of vitamin D had lower incidences of AMD.

The study's authors suggest that more research is needed, but there's no reason to keep these fine finned fellows from your plate since a 3.5-ounce piece of cooked salmon has 360 International Units (IU) of vitamin D, which is 90 percent of the

Daily Value recommended by the FDA (400 IU). The same amount of cooked mackerel has 345 IU, or just under 90 percent of the Daily Value, while 1.75 ounces of canned sardines has 250 IU and 3 ounces of tuna fish has 200 IU. A study from 2003 in the same journal revealed that patients in the early or intermediate stages of AMD who had a high fish intake had a lower risk of progressing to advanced AMD.

The king of vitamin D is another seafood-related item, but despite its containing 1,360 IU per tablespoon, or 340 percent of the Daily Value, I find it hard to recommend cod liver oil to anyone who still has functioning taste buds.

Memory Loss

IT MAY NOT BE AS LIKELY AS DEATH AND TAXES, but memory loss is right up there on the list of things you're probably going to have to deal with if you live long enough. You lose some brain cells here and there as you journey through life, and the natural chemicals that keep your brain well lubed and working properly diminish somewhat. So you're apt to misplace your keys or forget a name now and again.

Then in your senior years, you face an increasing risk of developing dementia. Although it's commonly associated with deteriorating memory, dementia is more than that. It can also change your behavior, personality, and ability to think clearly.

The most common cause of dementia in older people is Alzheimer's disease, which is marked by brain shrinkage and the appearance of physical signs in the brain called plaques and tangles. Plaques are clumps of protein that develop between brain cells, and tangles are strands within the cells that become twisted. Experts still haven't figured out what causes Alzheimer's, but once you hit 65, your risk of developing it doubles every 5 years.

Another common cause of age-related memory problems is multi-infarct dementia, also called vascular dementia. This results from either a series of small clogs in the vessels that feed blood to the brain or the rupture of a vessel. Keeping your blood vessels healthy and resistant to stroke will reduce your risk of this memory robber (and possibly Alzheimer's, too).

Healing Foods for Memory Loss

Fortunately, there's a lot you can do a lot in the kitchen, garden, and dining room to help protect your memory. Here are some ideas.

★★★**Black-eyed peas** More and more, we learn that homocysteine contributes to many maladies, and Alzheimer's may be one of them. According to the American Heart Association, this amino acid may be linked to coronary heart disease, strokes, and peripheral artery disease (a problem related to poor blood flow in the legs). Fortunately, a variety of plant foods, including black-eyed peas, may offer some protection.

A 2005 study involving older men, published in the *American Journal of Clinical Nutrition,* found that high levels of homocysteine and low levels of folate and vitamins B_6 and B_{12} indicated an increased risk of cognitive decline. A more recent study reported in the *Archives of Neurology* found that people who consumed adequate amounts of folate (400 micrograms or more a day) had a 50 percent lower risk of Alzheimer's. Another study of 3,000 adults of all ages found that nearly 20 percent were deficient in B_{12}, and memory loss can be one of the earliest symptoms of this deficiency.

As you can see, eating more foods rich in folate (a B vitamin also called folic acid) and vitamins B_6 and B_{12} is among the most important changes you can make in your diet. In addition to black-eyed peas, other good sources of folate (from strongest to weakest) include lentils, avocados, sunflower seeds, spinach, asparagus, and orange juice. A mixed bean soup containing just 1½ cups of black-eyed peas, chickpeas, lentils, lima beans, and pinto beans would provide more than the recommended daily intake of 400 micrograms.

FOODS TO WATCH

People who enjoy alcohol know about the double-edged sword of drinking: A little can be pleasant, but too much makes you feel terrible. The same goes for drinking and your cognitive health.

Light to moderate drinking has been associated with a lower risk of ischemic stroke—the most common kind, which is caused by blockages in blood vessels—and dementia. But if you drink more than a moderate amount, your risk of both these problems rises. Plus, in terms of your day-to-day memory, excessive drinking certainly isn't going to help you stay sharp.

If you're going to drink with an eye toward protecting your health, "moderate" means two drinks or less a day for guys and one a day for women. And from age 65 on, everyone should stick to one a day at most.

Good food sources of B_{12} include clams, beef liver, fortified cereals, and trout. For B_6, they include baked potatoes, chickpeas, and sunflower seeds.

★★★**Plant oils** Some research in animals has linked diets higher in monounsaturated and polyunsaturated fats and lower in saturated fats with improved cognitive performance. With this in mind, researchers reporting on a study in the *Archives of Neurology* gave 815 older folks a questionnaire about their food intake, then checked back with them a few years later. They found that a diet higher in saturated fat (found in meat, butter, and high-fat dairy foods) and trans fats (found in baked snack foods, margarine, and shortening) was associated with a higher risk of Alzheimer's. Conversely, unsaturated fats may have a protective effect.

This may be because eating trans fats decreases high-density lipoprotein ("good" cholesterol) and raises low-density lipoprotein ("bad" cholesterol), while eating unsaturated fats, such as those found in many plant oils, has an opposite, beneficial effect. Other research has shown a lower risk of Alzheimer's among people taking cholesterol drugs called statins, so a healthful diet's effects on your cholesterol may play a role in Alzheimer's disease.

Try to get more of your fat calories from a moderate amount of fats like those in olive, canola, peanut, and sunflower oils and avocados, peanut butter, nuts, and seeds.

★★**Citrus fruits** You just can't say enough about the protection that plant foods offer your mind and body. Some researchers believe that the protein fragments in the brain plaques that form in Alzheimer's create free radicals that cause damage in the brain. Antioxidant vitamins and other phytochemicals, such as polyphenols, found in fruits and vegetables may help protect your brain cells from damage.

A 2006 study involving more than 1,800 Japanese Americans found that drinking fruit and vegetable juice at least three times weekly was associated with a 76 percent reduction in Alzheimer's risk compared with those who drank juices less than once a week.

Another study, which followed 5,395 older Netherlands residents for several years, found that those with high intakes of vitamins C and E had a lower risk of Alzheimer's. The authors' theory was that the antioxidants could reduce free radical–related DNA damage, death of cells, and plaque development in the brain. Another study of 4,700 people, at Johns Hopkins University in Baltimore, found that those who took supplements of vitamins C and E were 64 percent less likely to develop Alzheimer's.

Supplements of vitamins C and E aren't the ideal way to get your antioxidants, though. Fruits and vegetables are good sources of C, plus they have thousands of other components that work together to achieve powerful antioxidant effects. The recommended daily intake for vitamin C is 75 milligrams for women and 90 milligrams for men; for vitamin E, it's 15 milligrams for men and women. Here are good sources of vitamins C and E, measured in milligrams.

Vitamin C

1 papaya—188

1 cup orange juice—124

1 cup cooked broccoli—101

1 cup strawberries—98

1 kiwifruit—71

Vitamin E

1 cup raisin bran cereal—13.5

1 cup canned tomato paste—11

¼ cup sunflower seeds—8

1 ounce almonds—7

1 cup canned spinach—4

★★**Grapes and tea** Resveratrol, a polyphenol found in grapes and red wine, has shown anti-inflammatory and antioxidant properties. That may be why modest consumption of red wine can lower your risk of heart disease and may also help ward off Alzheimer's. Population studies have associated moderate wine consumption with a lower Alzheimer's risk. Lab studies have shown that resveratrol reduces free radicals that result from a buildup of the "gunk" that creates cell-killing plaques in the brain.

Catechins, found in tea, may work synergistically with resveratrol—which means the sum adds up to more than the parts. Combining polyphenols may boost your protection from harm caused by plaques, according to a 2006 review in the *European Journal of Pharmacology*.

As you can see in "Foods to Watch" on page 265, drinking alcohol in excess has been linked to a greater Alzheimer's risk, so more red wine is not better. But if you enjoy the occasional glass and have several cups of green tea daily, your refreshment habits may just give you some brain protection. In addition, grapes contain a host of other chemicals that may help protect you from Alzheimer's, including some that may prevent those clumps in your brain, prevent blockages in your arteries, reduce inflammation and free radical damage, and protect brain cells.

★★**Pomegranates** Animal studies have demonstrated that drinking pomegranate juice may lead to better mental functioning. (It worked for the mice at least.) My database reveals that pomegranates contain salicylates, ellagic acid, polyphenols, and many other chemicals that act against inflammation, oxidation, and other harmful processes. Try some pomegranate juice today or dig into the seed-laden fruits themselves.

★★**Sage** Part of the botanical name of this spice, *Salvia officinalis,* comes from the Latin for "to save." If you want to save your memory, sage may help. Research with healthy young people found that those who took a sage oil extract performed better on a memory test an hour later than those who took a placebo.

In another study, albeit a small one, patients with Alzheimer's took either a tincture of sage or a placebo for 4 months. Those in the sage group showed improved mental functioning.

Sage may have an effect by blocking enzymes that break down a particular neurotransmitter in the brain. This neurotransmitter, acetylcholine, appears in lower amounts in people with Alzheimer's. Sage may also help protect your brain by discouraging the creation of free radicals and counteracting inflammation.

Include sage in recipes or simply add a teaspoon to a cup of hot water and let it steep for a few minutes, then strain and drink it.

★★**Turmeric** Population studies have hinted that people in India may have a much lower incidence of Alzheimer's because of the large amounts of turmeric they use in their cooking. This yellow-orange spice, derived from a root, has anti-inflammatory and antioxidant effects that may counteract the inflammation and oxidation found in Alzheimer's disease. It also, by the way, gives curry dishes a kick.

Mice who ate a diet containing curcumin (an active ingredient in turmeric) for 6 months showed 50 percent less plaque buildup in their brains. Other research found that a 2-month diet containing curcumin prevented memory deficits in rats. In a 2006 paper published in the *European Journal of Pharmacology,* the author states that curcumin should be able to get into the brain, where it can help prevent plaques from forming.

★**Blueberries** I can't promise that blueberries are magically going to protect your memory, but they may help, and they taste great. Animal studies have shown that diets containing blueberry extracts may improve mental performance. It's possible that the powerful antioxidants in blueberries could help keep your brain healthy.

★**Celery** In the summer of 2008, researchers reported that a compound called luteolin had shown promise for lowering levels of plaque-forming proteins in the brain. My database points to celery as a source of luteolin and many other components that could conceivably counteract risk factors for Alzheimer's, including atherosclerosis, inflammation, and oxidative damage.

So toss some celery into your cart the next time you wheel through the produce section. And while you're in the store, get some flaxseed to grind into your oatmeal, since flax also contains luteolin.

★**Garlic** According to research, aged garlic extract may help reduce the risk of cardiovascular disease and dementia by working as an antioxidant, reducing inflammation and cholesterol production, inhibiting blood clotting, decreasing homocysteine, and improving circulation. If you're concerned about memory loss, it's time to brush up on Italian, Asian, and other recipes that make liberal use of garlic.

★**Ginger** Although appearance-wise, it's kind of a homely root, ginger contains more than two dozen antioxidants and two dozen anti-inflammatory compounds. A 2004 laboratory study suggests that ginger extract can slow brain inflammation triggered by plaques. It's a long way between manipulating a few cells in a lab dish and protecting an actual brain, but it's reasonable to think that ginger could offer something helpful when it comes to preserving your memory. Enjoy some candied ginger, brew up some tea with ginger root, or just use the spice liberally in your recipes.

From the Herbal Medicine Chest

The herb ginkgo may have anti-inflammatory and antioxidant abilities that make it useful in treating Alzheimer's disease. It may also help neurotransmitters in the brain work properly. While some research has found a modest benefit for Alzheimer's, ginkgo may increase your risk of bleeding. This risk may be higher if you're taking aspirin, warfarin (Coumadin), or other blood-thinning drugs.

Menopause

WHAT A DIFFERENCE A DECADE MAKES. Even as I drafted the menopause chapter for *The Green Pharmacy*, it was clear that many scientists were already beginning to poke holes in the hormone replacement therapy (HRT) bubble. As I wrote then, I had misgivings about HRT. Although the female sex hormone estrogen evidently relieved hot flashes, vaginal dryness, and other discomforts of menopause, a good deal of research showed, even then, that it increased a woman's risk of getting breast cancer. Still, the vast majority of doctors prescribed HRT.

Many of those doctors were prescribing HRT, not for hot flashes, but for off-label uses—to reduce the risks for dementia, heart disease, and osteoporosis. Mrs. Duke never had a problem with hot flashes (married to a cold turkey like me), but she took HRT for some 2 to 3 years thinking it might reduce her risk of heart disease and osteoporosis. Then, around 2002, the flip-flop started when it was revealed that HRT did NOT protect against either condition. In 2003, researchers reported that, rather than preventing dementia, HRT doubled the risk. The number of women taking HRT dropped sharply because of a deservedly increased perception of risk. Ironically, in 2003, we saw the first big drop in breast cancer, thanks not to the "war on cancer," another quagmire, but to discontinuation of pharmaceutical HRT.

In February 25, 2008, *NBC Nightly News* further punctured the already deflated bubble with more bad news for HRT. The research showed that taking HRT for even a short period increased breast density, making mammograms more difficult and less reliable. The commentator cautioned that if you and your doctor decide that HRT is still right for you, insist on the lowest possible dose for the shortest possible period.

Back when I wrote *The Green Pharmacy*, before the HRT bubble burst, many complementary and alternative medicine practitioners, and herbalists like me, were suggesting using phytoestrogens as a safer alternative to HRT. And by 2002 there was evidence that the phytoestrogens prevented heart disease and osteoporosis whereas HRT did not. But as almost always, there were no third-arm clinical trials to prove that phytoestrogens were better than HRT and placebo for heart disease, dementia, hot flashes, and osteoporosis. Naturally, some soy industry–supported

FOODS TO WATCH

Some foods are classic triggers for hot flashes. When it comes to temperature and spiciness, hot foods are likely to bring on a hot flash, says Mary Jane Minkin, MD, clinical professor of obstetrics and gynecology at Yale University School of Medicine and author of *A Woman's Guide to Menopause and Perimenopause*. It's a good idea to avoid hot beverages, such as coffee or hot soups. The same goes for spicy foods, such as hot wings and some Asian and Mexican food.

Red wine is another classic trigger of hot flashes. If you're going to drink wine, go for a white variety.

studies hinted that soy (which attains my highest synergy score for menopausal difficulties) may be helpful. For more than a decade, I have stridently argued and shown, along with my chemical colleague Peter Kaufman, PhD, and his associates, that most of our more edible legumes have many of the same phytoestrogens as soy, often at even higher levels.

Healing Foods for Menopause

★★★**Pomegranate** I suspect the pomegranate might ease menopausal symptoms even be better than HRT. The ancient Biblical fruit probably contains a wider variety of phytoestrogens than any other plant, according to Robert Newman, PhD, and Ephraim Lansky, MD, in their book *Pomegranate: The Most Medicinal Fruit.* They call pomegranate seed "a rich source of safe bioactive phytoestrogens that may help women maintain their reproductive and menopausal health."

Pomegranate seed oil has been said to contain more estrogen than any other plant source, and may also even contain testosterone. But the reports of testosterone need confirmation. My sources say pomegranate contains apigenin (with progesteronic activity), coumestrol, daidzein, estradiol, estriol, estrone, genistein, kaempferol, luteolin (58 percent as potent as genistein), naringenin, quercetin, sitosterol, and stigmasterol. Some are strong human-identical hormones. Some are very weak phytoestrogens. Pomegranate may contain as much as 17 parts per million (milligrams per kilogram) of human-identical estrone, as well as 0.017 to 0.76 milligrams of coumestrol per kilogram. Some of these may bind to the beta-estrogen receptor, which should raise a warning flag for women targeted for estrogen receptor–positive breast cancer.

This leads me to guess that pomegranate might have the desirable effects of HRT but few or none of the undesirable effects, except for those estrogen receptor–positive women. Almost a decade ago, I calculated that a single estrone-rich pomegranate fruit could be as potent as 2 days of HRT pills. Today I confirm that possibility.

★★**Black bean** For an alternative to soy beans, try eating black beans to reduce your hot flashes. They contain about the same amount of phytoestrogens, and they can be cooked into great-tasting soups or sprinkled into salads.

Hot flashes and other menopausal symptoms are rare in vegetarian cultures, especially among people who consume a lot of legumes, such as black beans, mung beans, and soybeans. The reason may be the phytoestrogen compounds, including isoflavones, lignans, phytosterols, and saponins. In addition to acting like estrogen in women whose own sex hormone production has declined, phytoestrogens also appear to reduce the risk of estrogen-linked cancers, such as breast cancer. Animal experiments show that phytoestrogens are extremely effective in preventing tumors of the breast tissue.

★★**Flaxseed** Another source of phytoestrogens, flaxseed seems to help relieve hot flashes and sleep problems, two common menopausal problems. Flaxseed contains a large amount of estrogenic lignans that may have antioxidant properties, which means they may help menopausal women fight cancer.

In a recent phase II pilot study at the Mayo Clinic in Rochester, Minnesota, 28 women with frequent hot flashes (14 or more a week for more than a month) ate 40 grams of crushed flaxseed per day (4 tablespoons sprinkled on food or mixed with liquids) for 6 weeks. By the end of the study, the women's hot flashes decreased by an average of 57 percent and the frequency of their hot flashes decreased by 50 percent. The women also reported greater quality of life and less fatigue, anxiety, and anger.

Although the flaxseed seemed to reduce their hot flashes, many of the women in this study reported gastrointestinal problems. So the researchers recommend starting with smaller servings of flaxseed and gradually increasing the amount.

You might try adding a tablespoon of ground flaxseed to your cereal or on top of your salads, or bake it into bread and muffins.

★★**Soy** It's clear that soy has the best evidence base among the legumes I have reviewed for menopause. That's probably because soy has been more intensively studied, thanks to the soy industry. One review of studies on nonhormonal therapies for hot flashes in menopause found that prescription antidepressants (selective serotonin reuptake inhibitors and venlafaxine) reduce hot flashes 19 to 60 percent while soy isoflavones reduce hot flashes 9 to 40 percent in some trials, often no better than placebo.

The herbs black cohosh and red clover, commonly recommended as a remedy for hot flashes, also have had inconsistent results, with some trials showing benefit and some no difference compared with placebo. Soy isoflavones, black cohosh, and red clover were well tolerated in clinical trials. Other herbal agents commonly recommended for menopausal symptoms include dong quai, evening primrose oil, ginseng, and wild yam, with few published data on their effectiveness. Of these, only the soy shows up in supermarkets.

A survey by Tieraona Low Dog, MD, herbal expert and author of *Complementary and Integrative Approaches to Women's Health—A Clinical Guide,* was equally unkind to soy, based on the results of six clinical studies on isoflavone extracts. One study even challenged the long-term safety of high-dose soy isoflavone extract (150 milligrams per day for 5 years) on the uterine endometrium. Soy isoflavone extracts appear to have "minimal to no effect."

My conclusion: soy money talks like Big Pharma money talks. The therapy that has the most research money behind it gets the most press and hence the higher scores.

★**Celery and herbs in the celery family** Celery and dill, fennel, and anise, all tasty herbs of the celery family, are four more in the long list of mildly estrogenic herbs, due to the gently estrogenic phytochemical anethole. They all have some 40 to 50 phytochemicals. The gentle estrogenic compounds are a mix of various frequently recurring mild estrogens: anethole apigenin, kaempferol, luteolin, and quercetin. I think of it as a very healthful tea that is good for what ails you.

★**Walnut** Walnuts contain high amounts of omega-3 fatty acids that may help prevent serious health problems, such as heart disease, cancer, and rheumatoid arthritis. They also play a role in improving mood and sharpening memory, which can help during menopausal moments. Even better, a recent review of studies on dietary omega-3 fatty acids for women concluded that omega-3 fatty acids could help prevent postmenopausal hot flushes and premenstrual syndrome.

Flaxseed is also a good source of short-chain omega-3's—as are, of all things, the chia pet seeds. Many bean species have some alpha-linolenic acid at lower levels. Of course, fish, especially salmon, tuna, mackerel, lake trout, herring, and sardines, is high in two kinds of omega-3 fatty acids: eicosapentaenoic acid (EPA) and docosahexaenoic acid (DHA). How about a dinner of walnut-encrusted salmon with a three-bean salad? I'll not suggest you graze your chia pet.

From the Herbal Medicine Chest

Licorice (Glycyrrhiza glabra) contains natural estrogenic compounds. Like the isoflavones in soy, glycyrrhizin, the active ingredient in licorice, appears to reduce estrogen levels in women when they're too high and increase the levels when they're too low.

If you'd rather get your licorice from candy, make sure to read the label. Although many health food stores carry candies made from pure licorice, most licorice candy sold in the United States contains extracts of licorice plus anise, a spice that produces a licorice-like flavor. Anise contains a weak phytochemical (anethole) that is less estrogenic than glycyrrhizin.

Licorice and its extracts are safe to use in moderate amounts, but if you're planning to use licorice long term or in larger amounts, watch out for potential side effects, such as headache, lethargy, sodium, water retention, excessive loss of potassium, and high blood pressure. If you like licorice, it's hard to stop munching on it, but you'll just have to control yourself. A safe daily dose is said to be 5 grams, or less than a quarter-ounce.

Menstrual Cramps

MENSTRUAL CRAMPS AFFECT MORE THAN HALF OF ALL WOMEN who have menstrual periods. Approximately 5 to 15 percent of them have cramps so painful it interferes with daily activities. You can blame menstrual cramps on the hormone-like chemicals known as prostaglandins produced by the uterus. Prostaglandins make the uterine muscles contract and shed the lining that has built up during the menstrual cycle.

Some women make more prostaglandins or are more sensitive to them than other women. So they may have stronger, more frequent, and more painful uterine muscle contractions, causing cramps during the first day or two of their period. Menstrual cramps may also come with nausea, vomiting, diarrhea, headaches, weakness, and even fainting.

Nonsteroidal anti-inflammatory drugs (NSAIDs), such as aspirin and ibuprofen, are the usual treatment to decrease prostaglandin activity. But, like some women, you may find the usual painkillers don't relieve the pain. Rest and a heating pad or hot water bottle to the lower abdomen or back may help. In addition, a well-balanced diet and the following food remedies work well for some women.

Healing Foods for Menstrual Cramps

★★★**Walnut, flax, hemp, chia, chiso** These foods contain omega-3 fatty acids, which may help relieve some cramping. They are good sources of the short-chain omega-3 fatty acids (alpha-linolenic acid). But the higher-chain fatty acids found in such fish as mackerel, lake trout, herring, sardines, albacore tuna, and salmon may be the better choice. Many studies suggest that fish oil from cold-water fish has a positive effect on pain symptoms. These cold-water fish are high in the omega-3 fatty acids, eicosapentaenoic acid (EPA) and docosahexaenoic acid (DHA), that reduce inflammation and pain. This may help ease menstrual cramps.

In one study, scientists at the Division of Adolescent Medicine, Children's Hospital Medical Center, Cincinnati, Ohio, randomly assigned 42 adolescent girls who had menstrual cramps to two groups. In the first group, 21 girls took fish-oil supplements (1,080 milligrams of eicosapentaenoic acid, 720 milligrams of docosahexaenoic acid, and 1.5 milligrams of vitamin E) daily for 2 months, followed by a placebo for 2 more months. Another group of 21 girls took a placebo for the first 2 months, followed by fish-oil supplements for 2 more months. After 2 months of treatment with fish oil, the girls experienced markedly reduced symptoms.

Along with eating more fish, you might be wondering about fish-oil supplements. If my daughter was looking for a fish-oil supplement, I'd suggest krill oil from Antarctic krill (a zooplankton crustacean).

★★**Broccoli, kale, collard greens, bok choy, and other members of the cabbage family** These foods may help prevent the muscular contractions that cause cramping because of their calcium content, says research psychologist James G. Penland, PhD, a research psychologist and professor at the US Department of Agriculture Human Nutrition Research Center, University of North Dakota.

When most people think of calcium, they think dairy foods, and you can certainly get the recommended amounts of the mineral from foods such as low-fat yogurt and skim or low-fat milk. Keep in mind, though, that some doctors believe the estrogen content in cow's milk can worsen premenstrual symptoms. If you suspect your symptoms might be related to cow's milk, try leafy greens instead. On a dry-weight basis, leaves are our best sources of calcium. Other foods that contain calcium include almonds, black beans, navy beans, broadbean, watercress, licorice, savory, red clover shoots, thyme, Chinese cabbage, basil, celery (seed), and dandelion.

★★**Ginger** Ginger tea is a trustworthy remedy for menstrual cramps. Even Eclectic physicians—who advocated the use of botanicals, particularly Native American herbs—prescribed ginger for painful menstruation early in the 20th century. Famous Eclectics H.W. Felter, MD, and J.I. Lloyd, PhD, said that ginger tea was a popular

FOODS TO WATCH

Although scientific evidence is inconclusive, some women find that reducing their intake of salt, sugar, and caffeine eases cramping during the week before their period. Limiting salt may also help reduce bloating.

and efficient remedy for "relieving the pangs of disordered menstruation." Used as an agent to stimulate menstrual flow from Venezuela to Vietnam, ginger contains at least six analgesic and six anticramping compounds.

You could slice up fresh ginger root to make a tea and add a few drops of honey and lemon to taste. Or mix it with other herbs known for easing menstrual cramps, such as chasteberry and clover flowers. Red clover (*Trifolium pratense*) is rich in phytoestrogens, plant chemicals that act on the body in the same way as the female hormone estrogen. Herbalists believe that phytoestrogens help minimize menstrual cramps by bringing the body's hormone levels into better balance.

★**Guava, bell pepper, and thyme** These foods are surprisingly high in fiber, which may have a positive effect on menstrual cramps. A small Japanese study looked at the associations of menstrual cramps and intakes of dietary fiber, soy, and fat to evaluate their biological effects on estrogens or prostaglandin production. The researchers concluded that women who ate more fiber had significantly less menstrual pain than women who did not.

From the Herbal Medicine Chest

Black haw (*Viburnum prunifolium*) Related to honeysuckle and elderberry, black haw is a spreading shrub with clusters of white flowers. This herb (also known as cramp bark) was recognized as a treatment for menstrual cramps in most pharmacology reference books through the 19th century. The bark contains at least four substances that help relax the uterus. Two (aesculetin and scopoletin) also help relieve muscle spasms. With so much folklore and science to recommend it, black haw would be one of the first remedies that I'd suggest to my daughter if she came to me complaining of cramps.

Nausea

A FRIEND AND COWORKER, a registered nurse at the USDA, once asked me what to take for nausea, hinting that she was asking on behalf of a friend. Without even thinking, I immediately suggested ginger. Six months later, she casually said the ginger had worked. I then realized that she herself had been receiving cancer chemotherapy and coping with its nauseating side effects. That was several years before I saw published studies showing that ginger was helpful in chemotherapy-induced nausea. As a responsible grandmother, my friend would probably have rejected my second suggestion, marijuana, which I truly think is the best thing out there for that kind of nausea.

Beyond chemotherapy, there are a number of other things that cause nausea, that horrible gastric sensation that makes you feel like you're going to vomit. They include infections of the digestive tract (gastroenteritis), inner ear disorders, over-indulgence in alcohol or foods, intestinal parasites, morning sickness during pregnancy, emotional distress, toxic overloads of the liver, and motion sickness.

The word *nausea* comes from the Greek word *naus,* meaning "ship," suggesting that ancient Greek sailors struggled with seasickness. This kind of motion sickness results when your brain gets mixed signals—it feels as if it is sitting or standing still, yet it's actually moving in a boat, plane, or car. As a result, you feel tired, dizzy, and nauseated, which could lead to vomiting.

Controlling motion sickness is easy: Simply avoid the motion. But if you have to go in the boat, plane, or car, limit sensations of motion by positioning yourself carefully. On a ship, the most motionless part is the middle of the deck; on a plane, it's between the wings; and in a car, I believe it's the middle of the front seat. On one bus near the Amazon, I found the backseat to be the worst place for motion sickness; the front was much better.

Whether the cause is motion or something else, frequently, one good regurgitation is sometimes all it takes to relieve nausea. But in other cases, nausea persists even after the stomach has emptied, and though you try to vomit, nothing comes up—the dry heaves.

Sometimes eating will allay nausea. If you decide to try this, Sharon Walker, RD, director of nutrition at the Cancer Treatment Centers of America, who works with cancer patients dealing with nausea, suggests you eat small frequent snacks that are low in fat (fat is hard to digest). She also recommends avoiding spicy foods and foods with a strong odor. If you do vomit, drink fluids (but no milk or any other dairy product) to stay hydrated. Then, when the regurgitation stops, eat broth and unbuttered whole-grain toast, graduating to brown rice, potatoes, soups, steamed veggies, and yogurt.

Healing Foods for Nausea

For nausea or motion sickness that just won't quit—or to prevent the discomfort in the first place—here are some foods you can try.

★★★**Ginger** In *The Green Pharmacy*, ginger was numero uno for nausea, and it's still number one here. Ginger is a perennial plant native to the Orient but now widely cultivated in the tropics. It's the rhizome (the botanical term for an underground stem) of the ginger plant that contains the healing powers.

There are multiple studies to back up ginger's stomach-soothing abilities. One done at the UCLA Medical Center found ginger to be an effective remedy for nausea and vomiting due to either motion sickness or pregnancy. A British study found ginger to be better than both Dramamine and a placebo at relieving motion sickness. Research published in the *Journal of Travel Medicine* found that 500 milligrams of ginger prevented seasickness and the need for motion sickness medications in 1,741 tourists on a 6-hour whale-watching boat trip. A study done in Thailand showed that a dose of at least 1 gram of ginger was more effective than a placebo at preventing postoperative nausea and vomiting. And recent research shows that ginger appears to be as effective as metoclorpramide (Reglan, Clopra) for reducing nausea and vomiting caused by chemotherapy. As a bonus for chemotherapy patients, test-tube studies have shown that ginger may also provide some protection against cancer.

The pungent constituents of the ginger root—gingerols and shogaols—give ginger its tummy-taming powers. To harness these powers, food farmacists might either eat candied ginger; drink ginger ale, ginger beer, or ginger tea; swallow ½ to 1 teaspoon of crushed ginger; or take capsules or tincture of ginger. I've used ginger, and it works. Sometimes I munch it raw, but chances are that you'd prefer a few teaspoons in tea. If you buy a commercial product, make sure it contains real ginger by checking the label. Products containing ginger "flavoring" won't necessarily work.

★★★**Peppermint** Peppermint and ginger compete for my vote as best motion sickness and nausea remedy. Looking at morning sickness rather than motion sickness in a clinical situation, Canadian scientist Rachel Westphal found that peppermint worked as well for pregnant women as mixtures of peppermint and ginger or pure ginger did. With more than a half dozen gas-reducing carminatives (stomach-settling agents), more than a dozen gentle pain relievers, and even more sedative and tranquilizing compounds, peppermint offers a multiple whammy against tummy troubles.

Overall, peppermint seems to stop muscle spasms in the digestive tract, including those involved in vomiting. The oil found in peppermint leaves appears to block the transmission of nausea impulses from the brain to the stomach as well as sedate an irritated digestive tract. And the tannins in the mint help reduce stomach inflammation. You can easily make a cup of peppermint tea by steeping 1 to 2 teaspoons of dried leaves in a cup of boiling water for 10 minutes.

★★**Cinnamon** Cinnamon contains the antiemetic camphor and two carminatives (eugenol and safrole). It also contains chemicals called catechins, which help relieve nausea. This Old Testament herb also appears in folkloric traditions as a nausea

TravelTea

Before you head out on a potentially nausea-inducing excursion, I recommend you mix up some TravelTea. Generously cover a handful of peppermint (or other closely related mint species), shave in two small pieces of ginger, sprinkle on some powdered cinnamon, and add some of these other anti-nausea culinary herbs to taste: anise, hyssop, cilantro, coriander, fennel, nutmeg, rosemary, sage, sweet Annie, and tamarind.

remedy, and cinnamon toast or tea is one of the first things Mrs. Duke seeks in the morning when her digestion is upset. I suspect she'd join me in preventive ginger tea with cinnamon and peppermint if she ever lured me onto one of those cruises she so longs for and I so dread.

★★**Coriander** Although there is a little less scientific evidence supporting coriander than there is for fennel (but about as many promising phytochemicals), it does contain the antiemetic camphor and the carminatives carvone and thymol. I wouldn't hesitate to add coriander to any stomach-settling preparation I was concocting.

★★**Fennel** I have often thought of the celery family as a stomach-settling family, and fennel, celery, and coriander are outstanding carminatives in this group. An Ayurvedic herb, fennel may appeal to Asian Indians, whose restaurants here in the United States often offer fennel seeds to settle the stomach and improve the breath. It could also improve the ride home for those prone to motion sickness. You can chew well up to 20 raw seeds, just the way they come in Indian restaurants, to settle the stomach. In addition to a strong supporting cast of phytochemical players (I won't name them all), fennel also contains the camphor.

★★**Oregano** A great culinary herb, oregano contains camphor plus carvacrol, carvone, eugenol, and thymol, carminatives that work in concert (synergistically) with a half dozen sedatives and dozens of painkillers.

★**Cayenne** In addition to spicing up a variety of foods, cayenne pepper is a proven remedy for motion sickness. At the first sign of motion-related nausea, take a teaspoon of cayenne dissolved in a teaspoon of olive oil.

★**Chamomile** We can infer chamomile's great reputation in folklore for treating nausea from the way it settled the tummy of the tumultuous Brer Rabbit. Linda

White, MD, coauthor of *The Herbal Drugstore*, recommends it for nausea in children. Costa Ricans take the tea for nausea, menstrual cramps, and stomachache. I'd be remiss if I didn't say that paradoxically, highly concentrated hot chamomile tea is reportedly emetic (it can make you throw up). I suspect, as with most herbs and pharmaceuticals, it will help some folks and not others.

★**Citrus fruits** To prevent motion sickness, some experts suggest sucking on a citrus fruit, or even a citrus peel, to make the mouth dry. One practitioner suggests sipping small amounts of lemon or lime juice, strong green tea, or ginger tea. I'd just combine them with as many of the above-mentioned spices as I could find in the pantry.

★**Dates** The sugar fructose is described as anti-nauseant and for that reason has been suggested for hangovers. Dates can contain more than 30 percent fructose, chicory roots, 22 percent; onion bulbs, 16 percent; tamarind and turmeric, 12 percent; orange, 2.4 percent; hops, 2 percent; and grapefruit, 1.2 percent.

★**Hempseed** Available online at $13 a pound, organic hempseed may contain a few of the chemicals that make cannabis (illegal in this country) a very effective three–star, evidence-based antiemetic. The plant does contain antiemetic camphor, and nutritionally speaking, the seeds are rich in protein and omega-3 fatty acids.

★**Honey** If ginger doesn't work for your nausea, Jim LaValle, ND, a pharmacist, naturopathic physician, and founder of the LaValle Metabolic Institute in Cincinnati, says that honey can settle your stomach, too. When nausea or nausea and vomiting strike, he suggests taking a teaspoon of raw honey each hour for a few hours.

★**Raspberry** Raspberry tea leaf is widely recommended for nausea associated with morning sickness, and some herbalists also suggest it for motion sickness. I have no problem with this. In fact, ginger and raspberry teas mix nicely.

★**Rosemary** With more than a half dozen stomach-settling carminatives, several compounds to calm anxiety, and more than a dozen phytochemicals to soothe pain, rosemary is worth adding to your TravelTea (see page 279). It's also a rich source of antiemetic camphor. I've often thought of the mint family, like the ginger family, as being stomach settlers, and sage and rosemary are outstanding in that regard.

★**Sage** With three carminatives to settle the stomach, several sedatives and tranquilizers to ease the mind, and more than a dozen phytochemicals to soothe aches and pains, sage may also have a place in your TravelTea. It's one of our richest culinary sources of antiemetic camphor (up to 0.93 percent).

★**Strawberry** Mike Adams, the Health Ranger, who often offers a whole string of foods and herbs for various ailments, gives strawberries a high score as a remedy for motion sickness. The leaves of the strawberry plant are also a wonderful remedy for stomach upset when dried and used in a tea. Use only 2 teaspoons of dried strawberry leaves to make the tea (avoid the stems) and steep for 20 minutes.

★**Tofu** Eating foods high in protein, such as tofu and other soy products, has been shown to help prevent and decrease nausea. In a study at Pennsylvania State University, participants who drank a good-tasting, 300-calorie protein shake 30 minutes before a motion sickness test had significantly fewer nausea symptoms than participants who drank water or a protein shake that wasn't as tasty. Therefore, the combination of protein and a pleasant taste seems effective for nausea control.

From the Herbal Medicine Chest

When his patients complain of nausea, Jim LaValle, ND, a pharmacist, naturopathic physician, and founder of the LaValle Metabolic Institute in Cincinnati, sometimes suggests they chew licorice. He particularly likes using deglycyrrhizinated licorice, or DGL. He says you can also try drinking licorice tea, so you might have a cup three times a day. If you are taking blood pressure medication, however, check with your doctor before taking any form of licorice.

Osteoarthritis

ARTHRITIC DISEASE—WHICH INCLUDES more than 100 different conditions—is the most common cause of disability in the United States. The most prevalent form is osteoarthritis. In fact, I have it myself. It's an incurable condition that starts with minor aches and pains and eventually leads to chronic pain, stiffness, swelling, and limited range of motion, usually in the knees, hips, spine, hands, and feet. My own first line of defense is to carry Zyflamend, an herbal supplement manufactured by New Chapter, with me in case of flare-ups.

As the American population has grown older and heavier, the incidence of osteoarthritis has skyrocketed. The most recent estimates, published in a 2008 issue of the journal *Arthritis and Rheumatism*, show that a whopping 27 million Americans have the disease—up from 21 million in 1995. That means that nearly 1 in 10

Americans are coping with distress that can dramatically affect quality of life and at worst lead to expensive joint-replacement surgery.

Obesity-related osteoarthritis has soared by 465 percent since 1971, which is partly due to a drastic increase in midlife obesity among baby boomers. About 30 percent of boomers are obese, while only 16 percent of their parents' generation were obese at midlife.

The financial toll of osteoarthritis and other musculoskeletal conditions—which include rheumatoid arthritis, fibromyalgia, carpal tunnel syndrome, gout, and back pain, among others—is an astounding $128 billion a year in lost wages and medical expenses. By the year 2030, it's estimated that 40 percent of American adults will be affected by some form of arthritic disease.

For about 25 percent of us, the most common source of pain is our joints, according to a nationwide survey of 1,200 adults conducted in 2005 by researchers at Stanford University School of Medicine.

Desperate for relief, many osteoarthritis patients try to manage their symptoms with high daily doses of over-the-counter nonsteroidal anti-inflammatory drugs (NSAIDs) such as aspirin and ibuprofen. Unfortunately, these can irritate the stomach lining and even cause severe gastrointestinal bleeding, which is difficult to manage and is often life-threatening. A widely cited study showed that NSAID-associated bleeding caused 16,500 deaths in the United States in 1999, a toll higher than that of AIDS.

When celecoxib (Celebrex) and other "super-aspirin" NSAIDs were introduced in the 1990s, they were widely touted as being safer than traditional NSAIDs. But recent research suggests that they are just as hard on the gastrointestinal system and may have serious cardiac side effects.

Healing Foods for Osteoarthritis

To help prevent osteoarthritis—or manage lingering or lessening pain—there are a number of food remedies that may prove useful.

★★★**Chile peppers** Hot peppers contain aspirin-like compounds known as salicylates, as well as a resinous and pungent substance known as capsaicin that triggers the release of opiate-like substances known as endorphins. When applied topically, capsaicin temporarily depletes substance P, a chemical in nerves that transmits pain sensations. Without substance P, pain signals have no way to travel. Dozens of studies show that capsaicin can temporarily relieve many painful conditions, including osteoarthritis.

You can buy a commercial topical cream containing 0.025 to 0.075 percent capsaicin and apply it to your arthritic joints three or four times a day. Or you

FOODS TO WATCH

can do what people outside the United States often do: buy a chile pepper, mash it, and apply it directly to affected areas. You can also mix mashed hot pepper with a skin moisturizer. Either way, you'll save money. A fresh pepper costs a few pennies, while a commercial capsaicin product such as Zostrix can cost up to $16.

No matter which method you choose, you may experience a burning sensation the first few times you use capsaicin, but it usually subsides with repeated use. Just be sure to thoroughly wash your hands after using it. Contact with your eyes, nose, or mouth may prove more painful than your arthritic joints.

Although capsaicin is best used topically, it may be helpful to add more peppers and pepper-derived hot sauces to your diet. Another option is taking a cayenne tincture (0.3 to 1 milliliter) three times per day. You also can make an infusion by stirring ½ to 1 teaspoon (2.5 to 5 grams) of cayenne powder into 1 cup of boiling water, letting it steep for 10 minutes, and taking 1 teaspoonful mixed with water three or four times daily.

I recently received a tip from a reader named Harriet Brennan, a retired nurse who had been taking the prescription NSAID diclofenac (Voltaren) for 13 years for her arthritis. She was able to dispense with the drug after trying a regimen that strikes me as a good herbal alternative to Celebrex. After removing the stems,

Harriett blends ½ pound of chile peppers with 2 cups of apple cider vinegar, then lets the mixture marinate for 3 weeks and strains it through cheesecloth. Once a day, she adds 16 drops of this pungent brew to a 24-ounce glass of green tea with ginseng. She reports that her doctor actually requested her to make a batch for some friends! And if that wasn't enough, the mixture may even have helped her lose more than 100 pounds. Capsaicin is thermogenic, which means it creates heat by burning more calories.

★★★**Ginger** Ginger contains high amounts of the enzyme zingibain, a powerful anti-inflammatory substance. According to some experts, it's even more potent than the bromelain in pineapple or the papain in papaya. It also contains at least four natural COX-2 inhibitors and, unlike prescription COX-2 inhibitors such as Celebrex, is associated with no serious side effects.

It's easy to get enough ginger in your diet to help reduce pain. You can take it as an herb in tea by steeping three or four slices in a cup of boiling water. If you prefer, you can get medicinal doses in tinctures or capsules. Andrew Weil, MD, professor at the University of Arizona College of Medicine in Tucson, recommends eating candied ginger with bits of antioxidant-rich dark chocolate. You can get medicinal doses by sprinkling ½ teaspoon of powdered ginger onto foods or by eating about an ounce (6 teaspoons) of fresh ginger every day.

In one study, Indian researchers gave a little more ginger (1½ to 3½ teaspoons) daily to 18 people with osteoarthritis and 28 with rheumatoid arthritis. More than three-quarters of these patients reported significant relief from pain and swelling and no side effects, even after consuming this much ginger for as long as 2 years.

★★★**Pomegranate** The ancient Greeks used pomegranate to treat arthritis, and this exotic tropical fruit has been revered through the ages for its ability to treat a wide range of conditions. But when I wrote *The Green Pharmacy* in 1997, I recommended pomegranate for only one condition: diarrhea.

Since then, researchers have shown that this gorgeous fruit—which is loaded with antioxidants and anti-inflammatory compounds—ranks as a true superfood. Evidence is mounting that it can help conditions as diverse as heart disease, cancer, and osteoarthritis.

In 2005, scientists from Case Western Reserve University in Ohio performed an intriguing experiment using tissue samples of human cartilage affected by osteoarthritis. After adding a water extract of pomegranate fruit to the culture, they found that it blocked substances that cause cartilage destruction. Specifically, it inhibited a pro-inflammatory protein called interleukin-1B, which stimulates the production of enzymes such as matrix metalloproteases, which are necessary for tissue remodeling. In healthy people, these enzymes aren't harmful. But in conditions such as osteoarthritis, overproduction of these enzymes breaks down cartilage and causes joint damage and destruction.

According to the researchers, these results suggest that consumption of pomegranate could help protect cartilage from the harmful effects of an inflammatory protein, manufactured by the immune system, called interleukin-1B and slow or even halt the progression of osteoarthritis. They are conducting follow-up studies to see if pomegranate could even help repair damaged cartilage.

This is exciting research because pomegranate, unlike all of the drugs used to treat osteoarthritis, has virtually no side effects.

The researchers didn't recommend a specific dose of pomegranate fruit or juice, but I would recommend drinking one 8-ounce glass of 100 percent pomegranate juice a day. I'd also increase my consumption of other fruits and fruit juices rich in antioxidants and anti-inflammatory compounds, such as pineapple, papaya, and cherries. Intriguing recent research suggests that tangerines and cherries may help inhibit compounds associated with joint damage.

★★★**Tea** Tea contains at least seven different COX-2 inhibitors, including catechin, which helps reduce the inflammation associated with osteoarthritis and may even slow cartilage breakdown. It also seems to protect the bones. Women who routinely drink tea are significantly less likely than "tea-totalers" to develop osteoporosis. Compared to other varieties, green tea is especially rich in antioxidant compounds called phenols, which help protect the body from a multitude of disorders, including several cancers. For osteoarthritis, try drinking about five cups of tea a day.

★★★**Turmeric** This yellow curry spice is a rich source of curcumin, a strong antioxidant that protects against free radical damage. Curcumin contains natural pain-relieving COX-2-inhibitors, making it an attractive, side effect–free alternative to prescription COX-2 inhibitors such as Celebrex. It also reduces inflammation by reducing histamine levels and possibly stimulating the adrenal glands to produce more cortisone, the body's natural painkiller.

Human studies of curcumin have found that it can reduce the pain and stiffness associated with rheumatoid arthritis as well as help relieve postsurgical inflammation. I prefer a whole-foods approach whenever possible because as I've often said, I believe you get more healing power from whole foods than from individual components. I often add liberal amounts of curry to rice and other dishes and would consider adding other anti-inflammatory foods such as pineapple and papaya. Dr. Weil recommends adding a teaspoon of powdered turmeric to soups, stews, and other dishes. You can also can make tea with turmeric.

Curried Celery COX-2 Inhibitor

If you're contemplating taking a prescription COX-2 inhibitor such as Celebrex for osteoarthritis or any other inflammatory condition, you may want to consider this side effect–free food farmaceutical that I developed. It contains more than a dozen natural COX-2 inhibitors and is good for what ails you.

To make this warm curried soup, place four to eight stalks of celery (loaded with apigenin) into a pot and add a bit of diced cabbage, cayenne, chives, garlic (optional), resveratrol-containing grape leaves or Japanese knotweed spears (optional), and onion (a good source of quercetin).

Then add water to cover, some spices—turmeric, basil, ginger, rosemary, sage and/or thyme—and a generous amount of freshly ground black pepper (which contains piperine, a substance that makes turmeric more bioavailable), and bring to a boil.

For even more benefits, I'd chase this spicy dish with a cup of either green tea (which contains catechin and kaempferol) or chamomile tea (another good source of apigenin).

★★**Grapefruit** I prefer the darker red variety of grapefruit, which is so tasty that I can consume almost an entire fruit for breakfast. (Talk about whole foods!) Grapefruit—especially the darker red variety—contains three COX-2 inhibitors and loads of powerful antioxidants, such as lycopene (the source of the red pigment), limonoids, and naringin. Grapefruit is also one of the best sources of vitamin C, an essential nutrient for people with osteoarthritis. One cup of grapefruit sections contains 88 milligrams of vitamin C, which is nearly 1½ times the recommended daily amount.

★★**Oregano** The so-called pizza herb, a member of the mint family, contains dozens of anti-inflammatory and painkilling compounds. Among them are eight COX-2 inhibitors: apigenin, caffeic acid, eugenol, kaempferol, oleanolic acid, quercetin, ursolic acid, and rosmarinic acid. Of these, rosmarinic acid may be the most potent because it also has antibacterial and antiviral properties. Although many other mints—such as peppermint, rosemary, and biblical mint—may be useful for osteoarthritis, oregano stands out because it has the most antioxidant activity of any of the 100 different mints tested in scientific studies. I'd definitely add liberal amounts of this tasty herb to my pizza or any other food to help relieve the aches of osteoarthritis.

★★**Pineapple** This exotic fruit is rich in a number of substances that can help people with conditions such as osteoarthritis. Foremost among them is bromelain, an enzyme that helps reduce swelling and inflammation in many painful inflammatory conditions. Bromelain can also flush out compounds associated with arthritic conditions and help you digest fibrin, another compound implicated in arthritis.

This luscious tropical fruit also contains high amounts of manganese and vitamin C, both of which are essential for the formation of collagen, the tough, fibrous protein that builds connective tissues such as bone, skin, and cartilage. You can get 100 percent of the daily value for manganese (2 milligrams) from just 1 cup of fresh pineapple chunks or pineapple juice. A cup of fresh chunks also contains 24 milligrams of vitamin C, which is 40 percent of the Daily Value.

If you have osteoarthritis, vitamin C is essential. A 10-year study of 149 people with knee osteoarthritis, published in 2005 by researchers from Boston University, showed that those who consumed less than 150 milligrams of vitamin C per day tripled their rate of cartilage breakdown.

To get the maximum antioxidant punch from pineapple, try the "Gold" variety, which is imported from Costa Rica and contains four times as much vitamin C as other pineapples.

Unfortunately, recent research suggests that levels of bromelain in fresh pineapple and papain, a related enzyme in fresh papaya, may be too low to relieve a bad episode of osteoarthritis. While I would encourage enjoying these fruits—either whole or as juice—you'll probably need to take supplements to get effective levels. Naturopaths suggest taking anywhere between 250 and 500 milligrams of bromelain three times per day.

From the Herbal Medicine Chest

For relief from the aches and pains of osteoarthritis, you may want to try one or both of these herbs.

Pycnogenol This extract derived from the French maritime pine tree is a rich source of antioxidants and natural inflammation-fighting COX-2 inhibitors. In a 2007 study published in the journal *Nutrition Research,* researchers from the United States and Iran administered either 150 milligrams of Pycnogenol a day or placebos to 35 people with knee osteoarthritis. After 3 months, the Pycnogenol group had reductions of 43 percent in pain and 35 percent in stiffness and a 52 percent increase in physical function, while the placebo group showed no significant improvement. Those taking Pycnogenol were also able to decrease their use of over-the-counter and prescription anti-inflammatory drugs. Other research, including a study published in the *Journal of Inflammation,* shows that Pycnogenol can effectively counter joint destruction by preventing the immune system from releasing pro-inflammatory molecules called cytokines.

Stinging nettle (*Urtica dioica*) Nettle has a long tradition—especially in Germany—as a treatment for arthritis. That's because it contains many active painkilling and anti-inflammatory compounds, such as caffeic acid, ferulic acid, and scopoletin. Nettle can be taken orally or applied to the skin. Since the late 1990s, studies have shown that this herb reduces levels of inflammatory substances made by the immune system, such as tumor necrosis factor-alpha and interleukin-1B, and may be useful in treating osteoarthritis.

In a pilot study of 40 patients with arthritis, researchers studied the effects of either 50 milligrams of stewed nettle leaf combined with 50 milligrams of the commonly used arthritis drug diclofenac (Voltaren) or 200 milligrams of the drug alone. Because total joint scores improved equally in both groups, the researchers concluded that it might be possible to reduce the dose of arthritis drugs by 75 percent, reduce the risk of gastrointestinal bleeding, and protect against some of the newly discovered potential hazards of some COX-2 inhibitors such as (get this!) elevated levels of tumor necrosis factor-alpha and interleukin-1B!

Osteoporosis

IF EVER THERE WERE A CONDITION MADE for food-related interventions, it's osteoporosis. Study after study has yielded solid evidence that a variety of nutrients are helpful—excuse me, *required*—to maintain healthy bones.

But some experts say weight-bearing exercise may be almost as important or even more so. I'm convinced that both natural approaches (diet with whole foods and possibly with supplements, and exercise) are synergistically much better than the pharmaceutical approaches, one of which Mrs. Duke has been taking religiously because of her preosteoporosis condition.

A lot of people should pay close attention to the details on how to achieve a bone-building diet. According to the National Osteoporosis Foundation, 10 million

Americans have osteoporosis, and roughly 34 million more are thought to have low bone mass, which puts them at risk for the disease.

By 2020, given the aging population, more than 47 million people are expected to have low bone mass, leaving more than half of all Americans over the age of 50 at risk for developing osteoporosis.

This condition is nothing to sneeze at—literally. If you have osteoporosis, your bones may become so weak that simply coughing or sneezing causes a fracture. So can minor falls. The results of fractures can be severe. Wrist fractures, which are common in people with osteoporosis, may hamper you for just a little while. But two-thirds of people who fracture a hip never return to their normal levels of function. Fractures of the back can be extremely painful.

Paying attention to the steps for preventing and treating osteoporosis is something everyone should do, not just women or older folks. Getting an early start on preventing osteoporosis may make a big difference in your life later.

Note—the ratings in this chapter don't reflect the effectiveness of the suggestion, since they're all useful. But some are important enough to demand more of your attention, and these I gave a higher rating.

Healing Foods for Osteoporosis

★★★**Avocados** As our tastiest vegetable source of vitamin D, avocados may be useful for osteoporosis. The role of vitamin D in skeletal maintenance is well known. Your body is a little cavalier in the way it handles the valuable calcium you give it. Despite its importance to your bones, you absorb only about 30 percent of the calcium you take in. What a waste!

Fortunately, vitamin D helps improve your body's absorption of calcium by acting on your intestines. (In this regard, the vitamin works like a hormone.) Another interesting fact about vitamin D is that you don't even have to eat anything to get it. Your skin produces it when you're exposed to sunlight. Hence, weight-bearing exercise out in the sunshine can synergistically strengthen your bones against osteoporosis. Unfortunately, lots of people have trouble getting the vitamin this way. When you live in northern climes, you're not out in strong sunlight as much, especially in the winter. Older people and people with darker skin don't make vitamin D as well. And people tend to cover themselves in clothing and sunscreen these days when they're outside because of skin cancer concerns, which limits vitamin production.

That's why it's a good idea to get plenty of vitamin D in your diet. A meta-analysis that compiled the results of 25 studies found that vitamin D supplements reduced the risk of spinal fractures by about 37 percent (however, part of this reduction may have been due to the vitamin's improving the study participants' muscle strength, making them less likely to fall).

You don't want too much vitamin D, though. Since it's a fat-soluble vitamin, your body stores it up, and it's harmful in excess. The adequate intake for adults up to age 50 is 200 International Units (IU); for ages 51 to 70, 400 IU; and for older people, 600 IU. You can get 350 to 400 IU per day with only 10 grams of avocado, a pleasing and not too fattening prescription. Another ideal source of vitamin D—a cup of fortified milk—is also rich in calcium. It'll give you 98 IU of the vitamin. Sources of dairy such as cheese, ice cream, and the typical yogurt don't offer much vitamin D, however. Other good food sources include:

Salmon, 3 ounces	238 IU
Canned tuna, 3 ounces	136 IU
Sardines, 1 ounce	77 IU
Raisin bran, ¾ cup	42 IU

★★★**Low-fat dairy** Although some plants are good sources of calcium—and I'll list those in this section—many people are going to gravitate toward dairy foods when they need to boost their intake of this bone-building mineral. A list of nutrients that are needed for bone protection doesn't end with calcium, but it certainly starts with it. Your bones hold 99 percent of the calcium in your body, and although bones need calcium for strength, other parts of your body, such as your nerves and muscles, require calcium to operate properly, too. So if you're not consuming enough calcium to keep your internal processes running right, your body will make up for the shortfall by taking calcium from your bones.

Though people typically get concerned about osteoporosis after they've already gotten concerned about gray hairs, it's crucial to get a running start at protecting your bones much earlier in life. You hit your peak bone mass in late adolescence; I've read that the amount of bone mineral you store away during these years is roughly equal to the amount you lose through the rest of your adult life. If you don't build strong bones as a teen and young adult, you won't have as much bone mineral to see you through the following years.

Once you hit middle age, your bone loss begins or speeds up, and women hit a phase of particularly fast loss at menopause.

That's why it's so important to get plenty of calcium, no matter how old you are. One review of earlier research found that in 52 of 54 randomized trials, getting more calcium increased people's bone gain earlier in life, reduced bone loss later in life, or reduced the rate of broken bones. Unfortunately, most Americans aren't getting enough of this bone-building mineral. The average diet contains only 600 milligrams of calcium, which is far too little.

Adults up to the age of 50 need 1,000 milligrams a day, which rises to 1,200 milligrams daily in the following years. Milk and dairy foods are good sources of calcium, and that's where most Americans get it. However, a lot of people, especially those of nonwhite ethnic backgrounds, have lactose intolerance, which means they have trouble digesting dairy and thus avoid these foods. Even if you do have lactose intolerance, you may be able to drink up to a cup of milk twice a day accompanied with food, with fewer digestive problems. Or stick with cheese and yogurt.

Nowadays, with fortified foods you have more options for getting calcium. And some vegetables, such as broccoli and kale, contain calcium that your body absorbs well. Here are some good food sources of the mineral, measured in milligrams:

Sardines with bones, 3 ounces	324
Milk, nonfat, 8 ounces	302
Yogurt, nonfat, 8 ounces	300
Orange juice, calcium fortified, 6 ounces	Roughly 230
Cereal, calcium fortified, 1 cup	100 to 1,000
Cooked kale, 1 cup	94

On a dry-weight basis, other great plant sources of calcium include pigweed, lambsquarter, nettle, broad beans, watercress, licorice, marjoram, savory, red clover shoots, Chinese cabbage, and basil.

★★**Beans** You'll find that beans—including kidney beans, chickpeas, soybeans, and soybean-derived foods such as tofu—are a good plant source of protein. Protein plays many important roles in bone health. A protein called collagen forms scaffold-like structures that form a matrix that holds the minerals calcium and phosphate. Concrete walls have metal bars going through them that provide support with some flexibility; the matrix provides a similar role in your bones, since bones made just of minerals would crumble under the stresses they frequently endure. In addition, protein helps you produce hormones and growth factors that play a role in creating bone.

As a result, it's important to your bone health to get sufficient protein in your diet. The RDA for men is 56 grams of protein, and for women it's 46 grams. For reference's sake, half a salmon fillet has about 42 grams of protein. Legume protein may contribute to bone health in other ways. Urinary calcium excretion can be an indicator of bone mineral density and calcium balance. Some people blame the high rate of osteoporosis in western countries on the effect of too much animal protein, which causes calcium loss in the urine. Compared to animal protein, soy protein causes less urinary excretion of calcium. And soy scientists optimistically tell us that isoflavones in the food may also directly inhibit bone resorption.

On the other hand, eating *too much* protein may not be good for your bones. This is a controversial area, but some experts have promoted the idea that the more protein you eat, the more calcium you excrete in your urine. However, the research on the associations between vegetable and animal protein and bone health has had all kinds of conflicting results. It's probably wise for your bone health not to eat an excessively high-protein diet and to get plenty of your protein from plant sources, such as beans, rice, and soy.

★★**Carrots** Foods rich in vitamin A—such as carrots—are important for bone health. This vitamin is required during the bone remodeling process—but this is another nutrient for which more is not better. Too much of the form of vitamin A called preformed vitamin A, or retinol, has been linked to lower bone mineral density and higher risk of fractures. However, precursors of vitamin A called carotenoids, which are found in many fruits and vegetables and are turned into vitamin A as your body needs it, aren't detrimental for your bones.

The RDA is 3,000 IU for men and 2,330 IU for women. Avoid getting more than 10,000 IU of the retinol form daily.

Good sources include:

Beta-carotene

Carrots, cooked, 1 cup	26,571 IU
Spinach, canned, 1 cup	20,974 IU

Retinol

Cheddar cheese, 1 ounce	284 IU
Egg, fried	335 IU

Want to branch out and get some foods that are super sources of beta-carotene on a dry-weight basis? First we have that "weed" purslane again. It's off the charts. Then try barley grass, jujube, spinach, watercress, chives, mustard greens, and sweet potatoes.

★★**Cornmeal** How could a pan of cornbread help my bones, you may be asking yourself. Well, cornmeal is a good source of phosphorus, and you need a sufficient amount of this in your diet because it helps your body stock your bones with mineral. About 85 percent of the phosphorus in your body is located in your bones. This is one of those nutrients, however, for which getting more isn't necessarily better for your bones, a theme you'll see several times in this chapter.

Getting too much phosphorus and too little calcium may lead to bone loss. Given that sodas are high in phosphorus and low in calcium, and since we're a soda-guzzling nation and every soda you drink means a missed opportunity to drink milk, some experts have voiced concern about the effects of sodas on bone health. However, experts say that the ratio of phosphorus to calcium in your diet is probably more important for your bones than just the amount of phosphorus.

The recommended daily allowance (RDA) for men and women over age 30 is 700 milligrams. It's not wise to get more than 4,000 milligrams daily. If you have a high-phosphorus diet, be especially sure to get plenty of calcium.

Foods high in phosphorus include:

Cornmeal, 1 cup	860 milligrams
Halibut, half fillet	453 milligrams
Yogurt, plain, 8 ounces	356 milligrams
(also good source of calcium)	
Chicken breast, half	259 milligrams

For my vegetarian readers, other plant-based foods that are high in the mineral are beets, lambsquarter, tomatillo, flaxseed, and cowpeas.

★★**Enriched white rice** For bones of steel—well, *closer* to steel, anyway—you need some iron. This mineral is a component in several enzymes that help create the collagen in bone matrix. It also plays a role in turning vitamin D into its active form, which as you already read helps you absorb calcium. Animal studies have found critters that don't get enough iron have lower bone mass.

The RDA for adult men is 8 milligrams daily. Adult women up to age 50 need 18 milligrams a day (iron is lost during menstruation), and women over age 50 need 8 milligrams. Getting more than 45 milligrams daily is not advisable.

Good food sources of iron include:

Enriched white rice, 1 cup	10 milligrams
Soybeans, cooked, 1 cup	9 milligrams
White beans, canned, 1 cup	8 milligrams
Chuck roast, 3 ounces	3 milligrams
Chicken breast, half	2 milligrams

Caffeine. Excessive caffeine consumption can lead you to lose calcium in your urine. However, if you keep your intake of caffeine—found in sodas, coffee, and tea—moderate and get plenty of calcium in your diet, the caffeine shouldn't have much effect on your bones.

Sodium. Sodium in your diet causes your kidneys to excrete calcium. If you're not consuming enough calcium in your diet to make up for the loss in urination, where do you think your body will draw it from? That's right, your bones. People who eat a heavily salted diet might want to say farewell to their bones' calcium supply every time they urinate, because that's where a little bit goes.

Studies looking at groups of men and postmenopausal women found that those with higher salt intake have higher rates of bone loss, and other research suggests that people getting too little calcium and too much sodium have lower bone mineral density.

If you stick to the common guidelines for sodium consumption—no more than 2,400 milligrams a day—the sodium won't affect your bone health. Ensuring that you get plenty of calcium and potassium in your diet will cover for your sodium consumption, too.

Other notable sources of iron that I see in my database include dandelion, safflower, and thyme.

★★**Leafy greens** Although it's a nutrient in many leafy greens that doesn't get much attention, vitamin K helps in the process of bone formation. Population studies have linked higher vitamin K intake with lower rates of fractures, and other research has found that greater vitamin K intake is associated with higher bone density.

The RDA for people over age 30 is 120 units for men and 90 units for women. Leafy green vegetables—such as kale, collards, spinach, and beet, turnip, and mustard greens—are all high in vitamin K. This vitamin also is involved in the production of blood-clotting factors; as a result, if you're taking a blood-thinning drug, talk to your doctor about the appropriate amount of vitamin K in your diet.

Other plant sources include parsley, cabbage (the green outer leaves can have up to six times more than inner whitish leaves), watercress, soybean oil, and Brussels sprouts.

★★**Pineapple** A mineral found in certain foods that's not to be confused with magnesium is manganese. It plays a role in forming bone matrix and is a component in several enzymes found in bone. It's not known whether supplementation of manganese as an individual nutrient helps make your bones stronger, but supplements aren't a wise idea for people who are already getting plenty in their diets or people with liver disease.

However, it's easy to get plenty in your diet. The RDA for people over age 30 is 2.3 milligrams for men and 1.8 milligrams for women. A cup of whole-grain wheat flour contains 4.6 milligrams, and a cup of canned pineapple contains 2.8 milligrams. US Department of Agriculture scientists report that unrefined cereals, nuts, leafy vegetables, and tea are rich in manganese and that refined grains, meats, and dairy products are low. In my database, tea and cloves were highest; other good sources include fennel, spinach, and red clover.

★★**Plums and prunes.** Plums and their shriveled kin prunes—or, as they're now called, "dried plums"—are good sources of boron. This nutrient may help your bone health by improving your body's calcium absorption. Boron supplementation has been shown to markedly decrease the loss of calcium and magnesium in the urine among menopausal women. Research from 2002 found that dried plums may exert positive effects on bone in menopausal women. Fifty-eight women not receiving hormone replacement therapy were randomly assigned to eat 100 grams of the fruit daily for 3 months. The dried plums significantly increased the participants' serum levels of insulin-like growth factor I and bone-specific alkaline phosphatase activity.

There is no RDA for boron, but good food sources include avocados, nuts, and prune juice. Others in my database include quince, strawberries, peaches, cabbage, and asparagus. In addition, parsley, that dark green garnish so often thrown away instead of eaten, contains enough boron per 100 grams to be potentially helpful in preventing osteoporosis. I frankly think that salads and soups made from these dark green veggies might be the best approach to preventing osteoporosis.

★★**Potatoes** It seems like bananas get all the credit for being a high-potassium food, but another source that often goes unrecognized is the potato. Certain foods—such as meats—cause your body to become more acidic, and your body may have to draw material out of your bones to offset this effect. Getting plenty of potassium in your diet will help counterbalance this acidity, thus preserving your bones. Potassium also helps prevent loss of calcium in the urine: People eating less potassium in their diets lose more calcium with each trip to the restroom, and people who eat plenty of potassium keep more calcium where it does most good—in their bodies.

Research has found that women around the onset of menopause who have a potassium-rich diet have better total bone mineral density, and the elderly who get enough potassium have better bone mineral density in their hips and forearms.

Aim to get 1,600 to 3,500 milligrams of potassium daily. Eating 5 to 10 servings of fruits and vegetables each day should help you reach this goal. Here's one way to hit the target:

Baked potato	1081 milligrams
Tomato juice, 1 cup	556 milligrams
Orange juice, 1 cup	496 milligrams
Raisins, ½ cup	543 milligrams
Black-eyed peas, ½ cup	345 milligrams

Other good sources of potassium include lettuce, endive, mung bean, radish, Chinese cabbage, purslane, cucumber, and spinach.

★★**Tea** Another bone-building nutrient that you can find in a variety of food and beverages is fluoride. It stimulates new bone formation, but with fluoride, you don't want to get too little or too much. Excess fluoride intake actually causes brittle bones, so adding fluoride supplements on top of a healthy diet isn't necessary.

The RDA for people over age 30 is 4 milligrams for men and 3 milligrams for women. You shouldn't get more than 10 milligrams on a daily basis. Fluoridated drinking water, tea, and spinach are all sources of fluoride.

Research from 2002 found that tea had a protective effect on bone mineral density (BMD) in the total body, lower spine, and hips. Long-term, moderate tea consumption appeared to influence BMD more than short-term consumption of high amounts of tea, and no significant BMD differences were found between those who drank green, oolong, or black tea. The fluoride content of the tea may be responsible for its protective effects.

★★**Tomato paste** Copper isn't just used for coating pennies—it also plays a role in building bone. This nutrient is found in an enzyme that's required for collagen to form cross-links; thus, it's necessary for creating the matrix that forms a "scaffold" in the bone. The RDA is 900 micrograms for men and women over age 30. Amounts exceeding 10,000 micrograms daily aren't recommended.

This one's easy to get in a balanced diet. Two medium-size raw oysters contain 1.2 milligrams, which equals 1,200 micrograms. A cup of canned tomato paste contains just under a milligram. Consulting my database once again, I see that other sources of copper include cabbage, filberts, broccoli, black beans, collards, cucumber, cashews, and plums.

★★**Whole-grain wheat** Foods that are rich in the mineral magnesium are important for bone health, since more than half of the magnesium in your body is found in your bones. This nutrient helps ensure that your body processes minerals properly, and it seems to help create strong, good-quality bones.

Severe magnesium deficiency is rare among healthy people, but lots of Americans don't get as much as they should in their diets. The RDA for people over age 30 is 420 milligrams for men and 320 milligrams for women. Magnesium deficiency is found in nearly all patients with osteoporosis. I recommend turning to leafy greens, legumes, and whole grains for magnesium.

Good food sources include:

Whole-grain wheat flour, 1 cup	166 milligrams
Pumpkin seeds, 1 ounce	151 milligrams
Brazil nuts, 1 ounce	107 milligrams
Garbanzo beans, 1 cup	79 milligrams

Other good plant sources of magnesium include purslane—which many unenlightened sorts regard as a weed—green beans, poppy seeds, cowpeas, and spinach. I've been known to whip up a batch of magnesi-soup containing diced purslane, green beans, spinach, and nettles, with poppy seeds for flavoring.

★**Pepper** More than any other spice, black pepper has four compounds with anti-osteoporosis properties. So if you like pepper, you might consider sprinkling it on your avocado (assuming that every little bit helps).

Overweight

IN AMERICA, OBESITY IS a big problem—and big business.

I've read that Americans nowadays are spending $35 billion a year on weight-loss products. That's a lot of money to waste on pills and gimmicks that don't work. That's right—they're ineffective. I know this because statistics show the problem is getting worse. Over the past four decades, the prevalence of overweight and obesity in the United States has more than doubled, making two out of three of us vulnerable to all the health problems that carrying too much weight can bring! That's really a shame, because the key to losing weight is pretty simple: You have to eat and drink fewer calories than you expend through physical activity.

You can easily do that by eating reasonable portions of meals made up of mostly fruits, vegetables, legumes, whole grains, or nuts and by getting some physical activity every day—or at least on most days. Including the foods that follow can boost your weight loss even more.

Healing Foods for Overweight

★★★**Beans and other high-fiber foods** Losing weight isn't always a matter of eating less. In fact, sometimes you should eat more. For example, consuming greater amounts of beans, whole grains, and other plant foods can give your weight-loss program an extra edge.

Although your body can't digest the stuff, fiber is helpful in a weight-loss diet for many reasons. First of all, it's mostly present in plant foods, which are typically low in calories and fat and require more time and effort to eat than low-fiber, processed foods such as french fries, so there's less tendency to overeat them. Also, fiber is bulky and lingers longer in your stomach, so it helps you feel fuller.

Women should get 21 to 25 grams of fiber daily, and men need 30 to 38 grams. Studies have found that people who eat more fiber have lower rates of obesity. In addition, research shows that people who added 14 grams of fiber to their diets ate 10 percent fewer calories and lost 4 more pounds over roughly 4 months, with even more impressive results in obese people.

According to the USDA's handy-dandy nutrient database, the following are just a few good sources of fiber, measured in grams.

1 cup navy beans—19

1 cup lentils—16

1 cup oat bran—15

1 cup dates—14

1 raspberries—11

★★★**Cayenne** If your food is spicy enough, you're likely to sweat—and maybe even burn off a few calories—as if you've been working out. Research has found that by adding 6 to 10 grams of cayenne pepper to a meal or consuming 28 grams of the hot stuff in a day (6 grams is about a tablespoon), you may burn more calories and feel less hungry after meals. That's a lot of hot pepper, and it's possible that if you eat that much, you'll become so preoccupied with your burning mouth that you'll be too busy to think about being hungry. But it may be something to try.

★★★**Tea** In addition to fat-free milk, another good weight-loss beverage appears to be tea, particularly green tea. In a small 1999 study, men who took a green tea extract had greater energy expenditure and burned more fat over the course of a day than those who didn't take the extract. Taking caffeine didn't provide these benefits. As a result, the researchers believe that green tea encourages metabolism boosting and fat burning independently of the caffeine it contains. Another study found that men who drank a cup and a half of oolong tea daily for 12 weeks reduced their waist circumference and amount of body fat.

Research has found that green tea extract is thermogenic, meaning that it speeds up your metabolism, leading to more weight loss. This activity may be due to components in the tea, including epigallocatechin gallate, caffeine, myricetin, and quercetin. A 2008 study from Thailand found that green tea can reduce body weight in overweight individuals, partly because they're burning more energy and hence calories.

Replacing some of your daily sodas—diet or otherwise—with tea would appear to be a good idea if you're trying to lose weight.

★★**Almonds** Losing weight requires exercising plenty of restraint with food, so sometimes it's nice to go nuts. Eating almonds may be a tasty way to shed additional pounds. In a 2003 study reported in the *International Journal of Obesity*, 65 overweight and obese adults followed one of two diets for 6 months. Some ate a diet in which they got 39 percent of their calories from fat (most of which was "good" monounsaturated fat) and 32 percent of calories from carbohydrates—and they ate 3 ounces of almonds daily. The other group got 18 percent of their calories from fat and 53 percent from carbohydrates. Otherwise, each group took in the same low number of calories each day and the same percentage of calories from protein.

The almond group lost 62 percent more weight overall, 50 percent more off their waists, and 56 percent more fat mass than the other group. The nuts may have helped the higher-fat diet keep these people feeling fuller and more satisfied. But if you decide to snack on almonds, don't go overboard; an ounce (23 almonds) contains 163 calories.

★★**Broccoli and other chromium-rich foods** You may have seen advertisements promoting chromium picolinate as a weight-loss supplement. This is a combination of the trace mineral chromium and picolinic acid, a derivative of tryptophan, and we don't really know if it works. Various studies of the supplement have been inconclusive. Would eating reasonable amounts of chromium in food form help? Maybe, but it wouldn't hurt to try. Good low-calorie food sources, from best to good, include red wine, broccoli, grape juice, garlic, and potatoes (without butter or other fatty toppings).

★★**Dairy foods** Not only is calcium important for making your bones thicker, it may make your waist thinner, too. In an analysis of data from a national nutritional survey, researchers found that people with the highest calcium intakes had an 85 percent lower risk of being overweight. Another analysis of previous research found that each 300-milligram increase in daily calcium intake was associated with a 5- to 6-pound decrease in body weight in adults.

In addition, in a 2005 study, researchers put 32 obese adults on one of three diets for 6 months: a reduced-calorie diet with 400 to 500 milligrams of dietary calcium, the same diet with another 800 milligrams of supplemental calcium, or a reduced-calorie diet with 1,200 to 1,300 milligrams of calcium from three daily servings of dairy products. People on the standard diet lost 6.4 percent of their body weight, but people on the high-calcium diet lost 8.6 percent, and those on the high-dairy diet lost 10.9 percent! These differences were also seen in the total amount of fat people lost and the amount of fat they lost from their bellies.

Higher calcium intake may encourage your fat-storing cells to put away less fat and break down more of it. That's good for your weight. Calcium may also help by binding to fatty acids in your colon, keeping your body from absorbing them so the fat leaves your body in your stools.

Research indicates that calcium from dairy foods is more helpful than calcium from supplements, so try to include plenty of low-fat dairy foods in your diet each day. Good sources, measured in milligrams, include:

8 ounces yogurt—415

3 ounces sardines with bones—324

1.5 ounces cheddar cheese—306

8 ounces fat-free milk—302

½ cup firm tofu, made with calcium—204

Plant sources of calcium include soybeans, navy beans, turnip greens, and calcium-fortified orange juice.

★★**Eggs and other protein foods** When you have a snack or a meal, be sure to include a source of protein. Have an egg with your toast in the morning or some low-fat cheese with your crackers. Alternatively, load up on soy and beans and rice, which are good plant sources. Protein makes foods seem more satisfying and helps keep you feeling full for hours after you eat—which means you'll be less tempted to eat again for a while.

PMS

MOST PEOPLE KNOW PREMENSTRUAL SYNDROME (PMS) as a variety of vexations that occur for a week or two before a woman's menstrual period begins. The perpetual PMS jokes aside, only women in the throes of severe premenstrual pain know the true extent of the term. Estimates vary, but about 85 percent of menstruating women have at least one PMS symptom, according to the American College of Obstetricians and Gynecologists.

No one knows for sure, but most experts believe that changes in the levels of the sex hormones estrogen and progesterone during a woman's cycle may cause the problem. The higher the estrogen level, scientists say, the greater the risk of PMS. Each woman's experience of PMS is different. The US Department of Health and Human Services lists this curious assortment of symptoms:

- Acne
- Anxiety or depression
- Appetite changes or food cravings
- Breast swelling and tenderness
- Feeling tired
- Having trouble sleeping
- Headache or backache
- Joint or muscle pain
- Tension, irritability, mood swings, or crying spells
- Trouble concentrating or remembering
- Upset stomach, bloating, constipation, or diarrhea

Although high emotional stress can make symptoms worse, stress doesn't seem to cause the problem. Scientists believe serotonin, a chemical in the brain, may spark a severe and mostly psychological form of PMS, called premenstrual dysphoric disorder (PMDD). If you have this form, you know it can be excruciating. Symptoms affect about three to eight percent of menstruating women and can include these emotional symptoms:

- Difficulty sleeping
- Disinterest in daily activities and relationships
- Feeling out of control
- Feelings of sadness or despair, or possibly suicidal thoughts
- Feelings of tension or anxiety

- Food cravings or binge eating
- Lasting irritability or anger that affects other people
- Mood swings, crying
- Panic attacks
- Tiredness or low energy
- Trouble thinking or focusing

No single treatment has been found to work for every woman suffering from PMS, but if your symptoms are severe, speak with your health care practitioner. If your PMS is mild, dietary changes may help. Here are a few food strategies for easing the discomfort.

Healing Foods for PMS

★★★**Purslane, green beans, cowpea, and spinach** Calcium isn't the only mineral that affects brain chemistry. A number of studies indicate that women with PMS tend to have low levels of magnesium. If you're deficient in magnesium, you may have low levels of dopamine, a brain chemical that, like serotonin, helps regulate mood, says Melvyn Werbach, MD, assistant clinical professor of psychiatry at the University of California, Los Angeles, and author of *Healing Through Nutrition* and *Nutritional Influences on Illness*. A magnesium deficiency may also impair your metabolism of estrogen, another cause of premenstrual moodiness, according to Dr. Werbach.

Not eating enough vegetables puts you at risk for a magnesium deficiency. Many Americans with this condition have been found to suffer from a variety of conditions, such as asthma, diabetes, headache, hypertension, irregular heartbeat, migraine, and osteoporosis.

★★**Flaxseed, rape seed oil, walnuts, tofu** The western diet is typically higher in omega-6's, which throws the ratio with omega-3 fatty acids out of balance. These food sources of omega-3's can restore the balance and may even provide some relief from PMS. In a recent review of studies examining women's need for omega-3 fatty acids, scientists found that omega-3 fatty acids could play a positive role in preventing PMS (and postmenopausal hot flushes).

Omega-3 eggs are another highly recommended source. And if you eat fish, then consider mackerel, lake trout, herring, sardines, albacore tuna, and salmon—all high in two kinds of omega-3 fatty acids, eicosapentaenoic acid (EPA) and docosahexaenoic acid (DHA). Research suggests these fatty acids can reduce symptoms of

PMS—and as a bonus, they're good for your heart. If you prefer a fish-oil supplement, krill oil from Antarctic krill (a zooplankton crustacean) has been shown in a double-blind trial to be an effective treatment for PMS. In one study, krill oil was significantly more effective than regular fish oil in relieving emotional symptoms and breast tenderness related to premenstrual syndrome. The amount of krill oil used in this study was 2 grams per day for the first month. In the second and third months, the women took 2 grams per day beginning 8 days before their periods and continuing for 2 days after.

Vegetarians can get similar benefits from such omega-3 fatty acids as alpha-linolenic acid, found in such seeds as chia, chiso, flax, hemp, Inca peanut, and walnut. But almost always you'll be better off with the DHA and EPA fatty acids found in the fish. I have heard the same thing about supplemental gamma-linolenic acid (from borage, currant, evening primrose, and hemp seed oils).

★★**Low-fat yogurt** Studies suggest that a high intake of calcium and vitamin D may, in fact, not only lessen the severity of PMS symptoms but prevent them from developing in the first place.

Over a 10-year period, researchers at the University of Massachusetts at Amherst compared women who had PMS symptoms with those who had no symptoms or very mild symptoms. They concluded that women who ate or drank about 1,200 milligrams of calcium and 400 International Units (IU) of vitamin D daily had a much lower risk of developing PMS. Many studies have linked calcium and vitamin D to PMS relief; however, this study was one of the first to suggest these nutrients may actually prevent the condition.

Low-fat yogurt contains calcium that may reduce PMS symptoms in a number of ways. It may help prevent the muscular contractions that cause cramping, says research psychologist James G. Penland, PhD, who has conducted calcium/PMS studies at the US Department of Agriculture Human Nutrition Research Center in Grand Forks, North Dakota. Dr. Penland is convinced that the calcium content in foods affects certain brain chemicals and hormones known to affect mood.

If you're sensitive to cow's milk, you can always load up on other excellent sources of calcium, such as fortified orange juice, almonds, sesame seeds, collard greens, broccoli, kale, and bok choy.

Nondairy sources of vitamin D include salmon, sardines, tuna, mackerel, eggs, and fortified cereals. And, of course, you can get plenty of vitamin D from 15 minutes a day in the sunshine.

★★**Soy, peanuts, and other legumes** Tofu and other soy products contain genistein, a natural but weak plant estrogen (phytoestrogen) that limits the uptake of estrogen produced by the body. Although peanuts, black beans, and lima beans may contain more and different phytoestrogens, soybeans have gotten the most attention.

In a double-blind trial published in the *British Journal of Nutrition*, supplementing with soy protein (providing 68 milligrams of isoflavones per day) for two menstrual cycles was significantly more effective at relieving premenstrual swelling and cramping than a cow's milk protein placebo. Since some doctors believe the estrogen content in cow's milk can worsen PMS, the beneficial effect of soy protein may have been overestimated in this study.

Several recent studies of Korean women living in the United States also suggest that dietary intake of soy isoflavones has a positive affect on PMS symptoms. The researchers do say that further study and more accurate, objective measurements are needed to confirm the results.

Pneumonia

SERIOUS DISEASES OFTEN WAIT until you're down to strike—that is, when your immune system has become weak from fighting some other illness. True to form, pneumonia frequently—although not always—develops from a chest cold or the flu. And it can turn deadly. More than 60,000 people in the United States lose their lives to pneumonia each year.

People with taxed immune systems, such as those with chronic diseases and the elderly, have the highest risk of pneumonia, and surprisingly, a hospital stay can raise the risk even more. In 2004, 5.4 percent of deaths from pneumonia happened among hospital patients.

Because the infection grows deep in your lungs, the symptoms of pneumonia can be dramatic. You may feel chest pain and experience fever, chills, cough, and shortness of breath. Most doctors prescribe antibiotics for pneumonia, but these drugs won't work in all cases, first because antibiotic-resistant strains of the disease have developed and second because in half of all cases, a virus, not a bacterium, is the culprit. In rarer cases, fungi or other organisms cause pneumonia.

In my opinion, our government should be teaching us how to boost our immune systems with safe, preventive phytochemicals for protection against pneumonia, but since there aren't any government agencies or major associations of conventional medicine willing to offer this kind of advice, I'm leaping into the breach.

There are many promising foods for boosting your immune system, including bilberry, burdock, calendula, camu-camu, cantaloupe, cassia, chamomile, chickpeas, cinnamon, dandelion, elderberry, fenugreek, garlic, ginger, grapes, jujubes, oats, onion,

BronchoBuster Spread

To open up your sinuses and bronchial tubes, you may want to try my Broncho-Buster Spread, which incorporates some of the most important foods that relieve congestion. Combine chopped chile peppers, garlic, ginger, horseradish, mustard, onion, turmeric, and wasabi and use as a spread on crackers or bread. You could also make a piping hot tea with any or all of those ingredients.

oregano, shiitake, spinach, sweet potatoes, thyme, and turmeric. There is also a long list of herbs to relieve stress, which is important because stress lowers immunity.

Because pneumonia can be life-threatening, see your physician for treatment if you have any unusual symptoms in your chest or lungs. Immunity-boosting foods can help you avoid this illness, but if you do develop an infection, you need medical treatment. Also, be sure to get your doctor's permission before taking any herbs or supplements.

Healing Foods for Pneumonia

To protect yourself against pneumonia, you need a two-pronged defense. First, look in the Colds and Flu chapter on page 104 for advice on ways to combat those two conditions, either of which can lead to pneumonia. Then add some of the foods below to your diet to strengthen your immune system.

★★★**Elderberry** After successfully thwarting a flu that was making the rounds with a proprietary elderberry extract called Blockade, I decided to score it for anti-pneumonic activity. As discovered, the European elderberry—and probably our American variety as well—is an herbal shotgun, with more than a dozen antibacterial and antiviral compounds, plus nearly a dozen antifungal compounds.

★★★**Garlic** Garlic is practically a wonder food for treating infections, and natu-ropaths use it widely. It has more than 2,000 biologically active substances that give it medicinal properties. Chris Deatherage, ND, who lives and practices in rural Missouri, likes to combine garlic and hydrotherapy for acute illnesses like pneumonia and strep throat. Jill Stansbury, ND, of the National College of Naturopathic Medicine in Portland, Oregon, tells her students to use garlic to kill bacteria and viruses that cause bronchitis and gastrointestinal infections.

Ethiopian scientists have also studied the antibacterial properties of garlic on pneumonia-causing bacteria and concluded that it may be effective at fighting some strains of the disease.

★★★**Pomegranate** This tangy fruit scored as well as garlic in my database search for pneumonia-fighting properties. And a recent study on mice showed that pomegranate juice appears to help the lungs. The researchers induced tumors in mice and then gave half of them pomegranate. Those who drank the juice had marked reduction in tumor replication. The seeds and juicy flesh of the pomegranate fruit are full of antioxidants and help fight bacteria, viruses, and inflammation while boosting immunity.

★★**Citrus fruits** Because of their vitamin C content, eating oranges, grapefruit, tangerines, lemons, and limes can improve your immunity and make you more likely to fight off disease. Research has clearly shown that people who consume high amounts of vitamin C in their diets have healthier lungs. The vitamin boosts your immune system and helps protect you from viral infections. Some doctors even use very high doses of vitamin C supplements to treat pneumonia. I don't recommend trying to treat pneumonia on your own, but working to prevent it by getting plenty of vitamin C in your diet is a good idea.

The type of citrus fruit that scores highest in my database for vitamin C content was camu-camu, which grows on a bush in the Amazonian rainforest of Peru. It's followed by emblic, a berry-like tropical fruit; rosehips; bell peppers; cayenne; cashew apple, a fruit that's native to Brazil; pokeweed shoots, an herb native to eastern North America; vine spinach; Cherokee rose; guava; watercress; and sweet potato. Other sources include broccoli, papayas, kiwifruit, strawberries, cantaloupe, mangoes, tomatoes, green cabbage, and spinach. It also wouldn't hurt to take an additional supplement of vitamin C.

★★**Onions** Like garlic, onions have compounds that fight respiratory infections, including pneumonia. When I addressed 100 physicians at Flower Hospital in Toledo in 1995, one physician told a story of a Lebanese patient with a lung infection who had checked into a sanitarium several decades ago (when sanitariums were in vogue). After finding a load of onions, he ate several every day and was well within a month. Add plenty of onions and garlic to your meals, especially chicken soup.

★★**Oregano** This spice does more than add flavor to your spaghetti sauce. Lab studies show that it may also boost the immune system. It also fights bacteria and inflammation, helps relieve stress, suppresses a cough, acts as a decongestant, and helps clear the airways of mucus.

★**Basil** Who doesn't love a salad with sliced tomato, fresh mozzarella, and peppery basil topped off with a drizzle of olive oil? Basil scored well in my database to fight pneumonia, owing to its antioxidants and activities that fight bacteria and viruses and stimulate the immune system.

★**Celery** This flavor-packed vegetable is well known for stimulating the immune system to help fight disease. Celery is packed with antioxidants and compounds that fight bacteria, viruses, and inflammation.

★**Cinnamon** You may know that cinnamon extract helps people with diabetes control their blood sugar, but I also recommend using it to boost your immunity.

★**Ginger** It's known for settling nausea from motion sickness, chemotherapy, or pregnancy, but ginger also enhances your immune system. I like to make a tea by adding ginger shavings to boiling water.

★**Green and white tea** Green tea is full of antioxidants that rev up your immune system and help you stave off pneumonia and other diseases. Egyptian researchers found that drinking green tea while taking antibiotics improved the effectiveness of the antibiotics by up to three times. It worked by making the antibiotics more effective at killing bacteria and by making the bacteria more vulnerable to the antibiotic, even in cases where the strain of bacteria had become resistant.

Research is also shedding light on white tea as an immunity booster. In a study at Pace University in New York City, researchers found that white tea extract actually destroyed bacteria that can lead to pneumonia and other diseases such as staph infections. The extract worked even better than green tea at fighting bacteria and viruses in the body.

★**Rosemary** Like basil, rosemary is a culinary herb that scored well in my database for increasing immunity and fighting pneumonia. It's wonderful on chicken and lamb and in soups and stews.

FOODS TO WATCH

The foods listed below weaken rather than strengthen your immune system, so you should avoid them.

Too much alcohol. Alcohol interferes with your white blood cells' ability to fight infection. Drinking too much lowers your immunity and can make it harder for your body to fight an infection such as pneumonia.

Foods high in fat or sugar. Because pneumonia strikes when your immune system is down, focusing on immunity-building foods rather than foods with fewer nutrients (reaching for fresh fruits and vegetables rather than candy and cakes) will help your body fight off infection.

★**Turmeric** This spice is used in Traditional Chinese Medicine and Ayurvedic medicine as an aid for digestion, to relieve arthritis, to improve liver function, and to regulate menstrual cycles, and it also helps improve immunity and fight bacteria and viruses. In 2007, researchers discovered that a specific active ingredient in turmeric root called bisdemethoxycurcumin is what may be responsible for increasing immunity.

From the Herbal Medicine Chest

These herbs work particularly well for pneumonia.

Dandelion (Taraxacum officinale) Traditional Chinese Medicine calls for dandelion to treat pneumonia and other upper respiratory tract infections, and clinical trials have demonstrated that it works. I recommend cooking the greens and roots and drinking the juice that remains in the pot, called the pot liquor. Drinking tea made from the dried herb or taking capsules is also an option.

Echinacea (Echinacea spp.) Herbs like echinacea that stimulate the immune system can help with all types of pneumonia and infections. Six studies have even shown that echinacea is helpful for upper respiratory infections, but doctors don't know which of the several compounds in the herb are most active. If you have a lung infection, take 1 or 2 teaspoons of tincture in juice or tea several times a day.

Goldenseal (Hydrastis canadensis) Make goldenseal part of your overall plan for preventing and (with your doctor's permission) treating pneumonia. It contains two antimicrobial constituents, hydrastine and berberine. You can find tinctures of the herb at health food stores; follow the directions on the label. Goldenseal can be used along with barberry, goldthread, Oregon grape, and yellowroot because they have similar effects.

Poison Ivy, Oak, and Sumac

WHEN I THINK OF POISON IVY, I'm reminded of one of the reasons I went into botany. This anecdote is also in *The Green Pharmacy*, but since it made such an impression on me, it's worth repeating. Once, in one of the vacant lots on Mordecai Drive in Raleigh, North Carolina, where I played as a kid, I unknowingly used poi-

Mary Jo Bogenschutz-Godwin, or Mango Mary, as I sometimes call her, is my remote USDA database manager who has lived in Hawaii for more than a decade. Shortly after moving there from Beltsville, Maryland, she developed itchy pustules around her mouth, which she soon learned were caused by the mangoes growing abundantly in her new home state. Mango Mary would probably have the same problem if she ate cashew apples, pistachio nuts, or other tropical fruits in the poison ivy family. Appropriately, Carolyn Dean, MD, ND, and Chinese medicine guru Jeffrey Yuen recommend that you avoid mangoes if you are allergic to poison ivy.

son ivy as toilet paper. I discovered what I had done soon enough, though. It was a bad experience; I had anal pruritus for a week or so. It finally cleared up on its own, and luckily, I've suffered no more since then.

The rashes caused by poison ivy, oak, and sumac are severe allergic reactions that occur when the oils from any of these plants come in contact with or are inhaled by a sensitive person. There are 350,000 annual reported cases of poison ivy in the United States, and many more probably go unreported.

Healing Foods for Poison Ivy, Oak, and Sumac

Clearly, the best way to avoid the itch and sting of poison ivy, oak, or sumac is to avoid the weeds in the first place. Be careful to steer clear of plants that have three shiny leaves coming from a central stem. If, however, you unknowingly brush against one of their oil-bearing leaves and are unlucky enough to suffer a reaction, there are a few food remedies you can try. (Forgo the food remedies and see your doctor, however, if the rash is on your face or genitals, is oozing, or doesn't improve within a week.)

★★**Oatmeal** A classic remedy for easing the itch of chickenpox, oatmeal can apparently also relieve poison ivy, oak, and sumac. Nutritionist Molly Morgan, RD, owner of Creative Nutrition Solutions in Vestal, New York, suggests making a paste of oatmeal and spreading the concoction on the affected area to relieve the itching.

★★**Peppermint** Distinguished West Coast herbalist Christopher Hobbs mentions a combination that is new to this Easterner: peppermint oil in cosmetic clay with salt. Hobbs reasons that the salt and clay draw and dry, while the menthol reduces inflammation and cools by stimulating the skin's "cool" receptors. In the East, here in the garden, I advise my volunteers to try rubbing on peppermint if our local jewelweed (see "From the Herbal Medicine Chest" on this page) doesn't help.

★**Baking soda** Although more of a catalytic ingredient than a food, baking soda may help ease the itch of poison ivy. Chris Meletis, ND, an educator, international author and lecturer, and former dean of naturopathic medicine and chief medical officer at the National College of Naturopathic Medicine, suggests you dissolve some baking soda in water, put the mixture into a spray bottle, and spritz some on your skin periodically.

★**Onions** I mention these bulbs as my best source of the antihistaminic compound quercetin. While antihistamines aren't necessarily recommended for poison ivy, quercetin has several activities that may help alleviate the itch. The best source of quercetin is onion skins, which you can use to make a tea.

★**Water** Andrew Weil, MD, professor at the University of Arizona College of Medicine in Tucson, mentions a remedy that's new to me: run very hot water over the affected areas (realizing that heat stimulates, while cool assuages the itch) until the itch subsides. When it resumes, repeat with the hot water. This way, as Dr. Weil puts it, "the whole reaction will complete itself quickly, and your skin will return to normal much faster than it would otherwise."

From the Herbal Medicine Chest

Here are some herbs that may help prevent and/or reduce the discomfort of poison ivy, oak, and sumac.

Aloe (Aloe vera) One week after an Agricultural Research Services co-worker asked me what to do for poison ivy in the eye, I read in *EastWest* magazine that Christopher Hobbs, a distinguished West Coast herbalist, suggested using aloe vera in this sensitive area for cooling and drying up the rash. To apply it, slit open a fresh aloe leaf and dab some of the gel on the affected area.

Jewelweed (Impatiens capensis) Even the late pharmacognoscist Varro Tyler, PhD, who was pretty conservative, noted that of "100 different plants or plant products . . . used in the past to treat poison ivy . . . the most effective of these is probably jewelweed . . . . Internally, a decoction prepared from any part of the plant can be used; externally, the sap of the stem is applied to the affected area." Dr. Tyler cited clinical studies in which 108 of 115 people experienced dramatic relief from the itch of poison ivy in 2 to 3 days. The Herb Society of America suggests making ice cubes of jewelweed tea to apply to a poison ivy rash. I'd also add some mint and mountain mint for their menthol.

We have a big stand of jewelweed in the marsh below the Green Farmacy Garden. When I make my annual assault on the poison ivy that keeps coming back around my mailbox, I rub exposed parts of my body with wads of juicy jewelweed before I go out to do the weeding.

Soapwort (*Saponaria officinalis*) While I single out soapwort, I believe that any of the many soapy plants (containing saponins) could lessen the likelihood of a serious plant rash if crushed and used to rinse off affected areas of the skin. Other plants high in saponins include soapbark, rose leaves, gotu kola, horse chestnut, licorice, and Seneca snakeroot.

Prostate Enlargement

IF A MIDDLE-AGED OR SENIOR FRIEND of a certain age tells me he's waking at night to urinate and having trouble starting and stopping the flow of urine, my first thought is he's probably having prostate problems. Although it could be an infection of the prostate, bladder, or kidney, the problem is more likely prostate enlargement or benign prostatic hyperplasia (BPH), a noncancerous overgrowth of tissue of the prostate that often occurs as men age. The urethra runs directly through a man's prostate, so when an enlarged prostate squeezes the urethra, urinating becomes difficult.

An uncle of mine had his prostate operated on when he was older than 95 and died a few years later from complications of the surgery. If Uncle Tom were still with us, I'd recommend the "wait and see" approach used by conservative doctors. My own MD, after my last visit, told me to keep on doing what I'm doing; so far I have escaped prostate surgery.

BPH is the most common benign growth found in men, but the cause isn't well understood. Scientists at Johns Hopkins University now suspect that BPH may be linked to diabetes and obesity. Their recent research found that very obese men were 3.5 times more likely to have an enlarged prostate than normal-weight men of the same age. Having diabetes more than doubled the risk of developing BPH.

One reason may be that men who have diabetes or are extremely overweight often have higher levels of inflammation and free radicals, both associated with benign growth of the prostate gland and prostate cancer, the second leading cause of cancer death in US men. Having an enlarged prostate does not make you more likely to develop prostate cancer, according to the Prostate Cancer Foundation. With more than 200,000 new cases of prostate cancer diagnosed each year, however, the more strategies we can use to protect the prostate, the better.

Healing Foods for Prostate Enlargement

★★★**Pomegranate** While pomegranate juice isn't a substitute for medical treatment, researchers suggest including it as extra insurance. In early studies, the fruit's antioxidant and anti-inflammatory properties successfully shrank tumors in lab animals. Newer lab research at the University of Wisconsin–Madison suggests pomegranate may protect against prostate cancer and heal existing prostate cancer. Using human prostate cancer cells, the researchers found the higher the dose of pomegranate extract the cells received, the more cancer cells died.

The antioxidants in the juice may be the ingredient that protects healthy cells from free radicals. Flavonoids may help turn on genes that stop cancer cells from dividing or invading healthy tissues, or even help activate genes that make cancer cells commit suicide, say experts from the Linus Pauling Research Institute at Oregon State University in Corvallis.

When prostate cancer is present, levels of cancer markers (called prostate-specific antigens or PSAs) normally double every 15 months. But in a 30-year University of California, Los Angeles, study of 50 men who had undergone surgery or radiation for prostate cancer, drinking a daily 8-ounce glass of pomegranate juice slowed the rise of PSAs to 54 months, one-quarter their usual rate. PSA-doubling rates also slowed for men with early-stage prostate cancer who had chosen watchful waiting rather than surgery, radiation, or hormone treatment.

★★★**Pumpkin seeds** A handful of pumpkin seeds a day is the time-honored remedy for men trying to avoid BPH in Bulgaria, Turkey, and the Ukraine. Recent lab research corroborates this folk wisdom, finding that pumpkin seed oil alone significantly blocked prostate growth in rats.

A ½ cup serving of pumpkin seeds can contain as much as 8 milligrams of zinc, a mineral found to reduce the size of the prostate in several studies. Pumpkin seeds also pack prostate-friendly amounts of the amino acids alanine, glycine, and glutamic acid, reports Joseph Pizzorno, ND, president of Bastyr University in Seattle, and, with Michael Murray, ND, coauthor of *Textbook of Natural Medicine*. In a study of 45 men who took 200 milligrams of all three amino acids daily, the regimen significantly eased BPH symptoms.

A ½ cup serving of pumpkin seeds may contain 1,150 to 1,245 milligrams of alanine, 1,800 to 1,930 milligrams of glycine, and 4,315 to 4,635 milligrams of glutamic acid. That's about five to 20 times the recommended daily dosage. Other seeds that contain these beneficial amino acids include peanuts and sesame seeds (high in glycine), almonds, butternuts and peanuts (high in glutamic acid), and buffalo gourd seeds (generous amounts of all three).

★★**Brazil nut** Eat just one average-size Brazil nut a day and you'll ace the daily requirements for the mineral selenium, a potent antioxidant linked to low rates of cancer and heart disease. Among other nutrients, this nut that grows on enormous trees in the Amazon rain forest also contains vitamin E. A 2008 study in the journal *Prostate* suggests that selenium combined with vitamin E may be more effective than either is alone for preventing prostate cancer.

That's why, at age 79, I eat three Brazil nuts a day to help prevent three of the diseases competing for my attention: colon cancer, lung cancer, and prostate cancer. I'm also genetically targeted for BPH, but so far, no problems.

★★**Broccoli and other veggies in the broccoli family** One or more chemicals found in broccoli may help prevent prostate problems by interacting with a gene (*GSTM1*) associated with prostate inflammation and the growth of prostate cancer cells, according to a 2008 study at the Institute of Food Research, Norwich, United Kingdom. This experimental research presents the first evidence in humans to back up earlier observational studies that found men who eat three or more servings of cruciferous vegetables a week have 41 percent lower risk for prostate cancer.

Instead of eating large quantities of meat that might actually cause prostate cancer, I beef up my daily vegetarian soups with bags full of broccoli and other cruciferous fare (cabbage, cauliflower, kale, mustard greens, turnips, and watercress).

★★**Green tea** Japanese and Chinese men, known to guzzle green tea, have the lowest incidence of prostate cancer in the world. Scientists suspect the protection may come from a polyphenol and powerful antioxidant called epigallocatechin gallate (EGCG). In laboratory and animal studies, the EGCG in tea stopped both the development and the growth of prostate cancer cells.

In a case-control study of 130 men in southeast China, published in the *International Journal of Cancer*, cancer patients reduced their risk of recurring prostate cancer significantly when they drank more green tea, more often, and for a longer period of time. Scientists are now searching for a way to custom-tailor a pharmaceutical cocktail aimed at delaying prostate and other cancers. But why wait when you can custom-brew a beneficial beverage in your own low-tech kitchen?

★★**Tomato** Are tomatoes still the prostate's best pal? Scientists are still sorting that out. You've most likely heard of lycopene, the powerful antioxidant found in tomatoes that received much press attention. Lycopene is concentrated in the prostate gland. A few years ago, the FDA approved a label claim for tomato products that says, "Very limited and preliminary scientific research suggests that eating one half to one cup of tomatoes and/or tomato sauce a week may reduce the risk of prostate cancer."

Then a large study by the National Cancer Institute and the Fred Hutchinson Cancer Center announced that neither lycopene nor tomato-based products helped prevent prostate cancer. After examining the serum carotenoid levels (lycopene is one type of carotenoid) from 28,000 men enrolled in the Prostate, Lung, Colorectal, and Ovarian Cancer Screening Trial, the researchers concluded that even men with the highest intake of lycopene had no increased protection against prostate cancer.

Following that discouraging news, a German pilot study helped revive lycopene's prostate-friendly reputation, at least in men with BPH. Researchers looked at 40 men diagnosed with BPH who did not have prostate cancer. After 6 months, the men in the lycopene group had decreased PSA levels and their prostate did not enlarge. But among the men in the placebo group, PSA levels did not decrease and prostate enlargement progressed. The researchers concluded that lycopene inhibited progression of BPH.

To add a new twist to the tomato tug of war, researchers at the University of Illinois at Urbana-Champaign found that tomatoes are better at shrinking prostate tumors when they're eaten along with broccoli than when either food is eaten alone. The researchers implanted prostate cancer cells in lab rats and then fed them a diet containing 10 percent tomato powder and 10 percent broccoli powder made from whole foods. Other rats received either tomato or broccoli powder alone, a lycopene supplement, or finasteride (the drug commonly prescribed for BPH). Another group of rats was castrated. After 22 weeks, the tomato and broccoli group outperformed all other groups in shrinking prostate tumors, including but followed by the castration group.

The researchers did some conversions to figure out how a 55-year-old man concerned about prostate health can get the same positive effects, and came up with 1.4 cups of raw broccoli and 2.5 cups of fresh tomato daily, or 1 cup of tomato sauce, or ½ cup of tomato paste. As an example, they suggest putting broccoli on a pizza with ½ cup of tomato paste. Eating tomatoes is better than taking a lycopene supplement, they say, and cooked tomatoes may be more easily absorbed in the body than raw tomatoes.

★**Flaxseed** Flaxseed is high in omega-3 fatty acids and in a type of phytochemical called lignan, which has been shown in some studies to protect against prostate cancer. Like the plant-estrogen properties of soy, flax lignans have hormonal effects that may slow prostate cancer formation and growth, according to a small study at Duke University Medical Center.

In the study, men with prostate cancer who ate ground flaxseed as part of a low-fat diet (20 percent of calories from fat), reduced serum testosterone, slowed the growth rate of cancer cells, and increased the death rate of cancer cells. More research is needed to find out whether these results had more to do with the low-fat diet than the flaxseeds, but the researchers say combining the two may lower the risk of prostate cancer.

★**Prickly pear** The fruit (called tuna) and the stems (called nopalito) of this American desert cactus are edible and sold in stores in foods such as jam and nectars. On my last trip to Israel with the late Dan Palevitch, a well-known herbal medicine expert in Israel and professor at the Department of Agriculture at the Hebrew University in Rehovot, I learned that Russian immigrants in Israel sought this cactus, not for diabetes, as it is widely used in America, but for prostate problems.

Prickly pear contains at least three prostate-friendly phytochemicals: beta-sitosterol, linoleic acid, and zinc. A good combo for prostatitis might be prickly pear cactus, pumpkin seed, and saw palmetto. You might even try making a vegetarian "tuna" salad, or try nopalitoes with Brazil nuts and salsa (for the tomatoes with lycopene).

Psoriasis

PSORIASIS MAY APPEAR TO BE ONLY SKIN DEEP, but that doesn't mean it's not a major problem. It's a lifelong skin disease, and it's not called "the heartbreak of psoriasis" for nothing. Researchers at the University of Pennsylvania in Philadelphia found that it may raise heart attack risk by as much as 300 percent. To make matters worse, people with a severe form of the ailment have a 50 percent increased risk of death.

According to the National Institutes of Health, as many as 7.5 million Americans have one of the disease's five types. The most common is plaque psoriasis, which appears as raised red patches on the skin that are covered with a silvery buildup of dead skin cells, called scale. These patches can appear anywhere on the body, but they occur most commonly on the scalp, knees, elbows, and torso.

You can develop psoriasis at any time, but it's most likely to begin between the ages of 15 and 35. While no one knows for sure what causes it, it may be linked to an immune system glitch. Normally, skin cells form and push up to the surface, where they die and flake off. This process normally takes 28 to 30 days, but in people with psoriasis, the process is stuck in fast-forward. The cells move to the surface in just 3 to 4 days, where they pile up on the skin as the telltale white scales.

Although we may not know what causes psoriasis, we do know that some food remedies can help provide relief.

Healing Foods for Psoriasis

★★★**Carrots and other produce** Eating more fruits and vegetables can help prevent—and treat—psoriasis. Researchers in Italy found that the people who ate the most carrots, tomatoes, fresh fruits, and green vegetables were much less likely to develop psoriasis (or experience flare-ups if they already had it). In fact, people who ate three or more servings of carrots a week reduced their risk by 40 percent, those who ate two servings of fresh fruit a day reduced their risk by 50 percent, and those who ate seven or more servings of tomatoes a week reduced their risk by 60 percent. Because these are all sources of beta-carotene and vitamins C and E, the researchers think it's the antioxidant effects that provide protection.

Another benefit of produce is that it's high in fiber. Fiber escorts psoriasis-triggering chemicals out of the intestines.

★★**Chile peppers** Researchers in Rome found that the most frequent complaint of people with severe psoriasis is itching. One of several foods that can help ease the itch is hot pepper.

Chile peppers contain a chemical called capsaicin, which gives them their heat. Capsaicin was first shown to relieve the itching of psoriasis more than two decades ago. Since then, several studies have confirmed its effectiveness. Researchers don't know exactly how it does this, but putting capsaicin on the skin reportedly depletes stores of substance P, a neurotransmitter that's involved in the cause of psoriasis and itching.

You can buy several over-the-counter products that contain 0.025 or 0.075 percent capsaicin. Not surprisingly, the higher-strength cream is more effective.

While capsaicin cream often causes a burning feeling when you apply it, the sensation usually goes away after using the cream for a few days. As you might imagine, it would really burn if you got it in your eyes, nose, or mouth, so either wear protective gloves or apply it with an applicator and wash your hands thoroughly afterward. If the cream gives you more irritation than relief, stop using it.

FOODS TO WATCH

If you have psoriasis, you should be wary of the following foods, which may trigger or aggravate a flare-up.

Alcohol. According to the National Psoriasis Foundation, alcohol is a quadruple whammy where psoriasis is concerned. Heavy drinking can increase your risk of developing psoriasis in the first place, it may make it significantly worse, it can keep your treatment from working, and it can prevent psoriasis from going into remission.

Researchers in Finland found that men with psoriasis consumed twice as much alcohol (1.5 ounces) on a daily basis than men who were psoriasis free (0.75 ounce). Other studies have shown unusually high rates of psoriasis among people who abuse alcohol.

Fried and fatty foods. These foods promote inflammation, which is exactly what you want to avoid if you have psoriasis. Drive right on past the drive-throughs. Any food handed to you out of a window probably isn't going to help your skin.

Grapefruit juice. The foods you eat can affect the medications you take, and drugs for psoriasis are no exception. Grapefruit juice can increase the absorption level of cyclosporine, a drug used to treat psoriasis.

Also, it can be helpful to limit—or even eliminate—caffeine, alcohol, sugar, white flour, and products containing gluten. That's a pretty long list! You could keep a food diary, carefully noting what you eat, to track your symptoms and look for patterns.

High-protein foods. Several studies have shown that cutting back on protein-rich foods—such as meats and dairy products—may help alleviate psoriasis flare-ups. Anecdotally, some people report a decrease in their symptoms if they avoid pork and other fatty meats.

Tomatoes. Anecdotal reports suggest that some people with psoriasis do better when they avoid or eliminate tomatoes and tomato-based dishes from their diets. Perhaps the acids in tomatoes make psoriasis symptoms flare.

★★Flaxseed Another good source of omega-3's is flaxseed. Keep a bag of ground flaxseed on your countertop and sprinkle it liberally on foods such as cereal and salads.

★★Honey, olive oil, and beeswax For centuries, honey has been used as a natural sweetener and healing agent, and modern research has shown that it has antibiotic properties.

One study in the United Arab Emirates found that a mixture of 1 part natural honey, 1 part beeswax, and 1 part olive oil applied to the skin improved psoriasis in 60 percent of people.

★★Oats, milk, and apricot kernel oil Oats have been used for centuries to soothe dry, itchy skin, and many bath products contain colloidal oatmeal. (Colloidal means the oatmeal has been ground to a fine powder that will remain suspended in water.)

The National Psoriasis Foundation suggests this oatmeal bath: Pulverize 1 cup of oats and ¼ cup of powdered milk in a food processor or blender, then gradually mix in 2 tablespoons of apricot kernel oil. Place the mixture in a cotton bag, sock, or handkerchief, close the bag, and put it in the tub while it fills. Soak in the bath and squeeze the bag to release the preparation. (Be careful getting in and out of the slippery tub.)

★★Purslane Although the FDA classifies purslane as a weed, it's a popular vegetable and herb in China, Mexico, and Greece. Here's why people with psoriasis should add it to their diets: It has the highest amount of omega-3 fats of any edible leafy vegetable I know of.

Admittedly, purslane isn't the best-known source of omega-3's; that title goes to fish. A British study found that people with psoriasis who ate 6 ounces of fatty cold-water fish—such as salmon, mackerel, and herring—a day had a 15 percent improvement in itching and scaling within just 6 weeks. Experts think the omega-3's in fish reduce the production of inflammatory compounds.

You could try eating fatty fish high in omega-3's twice a week for healthier skin. But if you prefer to go the plant route, as I do, look for purslane at your local farmer's market or at some supermarkets as an individual leafy green or in bagged salad mixes. Enjoy it steamed like spinach or use the young shoots in salads. Come summer, it will be in all my daily vegetarian soups.

★★Turmeric In biblical times, this yellow-orange spice was used in perfumes. Today it's mainly used to add color and flavor to foods, but you may want to try it to relieve psoriasis symptoms. Studies have found that turmeric inhibits autoimmune diseases, such as psoriasis, by regulating inflammatory proteins that are secreted by the immune system. Rather than eating more turmeric in your foods, some authors suggest using curcumin (a compound in turmeric) in topical creams, emulsions, or ointments for psoriasis. Let me warn you, though, it's messy.

★★**Vegetable oil** Soaking in warm water can soften the plaques of psoriasis, but it can dry your skin and make itching worse. Adding oil can give you the benefits of the bath without the dryness. The best way to do this is to lie back in a warm bath, allow your skin to soak up some water, then add a few teaspoons of oil. (Be careful getting in and out of the slippery tub.)

★**Apple cider vinegar** Many ancient cultures derived vinegars from dates, figs, and other foods and used them for medicinal purposes. Apple cider vinegar, for example, has been used for generations as a disinfectant and soothing agent. According to the National Psoriasis Foundation, many people with psoriasis apply it to their skin, soak their fingernails and toenails in it, or mix it with their moisturizers.

Here's one remedy to try: Add 1 cup of apple cider vinegar to 1 gallon of water. Soak a clean, soft cloth in the mixture, wring it out, and apply it to your skin.

★**Baking soda** To soothe your itchy skin, dissolve ⅓ cup of baking soda in a gallon of water, then soak a clean, soft cloth, wring it out, and lay it over affected areas for several minutes.

★**Beets** Many people with psoriasis have congestion in the bowels and liver. Beet juice is wonderful to help detoxify the liver, but you probably won't like the taste of the stuff if you drink it straight. To mitigate the strong flavor, blend the juice of one beet with the juice of four carrots and a quarter of a lemon. Drink one glass of the juice every day.

★**Green tea** Researchers at the Medical College of Georgia conducted an animal study with green tea and found that it may have promise for treating inflammatory skin conditions such as psoriasis.

From the Herbal Medicine Chest

You may find the following herbs helpful in relieving psoriasis symptoms.

Calaguala (Polypodium aureum) The Latin American fern calaguala, though previously used for cancer, has been used more recently for psoriasis and dermatitis. Its beneficial effects, which have been observed in clinical use, have also been demonstrated in the lab. One study found that people who took calaguala extract showed measurable improvements in their immune responses.

Chamomile (*Matricaria recutita*) This herb contains anti-inflammatory compounds that can help relieve psoriasis flare-ups. Naturopaths say that chamomile is as good as—or even better than—cortisone when applied topically. Chamomile preparations are widely used in Europe for various skin conditions, including psoriasis. This calming herb contains flavonoids and essential oils that have significant anti-inflammatory and anti-allergic activities.

To make a chamomile compress, place 1 heaping teaspoon of chamomile flowers (sold in health food stores) in 1 cup of boiling water. Steep for 10 minutes, then strain out the herb. Soak a clean, soft cloth in the solution, then apply it to your affected skin.

Tea tree (*Melaleuca alternifolia*) The tea tree plant hails from the land down under. Its oil was first used in surgery and dentistry in the 1920s, and research shows it has antibacterial and antiseptic properties. Tea tree oil is a common ingredient in lots of creams, lotions, and potions, and the National Psoriasis Foundation reports that some of its members have success using it for scalp psoriasis.

You might mix a few drops of tea tree oil into a couple of tablespoons of herbal shampoo. But don't take this oil—or any essential oil for that matter—internally. They are extremely concentrated and can be poisonous.

Rheumatoid Arthritis

RHEUMATOID ARTHRITIS, OR RA—an incurable autoimmune disorder in which the body's immune system attacks healthy joint tissue—is a common scourge that, if left untreated, can cause crippling deformity.

Although it frequently affects the hands—usually both at the same time—it also can strike many other joints. The most common symptoms include joint pain, swelling, inflammation, and limited range of motion, but other symptoms can also include fatigue, fever, loss of appetite, enlarged lymph nodes, lumps beneath the skin, and muscle stiffness after sleep or inactivity.

The most recent estimates, published in a 2008 issue of the journal *Arthritis and Rheumatism,* show that 1.3 million Americans—about three-quarters of them women—have RA, a decline from an estimated 2.1 million in 1995. The reasons for the decrease are unclear, but one may be that doctors now use a more specific and restrictive definition to identify people who have the disease.

One thing, however, is clear. The average age at which people are diagnosed with RA has steadily increased, suggesting that it's becoming a disease of older adults.

Conventional treatment has improved in recent years with the widespread use of disease-modifying anti-rheumatic drugs (DMARDs), such as methotrexate, and biologic response modifiers, such as adalimumab (Humira), which reduce the rate of damage to bone and cartilage. But such drugs can have serious side effects, including liver damage and bone-marrow toxicity.

Healing Foods for Rheumatoid Arthritis

To help prevent rheumatoid arthritis, I'd start with the Mediterranean diet, which is rich in fruits, vegetables, fish, olive oil, and moderate amounts of wine, all containing high concentrations of antioxidants and anti-inflammatory compounds. If you already have RA, switching to this diet for just 12 weeks may reduce pain, stiffness, and hand weakness by up to 38 percent, according to a 2003 study published in the *American Journal of Epidemiology*. Here are some of the benefits you may get from the Mediterranean diet's individual components, as well as some other foods.

★★★**Fish** Cold-water fish—such as Spanish mackerel, trout, salmon, bluefin tuna, halibut, and pollack—are a rich source of anti-inflammatory omega-3 fatty acids, the most important of which are eicosapentaenoic acid (EPA) and docosahexaeonic acid (DHA). Canned fish such as salmon, herring, sardines, and chunk light tuna are also good.

Fish is an essential part of the Mediterranean diet, which limits consumption of pro-inflammatory animal protein, especially red meat. Human and animal studies show that fish and fish oil help decrease inflammation-inducing cytokines, proteins that help incite the joint swelling, pain, and tenderness of RA. For example, one Danish study showed that people with RA who ate an average of 4 ounces of fish a day for 6 months experienced a significant decrease in morning stiffness, swollen joints, and pain. They also were able to reduce their dosages of conventional arthritis medications.

Andrew Weil, MD, professor at the University of Arizona College of Medicine in Tucson, suggests that people with arthritis eat at least three servings of fish a week and supplement that with 2 or 3 grams of fish oil a day.

But fish isn't the only good source of omega-3's. You can also get high amounts from plant sources such as canola oil, flaxseed, dark greens, and walnuts.

★★★**Turmeric** This yellow curry spice is a rich source of curcumin, a strong antioxidant that protects against free radical damage. Curcumin contains natural pain-relieving COX-2-inhibitors, which makes it an attractive, side effect–free alternative to prescription COX-2 inhibitors such as celecoxib (Celebrex). It also reduces inflammation by lowering histamine levels and possibly by stimulating the adrenal glands to produce more cortisone, the body's natural painkiller. Lately, I've had two students who switched from Celebrex to either curcumin or curried celery (see my Curried Celery COX-2 Inhibitor recipe on page 286) and thought it was a good tradeoff.

Human and animal studies of curcumin have found that it can reduce the pain and stiffness associated with RA. In a 2006 study published in the journal *Arthritis and Rheumatism,* researchers from the University of Arizona showed how turmeric prevented rheumatoid arthritis in an animal model of the disease. The study demonstrated that an oil-depleted extract containing the three major curcuminoids—which is similar to commercially available turmeric dietary supplements—blocked the protein NF-KB, which switches on genes that produce joint-damaging substances. The findings suggest that the extract works the same way as drugs under development for blocking NF-KB, but presumably with far fewer side effects.

Because I prefer a whole-foods approach, I often add liberal amounts of turmeric to rice and other dishes and would consider adding other anti-inflammatory foods such as pineapple and papaya. Dr. Weil recommends adding a teaspoon of powdered turmeric to soups, stews, and other dishes. You can also make tea with turmeric.

Unfortunately, it's difficult to get medicinal doses of curcumin from your diet alone. According to naturopaths, that dose is 250 to 500 milligrams of pure curcumin a day between meals, which translates into 5 to 25 teaspoons of dried turmeric a day. That's a good deal more than even a curry fan like me would want to add to my food. I would recommend adding as much turmeric as possible to your diet to help prevent pain and taking turmeric supplements—standardized to 90 to 95 percent curcumin—to help relieve acute pain.

★★**Chile peppers** Hot peppers contain a resinous and pungent substance known as capsaicin, which is number one among my painkillers. When applied topically, capsaicin temporarily depletes substance P, a chemical in nerves that transmits pain sensations. Without substance P, pain signals can no longer be sent. Dozens of studies show that capsaicin can temporarily relieve many painful conditions, including RA.

COX-2-Inhibiting Chile Drink

I've gotten several good responses to my curried alternatives to prescription COX-2 inhibitors (see the Osteoarthritis chapter on page 281). Here's one I really like.

Dear Dr. Duke,

I have benefited so much from your books that I would like to share with you the hot drink which I concocted as a tasty way to take enough turmeric to treat my arthritic fingers. I credit this drink with straightening two fingers on my right hand, which had seemed destined to be permanently curled and twisted. Not only have the fingers straightened and become flexible but the joints are no longer swollen and painful. What a pleasure!

Here's the reader's recipe. You can adjust the proportions to suit your taste. In 1 cup of hot water, add a few grinds of black pepper, ¼ teaspoon of cumin, ½ teaspoon of chili powder, 1 teaspoon of turmeric, and a generous squirt of ketchup. While the mixture is still hot, stir occasionally, sip slowly, and enjoy!

You can buy a commercial topical cream containing 0.025 to 0.075 percent capsaicin and apply it to your arthritic joints three or four times a day. Or you can do what people outside the United States often do: buy a chile pepper, mash it, and apply it directly to your swollen joints. You can also mix mashed hot pepper with a skin cream such as cold cream. Either way, you'll save money. A fresh pepper costs a few pennies, whereas a commercial capsaicin product such as Zostrix can cost up to $16.

No matter which route you choose, you may experience a burning sensation the first few times you use capsaicin, but it usually subsides with repeated use. Just be sure to thoroughly wash your hands after using it. If you get any in your eyes, nose, or mouth, it may be almost as painful as your arthritic joints.

Although capsaicin is best used topically, it may be helpful to add more peppers and pepper-derived hot sauces to your diet. Another option is taking a cayenne tincture (0.3 to 1 milliliter) three times a day. You also can make an infusion by stirring ½ to 1 teaspoon (2.5 to 5 grams) of cayenne powder into 1 cup of boiling water, letting it steep for 10 minutes, and taking 1 teaspoon mixed with water three to four times daily.

★★**Fruits and vegetables** In a 2005 study published in the *American Journal of Clinical Nutrition,* researchers from the University of Manchester in the United Kingdom presented data showing that an inadequate intake of vitamin C and a pigment called beta-cryptoxanthin—both of which are found in brightly colored fruits and vegetables—can increase the risk of RA. When they compared 88 new patients who had inflammatory arthritis with 176 disease-free individuals, they found that the average intake of beta-cryptoxanthin was 40 percent lower in the arthritis patients. They also found that people who ranked in the top third for consumption of beta-cryptoxanthin were only half as likely to develop inflammatory arthritis as those in the bottom third.

Some of the best sources of beta-cryptoxanthin include green grapes, broccoli, green beans, celery, Brussels sprouts, cucumbers, lettuce, scallions, and butternut squash.

The results of the study also confirmed researchers' earlier finding that a diet lacking in fruit—especially vitamin C–rich fruits such as oranges and grapefruit—can up to triple the risk of developing inflammatory arthritis. You may want to increasine your intake of the above-mentioned fruits and vegetables or drinking at least one 8-ounce glass of orange juice a day to boost your beta-cryptoxanthin levels.

★★**Green tea** The incidence of RA is far lower in countries where green tea is part of daily life—especially in Asia—than it is in the United States, suggesting that regular consumption can help prevent it. Now, laboratory and animal studies show that green tea—a rich source of anti-inflammatory catechins—can actually help slow cartilage breakdown and decrease chronic inflammation in people who already have the disease.

If I were at risk of developing RA—or already had it—I would drink the human equivalent of the amount of green tea used in this study: four cups a day.

★★**Olive oil** Loaded with healthy monounsaturated fat, olive oil has well-documented cardiovascular effects, but it also can help prevent and even treat RA. In a study published in the *American Journal of Clinical Nutrition,* Greek researchers assessed the diets of 145 RA patients and 188 healthy control participants. It turned out that the risk of RA was 2.5 times higher in people who consumed the least amount of extra-virgin olive oil throughout their lives than in those who consumed the most. Because it's made from the first pressing of perfectly ripe olives, it has the richest taste of all olive oils. Studies suggest that it may be especially useful in preventing RA because it contains higher amounts of inflammation-reducing monounsaturated fat and disease-fighting polyphenols. If you already have RA, switching to olive oil as your primary fat is a smart idea. Some studies have shown that extra-

FOODS TO WATCH

The typical Western diet—including high consumption of red meat and low consumption of fruits, vegetables, and fish—can increase your risk of developing rheumatoid arthritis (RA), according to recent studies at the University of Manchester in the United Kingdom.

In a 2004 study published in *Arthritis and Rheumatism,* researchers compared the dietary habits of patients with inflammatory arthritis to those of healthy, disease-free people. They found that those who ate the most hamburgers, steak, and other red meat had a doubled risk of developing RA. The possible reason: red meat contains high amounts of collagen, a major component of joint tissue. In people susceptible to RA, this may lead to collagen sensitization, meaning that your immune system may begin to attack collagen as if it were a disease-causing invader in your body.

So if RA runs in your family—or you already have it—I'd strongly recommend cutting back on red meat.

I'd also be wary of coffee. Some studies show that people who drink four or more cups a day are twice as likely to test positive for rheumatoid factor, an indicator of RA. People who drink 11 or more cups a day were 15 times more likely to test positive for rheumatoid factor. Other studies suggest that the coffee-associated risks are even higher in people who people who drink decaf than in those who prefer high-test.

virgin olive oil—in amounts as little as 2 tablespoons a day—can have anti-inflammatory effects that rival those of ibuprofen.

★★**Wine** People who eat a Mediterranean-type diet often drink moderate amounts of wine, especially during meals. They especially like red wine, which contains high amounts of anti-inflammatory compounds such as quercetin, resveratrol, and saponins. Because these compounds help lower cholesterol, prevent harmful low-density lipoprotein from sticking to artery walls, and lower the risk of blood clots, red wine seems to be one important element in the Mediterranean diet's ability to lower the risk of heart disease.

However, all alcoholic beverages, not just wine, seem to help protect against RA, according to research presented at EULAR 2007, the Annual European Congress of Rheumatology, in Barcelona, Spain. In an analysis of 1,204 RA patients and 871 healthy control participants, Swedish researchers found that people who consumed three or more drinks a week (with one drink equaling 4 ounces of wine, 12 ounces of beer, or 1 ounce of spirits) had a 50 percent lower risk of developing RA than teetotalers. Consuming 10 drinks a week was even more protective.

A 2006 animal study published in *Proceedings of the National Academy of Sciences* also showed that alcohol consumption—in levels too low to cause liver toxicity—prevented mice from developing collagen-induced arthritis, an animal model of rheumatoid arthritis.

Such research suggests that moderate alcohol consumption—no more than one drink a day for women and no more than two a day for men—may be helpful in alleviating RA symptoms.

★**Kiwi and related fruits** In Korea, scientists have studied the effects of kiwifruit and other fruit juices on antioxidant concentrations in the blood. Low levels have been implicated in a number of disorders, including RA. In a study published in a 2005 issue of the *Journal of Medicinal Food*, researchers measured the effects of nine different juices—kiwi, apple, orange, grape, peach, plum, melon, watermelon, and pear—on free radical levels of the bloodstreams of a small group of men. With the exception of pear, all the juices showed potent antioxidant effects.

From the Herbal Medicine Chest

If I had rheumatoid arthritis, I'd try using boswellia, which is extracted from the gummy resin exuded by a branching tree that grows in the dry, hilly areas of India. This extract contains anti-inflammatory boswellic acids, the most active of which are terpenoids. Its actions seem similar to those of non-steroidal anti-inflammatory drugs, but without side effects such as stomach irritation and gastrointestinal bleeding.

Many doctors recommend that their arthritis patients take extracts standardized to contain 37.5 to 65 percent boswellic acids. The usual dosage is 150 milligrams of boswellic acid three times a day for 8 to 12 weeks. So if you buy an extract containing 37.5 percent boswellic acids, that means you would need to take 400 milligrams of extract three times a day in order to see a beneficial effect.

Shingles

FOR ANYONE WHO HASN'T SUFFERED from the condition, shingles might make you think of the work involved with putting a new roof on a home—but for those in the know, reroofing a house in midsummer heat might be preferable to the uncomfortable blisters and pain that accompany the disease.

Shingles, also called herpes zoster, is caused by the same virus that causes chicken pox, and anyone who has ever had chicken pox is at risk of developing shingles later in life. This happens because once the chicken pox have run their course, the virus is believed to lie dormant within the nervous system. If the virus becomes reactivated in later years—and no one is sure why this happens since it remains inactive in most people—it travels up the nerves to the skin and the virus starts to multiply.

The first clue of a shingles outbreak is a burning pain or itch in one specific part of the body. In a few days, chicken pox–like blisters form in one location; they often spread out in a band on one side of the torso and reaching around the waistline. The blisters heal after a few weeks, but in some people the pain associated with shingles sticks around for weeks or months after the blisters.

You're most at risk of shingles if you have a suppressed immune system, such as those undergoing chemotherapy for cancer, receiving an organ transplant, or living with HIV. Shingles is contagious for those who haven't had chicken pox, and anyone who catches the virus from you will develop chicken pox, not shingles—although the virus will then stay dormant in them.

The FDA approved a varicella zoster virus vaccine (Zostavax) in 2006 for use in those over age 60 who have had chickenpox, and the National Institute of Neurological Disorders and Stroke reports that the expected number of cases of shingles has been halved as a result. Those who took the vaccine and still developed shingles typically had fewer complications and less severe outbreaks. Aside from vaccines, though, you might consider the following.

Healing Foods for Shingles

★★**Chile peppers** Surprisingly enough, I'm not going to suggest that you eat these peppers; instead you're going to wear them, or at least part of them. The active ingredient in chile peppers—the substance that gives it a kick—is capsaicin, and when applied to the skin it can block pain signals from nerves located just under the surface.

Note that you don't just cut open a pepper and slab it on your ribcage. The capsaicin needs to be diluted first. The FDA has approved the use of capsaicin in topical ointments, and a number of those are on the market, but you can also create your own soothing cream by mixing enough powdered red pepper into a white skin lotion that the lotion turns pink. Dab the lotion onto the affected spots, then wash your hands thoroughly so that you don't place any capsaicin on sensitive parts of your body. Test this lotion in a small area of skin before applying it all over, and discontinue using it if your body seems irritated.

★**Black currants, guava, and kiwi** A 2005 study in the *International Journal of Epidemiology* examined the role of seven micronutrients—vitamins A, B$_6$, C, and E; folic acid; zinc; and iron—on the risk of developing herpes zoster. The only direct connection found was an increased risk of shingles for those with a decreased intake of vitamin C.

The FDA recommends 60 milligrams of vitamin C daily, and you can easily meet that requirement depending on the fruits and vegetables you choose to eat. Black currants, for example, contain 180 milligrams of C in 100 grams, while a single guava boasts 125 milligrams and a lone kiwi has 70 milligrams.

Keep in mind that you can get too much of a good thing when it comes to vitamin C. According to the US National Library of Medicine, taking more than 2,000 milligrams of vitamin C per day can lead to diarrhea and upset stomach, so don't start adorning all your meals with black currants.

★**Oatmeal** As with the chile peppers, the oatmeal is intended for something other than eating. Specifically, if you currently have shingles with developed blisters, you can add oatmeal—or, even better, colloidal oatmeal, which is ground to a fine powder and not meant for eating—to a warm bath, then take a long soak. Bathing in this solution should help relieve the itches that come with blisters. Watch your step when getting out because the oatmeal creates a slick surface, and pat yourself dry instead of rubbing to avoid irritating your skin.

★**Red and green peppers and broccoli** If you favor veggies over fruits, then the optimal choices that you could make for vitamin C would be sweet red and green peppers. One medium red pepper contains 152 milligrams of vitamin C, while a green pepper of the same size has 95 milligrams. One cup of broccoli features 81 milligrams of vitamin C.

★**Strawberries, oranges, lemons, cantaloupes, and grapefruit** Vitamin C is also present in more traditional fruits such as those listed above, although the quantities aren't as high. A single medium strawberry hides 7 milligrams of vitamin C, which means that a cup's worth of whole strawberries holds 84 milligrams. One orange has

83 milligrams of vitamin C, while half a grapefruit has 45 milligrams, an eighth of a cantaloupe has 25 milligrams, and the juice of one lemon yields 21 milligrams.

★**All fruits and veggies!** While the study from the *International Journal of Epidemiology* didn't find connections between other micronutrients and a lowered risk of developing shingles, it did find a connection between the intake of all types of fruits and vegetables and shingles. In particular, those who ate no more than one portion per day had almost three times the risk of shingles as those who consumed the most. When compared separately, fruit had a stronger impact on lowering the risk of shingles than vegetables.

The study even noted that taking nonprescribed supplements of micronutrients did not provide increased protection against shingles, possibly because the supplements don't contain the full range of nutrients found in whole fruits and vegetables.

Sinusitis

YOUR SINUSES ARE CAVITIES behind your forehead, cheeks, and eyes. When they're healthy, they're empty and free of mucus. But when they become blocked with congestion from a cold or the flu, they fill with fluid and can become infected by bacteria or other organisms. When that happens, sinus pressure can be so painful that it feels as if you've been punched in the face.

Sinusitis is extremely common: More than 30 million adults and children have it each year. The infection may last only a couple of weeks or take months to clear up. In addition to sinus pressure, you'll probably experience a stuffy nose—possibly with thick secretions—postnasal drip, sore throat, headache, cough, fatigue, and possibly a fever.

FOODS TO WATCH

You may be surprised to learn that food allergies, along with cigarette smoking, can cause sinus congestion.

Any food that you're allergic to—whether it's peanuts, wheat, milk, or fish—can stop up your sinuses and lead to inflammation. Food allergies cause an immune reaction that can trigger the production of mucus. Any food can cause an allergy, so it's important to avoid those you know you're allergic to.

Thankfully, only a small number of colds lead to sinusitis, but some people are susceptible and get it more frequently. Doctors prescribe decongestants, corticosteroid sprays, and pain relievers for sinusitis. Your doctor may also suggest using a saline nasal spray. If he thinks you have a bacterial infection, he'll prescribe an antibiotic.

I prefer to get relief from eating foods that boost my immunity and reduce congestion.

Healing Foods for Sinusitis

These foods specifically work on nasal congestion, but because colds and respiratory infections can lead to sinusitis, you may want to follow the suggestions in the Colds and Flu chapter (page 104) as well.

★★**Citrus fruits or juice** The vitamin C in citrus fruits boosts your immune system and helps defend against viral infections. Protect yourself by drinking citrus juice or lemonade or eating oranges, grapefruit, or nectarines. If you're looking for other sources of vitamin C, try guavas, chopped red bell peppers, papayas, broccoli, strawberries, cantaloupe, tomato juice, mangoes, potatoes, cabbage greens, and spinach. It also wouldn't hurt to take a vitamin C supplement.

★★**Cruciferous vegetables** Crucifers, which include all the members of the cabbage and mustard families, would make a good addition to your SinuSoup. They open up the sinuses, and as a bonus, they have antiseptic and anticancer properties as well. Broccoli, brussels sprouts, cabbage, collard greens, cress, kohlrabi (a cabbage with a turnip shape), radishes, and turnips fall into this category.

★★**Garlic and onions** At home, I enjoy my SinuSoup, a concoction specially designed to keep my sinuses clear. It includes garlic, onions, and all the hot spices I can find around the house, such as curry, horseradish, hot pepper, mustard seed, and black pepper. Garlic and onions have high amounts of quercetin, which can reduce inflammation and act like an antihistamine to lessen congestion.

★★**Oregano** This culinary herb is full of antihistamine, antiseptic, and antioxidant compounds, and it's an herb I like to turn to for sinus relief. This year, after the first full moon of spring, my nose began to feel stopped up, so I went out into my frostbitten garden to pick some old, dried-out oregano. It was still aromatic and medicinal. I boiled it with celery and lemon juice to make a concoction I call

AcelerADE. By combining three powerful foods in one drink, I managed to get 10 antihistamine compounds from the oregano, 12 from the celery, and at least 15 from the lemon.

However, if you have only oregano on hand, make a hot tea from the herb and inhale its aroma once you've poured it. You can also add oregano essential oil to a lotion or vegetable oil for massage.

★★**Mints and menthol** In the summer, I like to drink mentholated teas and inhale menthol to clear my sinuses. I've even been known to put aromatic mints into my nose if I have sinusitis, which sometimes hits me following a bout of hay fever. I even have a picture somewhere of a New Zealand doctor visiting the Green Farmacy Garden in the December snow and stuffing a weedy mint called ale hoof up his nose. Menthol, present in many mints, and the ubiquitous chlorophyll, which is found in all green plants including green mints, may help clear the sinuses. You may also realize benefits from drinking peppermint tea and eating peppermint candy, gum, jelly, and sauces. Since I know it's unseemly, I won't suggest that you stuff a mint up your nose (but it works).

★★**Saltwater** It's not to drink but rather to rinse your sinuses as part of a nasal douche. Andrew Weil, MD, professor at the University of Arizona College of Medicine in Tucson, recommends dissolving ¼ teaspoon of salt in a cup of warm water to use this way. Be sure to use kosher or sea salt rather than table salt since table salt contains chemicals that can be harmful if used every day.

Add the saltwater to a bulb aspirator or neti pot (a small teapot-shaped pot that you can find in many drugstores), then bend over a sink, tilt your head to one side, and pour the water into the nostril that's facing up. The water will flow out of your other nostril, helping to break up mucus so it's easier to blow your nose. Do this rinse when you have sinusitis, a cold, or allergies. Some people even do it every day to avoid congestion.

The saltwater helps release mucus from the sinus cavities, and having less mucus means the cavities are less likely to become infected. I wouldn't hesitate to add anti-septic mint herbs to the rinse as well.

★**Fruits, vegetables, and beans** Flavonoids, phytochemicals that are packed into fruits, vegetables, and teas, work in the body to prevent the release of histamine, the chemical that causes sinus congestion and allergy symptoms. Many fruits and vegetables also contain vitamin A, which may protect against viral infections. Be sure to get plenty of blackberries, blueberries, red grapes, raspberries, strawberries, plums, red cabbage, red onions, apples, apricots, parsley, thyme, oregano, chile peppers, lemons, onions, kale, leeks, broccoli, and beans. Red wine, green and black tea, and dark chocolate also contain flavonoids.

★**Horseradish and other hot spices** I put it in my SinuSoup and recommend it to anyone trying to fend off sinusitis. All hot spices, including chile powder, ginger, and pepper, can open the sinuses.

★**Pineapple** Some naturopaths say the enzyme bromelain in pineapple may help to clear up a nasty case of sinusitis. There hasn't been much recent research on bromelain for this use, but a couple of studies from the 1960s reported that it relieved symptoms. The studies used enteric-coated bromelain supplements. But whether or not bromelain actually helps with sinusitis, there's another reason to eat pineapple: a cup of chunks contains 79 milligrams of vitamin C, a powerful ally in avoiding infection.

★**Tea** Tea comes in second to onion for content of quercetin, which is an antihistamine that helps unclog stuffed sinuses. You'll also find quercetin in sunflowers, apples, cranberries, garlic, kale, cabbage, and cayenne.

From the Herbal Medicine Chest

Herbs can fight infections and specifically help reduce congestion from sinusitis. Here's what I recommend.

Eucalyptus (*Eucalyptus globulus*) Eucalyptus works as an anti-inflammatory, antioxidant, and decongestant to improve sinus problems. In 2004, researchers gave 76 people with sinusitis capsules containing cineole, the major ingredient in eucalyptus oil. Another 76 people with sinusitis received a placebo. After 7 days of taking 100 milligrams of cineole three times a day, most of those in the cineole group—92 percent—reported improvement in more than half of their symptoms. In the group taking a placebo, only 45 percent reported a similar improvement. Ultrasound scans confirmed that 95 percent of those in the group taking cineole had no more swelling or fluid in their sinuses, while only 51 percent in the placebo group showed the same improvement.

You can inhale eucalyptus by rubbing the essential oil mixed with vegetable oil on your temples or by adding a small amount to a bath. Be careful not to swallow any of the oil because it can be toxic.

You could also crush eucalyptus and peppermint leaves, wet them with water, and rub them on your chest or gently push them into your nostrils. I also recommend drinking a tea made with eucalyptus and any kind of mint leaves.

Goldenseal (*Hydrastis canadensis*) and echinacea (*Echinacea spp.*) These two herbs are often combined in herbal preparations to boost the immune system, and both are known as powerful antibiotics that fight infection. You can take them in capsule form or drink them in tea.

Siberian ginseng (*Eleutherococcus senticosus*) and andrographis (*Andrographis paniculata*) Research suggests that taking these two herbs can be a substitute for antibiotics in treating sinus and throat infections. In a study, researchers gave half of the 185 participants with sinusitis or upper respiratory infections 12 tablets a day containing 85 milligrams of andrographis and 10 milligrams of Siberian ginseng for 5 days. The other half received a placebo. Those who took the herbs had significant improvements in headache, sore throat, runny nose, and fatigue.

Skin Problems

DASHING THROUGH THE SNOW, in a one-horse open sleigh, o'er the fields we go, itching all the way . . .

Winter, for all its wonders, can be quite the itching season. According to the National Health Interview Survey, at least 81 million Americans—one in four of us—experience dry, itchy, or scaly skin during the winter months. It's caused by overheated homes and offices; cold, dry air; and exposure to the winter sun. Dermatologists call it dermatitis—literally an inflammation of the skin—or eczema.

Of course, dry winter air isn't the only cause. Contact with certain chemicals or allergenic plants can cause similar symptoms, and about 3 percent of the population has a particular form of the condition called atopic dermatitis, or atopic eczema. This type causes the skin to redden and blister and become oozy, scaly, brownish, and/or thickened. It usually itches.

Healing Foods for Skin Problems

★★★**Honey, olive oil, and beeswax** Besides being used as a sweetener, honey has served as a folk remedy for generations. Research has shown that it has antibiotic properties.

One study in the United Arab Emirates found that applying a concoction of natural honey, beeswax, and olive oil to the skin improved dermatitis significantly in 8 out of 10 people after 14 days.

★★★**Oatmeal** This is a classic folk remedy for irritated skin. Add 1 cup of oatmeal to a warm bath and soak for 10 to 15 minutes to soothe itchy skin. Don't use hot water, though; it can make the itching worse.

You can also use oatmeal instead of soap. Wrap a handful of oatmeal in a soft cloth or handkerchief and place a rubber band around the top, then dunk it in water, wring it out, and use it as you would a washcloth.

FOODS TO WATCH

About 10 percent of the time, dermatitis is triggered by foods. This happens more often among infants and young children with asthma. If you suspect a particular food is a trigger, eliminate it from your diet.

Foods that have been known to worsen eczema include eggs, milk, peanuts, soy, wheat, and fish. Some people report that chocolate, coffee, alcohol, tomatoes, and sugar can trigger a flare-up.

Also watch out for Margaritas (just kidding, sort of). When certain plant compounds come into contact with skin, they make the area sensitive to light, causing a red, swollen, itchy rash similar to sunburn or a poison ivy rash. This condition is called phytophotodermatitis. During the summer, lime juice is the common cause of the condition, which is why some doctors call it Margarita dermatitis. The sensitizing compound is also found in celery and parsley. Treat the condition as you would a poison ivy rash, with cool compresses and over-the-counter creams.

Dairy foods are other offenders. While putting milk on your skin may soothe it, drinking it may do just the opposite. "Probably the biggest food we see impacting skin is cow's milk," says Joel Schlessinger, MD, a board-certified dermatologist and immediate past president of the American Society of Cosmetic Dermatology and Aesthetic Surgery. "There is mounting evidence that milk, and the hormones it contains, may be increasing the severity of acne and the longevity of it as well, causing more adult acne. Soy milk might be a better choice."

★★★**Olive oil** Little did I know when I anointed my body with olive oil that I was not only following a biblical dictum but also using one of the best medicines for many kinds of dermatitis. Olive oil has five anti-dermatitic compounds (aesculin, apigenin, esculin, quercetin, and rutin) to accompany dozens of anti-inflammatories. You might try mixing up an oil of olea—olive oil with a little walnut oil and avocado oil and a few calendula petals—and apply it topically.

★★**Avocados** Rich in vitamins A, D, and E, all of which are great for healthy skin, avocado oil may be helpful whether applied topically or eaten.

★★**Cucumbers** These pale green vegetables are kin to watermelons, zucchinis, pumpkins, and other types of squash. Cucumbers were very popular in the ancient civilizations of Egypt, Greece, and Rome, where people ate them and used them for their skin-healing properties.

If I had a skin problem, I'd peel some cucumbers, puree them in my blender, and apply the puree directly to the affected area, leaving it on for 15 to 60 minutes. If you wish, you could add an avocado. Its oil is patented as a treatment for some forms of dermatitis.

★★**Flax** In the Roman Empire, flax was treasured for its healing properties. In modern times, it fell out of favor because its omega-3 fatty acids give it a short shelf life. Yet ironically, those fatty acids are what make flax so useful for so many things, including skin problems. Forty to 65 percent of flax oil is composed of an omega-3 called alpha-linolenic acid.

Try taking 1 tablespoon of flaxseed oil a day or sprinkling 2 tablespoons of ground flaxseed on your food. Instead of flaxseed, I add Nutiva hemp seed to my cereals and soups, but it works on the same principle.

Another great source of omega-3's is fish, particularly fatty fish that live in cold waters, such as salmon and sardines. Interestingly, researchers in Mexico found that 1-year-olds whose mothers had eaten fish 2½ times a week during their pregnancies had a 37 percent decrease in their risk for eczema compared to 1-year-olds whose mothers ate fish only once a week.

Experts recommend eating fatty fish such as salmon, mackerel, and albacore tuna twice a week for healthier skin.

★**Cauliflower and other foods high in vitamin B$_6$** One of the symptoms of a vitamin B$_6$ deficiency is dermatitis. If I were bothered by this condition, I'd eat more cauliflower, watercress, spinach, bananas, and okra, which are all good sources of the vitamin.

★**Chile peppers** Capsaicin is the chemical in chile peppers that makes them hot. Salves containing 0.025 percent capsaicin, which is about the strength of a reasonably hot pepper, have been shown effective for the especially itchy skin of psoriasis, so it may do the trick for plain old itchy winter skin, too.

Commercial preparations usually contain 0.025 percent or 0.075 percent capsaicin. You can make your own salve by crushing a hot red pepper and mixing it with your favorite skin moisturizer.

While capsaicin can cause a burning sensation on your skin, you should become less sensitive to it over time. Use an applicator or rubber glove to apply it, and wash your hands thoroughly afterward. If the treatment causes more irritation than relief, stop using it.

★**Milk** A tall glass of cool milk may do the trick to soothe your itchy skin—but don't drink it! Pour it onto a gauze pad or clean, soft cloth and apply it to your skin for 2 to 3 minutes. Resoak the cloth and reapply, continuing the process for about 10 minutes. The cool compress can help soothe skin and relieve itching.

From the Herbal Medicine Chest

Herbalist Leslie Tierra praises calendula tincture as "hands down, one of the best herbs for any skin problems." High praise indeed. It's useful for bacterial and fungal infections, mothers find it wonderful for diaper rash, and Tierra used it on her son when he had chickenpox.

A good—and easy—way to use this herb as a skin treatment is to buy a commercial calendula flower ointment and apply it to your skin as needed.

Sore Throat/Laryngitis

DURING THE 2008 PRESIDENTIAL RACE, the candidates were reportedly given strict rules by their doctors: remain quiet whenever you can; drink extra fluids; and whatever you do, don't whisper. Whispering stresses your vocal cords, and the candidates were speaking so much while campaigning that they were at serious risk for laryngitis.

Not surprisingly, they turned to natural solutions to protect their voices. The *Wall Street Journal* and the *New York Times* reported that Sen. Barack Obama enjoyed hot water with lemon, honey, and ginger to save his voice. Sen. John McCain reportedly swallowed a tablespoon of olive oil before debates.

As you can imagine, if the candidates hadn't taken these preemptive measures, they may have developed a serious case of hoarseness. But laryngitis, in which your vocal cords become inflamed and irritated, can be a sign of an infection. Your vocal cords are in your voice box, or larynx. When you speak, they open and close to form sounds. If they're inflamed and swollen, the sounds they make will be distorted and hoarse and in some cases may be barely audible.

A sore throat, on the other hand, doesn't directly affect your vocal cords but does make talking and swallowing painful. It sometimes serves as a warning, often being the first sign that you're coming down with an illness. Most sore throats are due to a viral infection, such as a cold, the flu, or measles, but sometimes they can come with a bacterial infection such as streptococcus (strep throat) or tonsillitis. And infections aren't the only cause. Even allergies, dry air, pollution, and acid reflux can make your throat hurt.

If you have a sore throat with a fever, see your physician. It could be strep, and that needs to be treated by your doctor because it could lead to rheumatic fever. Otherwise, sore throats usually go away on their own in about 5 to 7 days.

Typically, people suck on lozenges to get relief from a sore or hoarse throat, but all that does is anesthetize the nerve cells in your throat to temporarily relieve the pain. A better choice might be to soothe the inflamed tissue with foods and herbs.

Healing Foods for Sore Throat/Laryngitis

A chronic sore throat or laryngitis deserves a trip to your doctor to make certain it's not a sign of something more serious. But if it's not chronic, try these foods that work directly on the tissue of your larynx to soothe it. If your throat pain is caused by a cold or the flu, see that chapter for more remedies.

★★★**Cardamom** Since cineole is both anti-laryngitic and anti-pharyngitic, and since cardamom is by far the richest source of cineole I've found, it's a logical candidate for treating a sore throat.

★★★**Garlic** As "Russian penicillin" and my *numero uno* antiseptic and immunity booster all rolled into one, garlic is one of the first things I try for any inflammation in the respiratory tract.

Garlic can be made into a tea and used as a gargle. I suspect that garlic relatives such onion and leek would do almost as well, especially since onion is richer in quercetin than garlic. To cure a sore throat, the Jews of Kochin (an ancient Jewish settlement in India) used a decoction of onion and lemon juice.

★★★**Ginger** Like garlic, ginger is great for sore throats and can be added to lemon juice, vinegar, and honey and used as a gargle. I enjoy ginger honey as mentioned

There are probably plenty of things you don't feel like eating or drinking when you have a sore throat or laryngitis. Here are some in particular you should avoid.

Caffeinated drinks. Getting plenty of fluids is important when you have a sore throat, but soda and other drinks with caffeine dehydrate you. It's better to choose water, soup, broth, or even ice chips.

Excessive alcohol. Drinking a lot of alcohol can irritate your throat and vocal cords, which can then lead to laryngitis.

Foods that cause acid reflux. Stomach acid that backs up into your esophagus can also irritate your throat and make it sore. It can even lead to laryngitis, so it's important to avoid foods that trigger reflux, especially acidic foods such as tomatoes and high-fat, heavy foods such as french fries and rich sauces.

by famed cook and herbal columnist Sue Belsinger and prepared and sold by New Chapter.

Since I like ginger with pineapple juice, I might also combine both with several of the high-cineole herbs listed below to make what I call Cineolade, which contains the expectorant cineole, reportedly useful for laryngitis. Plants with high concentrations of cineole include basil, bee balm, cardamom, cinnamon, eucalyptus, fennel, ginger, hyssop, lavender, lemon leaf, lemon verbena, nutmeg, peppermint, rosemary, spearmint, sweet Annie, tansy, tarragon, turmeric, and yarrow.

★★★**Pomegranate** This Biblical fruit—perhaps the "apple" of the garden of Eden—has a long history of use for sore throat, from the Andes to India. It's a broad-spectrum antiseptic, and it contains at least nine immune-boosting compounds. You might try sipping the juice throughout the day, alternating with water.

★★★**Sage** While I'm not sure how it would taste, I'd mix some sage with more promising anti-pharyngitics like garlic, ginger, and onion and maybe even some oil, honey, or vinegar. Or I'd make a sage tea with lemon juice and honey.

A 2006 clinical study supported my conviction that sage could be sagely used for sore throat relief. Researchers sprayed a 15 percent sage solution into the sore throats of study participants, then checked their pain levels every 15 minutes for 2 hours after the first application. Results showed that the patients enjoyed significant pain relief with few, if any, mild side effects.

★★★**Thyme** My friend Martha Libster, RN, author of *Delmar's Integrative Herb Guide for Nurses,* has noted that patent medicines for laryngitis, sore throat, bronchitis, and whooping cough contained thyme. The herb helps remove mucus from the respiratory tract, works as an antiseptic, and boosts the immune system.

Here's one way to reap the benefits of thyme: Make a decoction by boiling or simmering the herb in water for 10 to 20 minutes. If you like, you can improve it by adding lemon and honey while it's hot. Let the mixture cool, then gargle with it. You can also enjoy thyme as a tea, especially if you drink it about a half hour after eating a hot spice such as garlic, hot peppers, horseradish, or wasabi.

★★**Fluids** The Mayo Clinic tells patients with sore throats to drink twice as much as usual because fluids thin the mucus in the throat and make it easier to clear. Adding moisture to the air with a humidifier can also bring relief.

★★**Honey and lemon juice** Barack Obama isn't alone in turning to this concoction for relief; it's a traditional remedy for a sore throat and laryngitis. The Mayo Clinic recommends stirring lemon juice and honey into a glass of hot water and letting it cool before drinking. The lemon helps clear mucus, while the honey coats your throat.

★★**Horseradish and mustard** In addition to garlic and ginger, hot spices such as horseradish and mustard can help relieve laryngitis.

★**Aniseed** The German Commission E, a government agency that evaluates the safety and efficacy of medicinal herbs, recommends anise for respiratory problems and cough with phlegm because it helps break up congestion. I suggest crushing 1 to 2 teaspoons of aniseed, pouring boiling water over it, and letting it steep for 10 to 15 minutes. Be sure to strain it before drinking. If you don't have high blood pressure or low potassium levels, you might add licorice to this tea.

★**Frozen fruit or fruit ices** Try frozen peeled bananas, grapes, strawberries, blueberries, or melons as a soothing treat for your throat. Fruit ices, ice pops, and ice chips may also help. The American Cancer Society recommends cold and frozen foods for a sore throat.

★**Olive oil** It wouldn't hurt to try Sen. McCain's remedy of downing a spoonful of olive oil to prevent laryngitis. If I can manage to swallow a tablespoon of fish oil (I can), I can certainly get down a teaspoon of olive oil. (Having thought about it for less than a minute, I abandoned my boring computer for an interesting kitchen and took a tablespoon of my garlic/olive oil/balsamic vinegar salad and bread dressing. It's not bad, but it's even better on whole-grain toast, buttered or unbuttered.) Olive oil is a folk remedy without much research behind it, but it's a healthy source of monounsaturated fat, so it won't hurt to take a spoonful.

🌿 *From the Herbal Medicine Chest*

Certain herbs can work wonders for a scratchy, irritated throat. These are among my favorites.

Horehound (*Marrubium vulgare*) Horehound is one of the first herbs I recommend for throat problems. The German Commission E, a government agency that evaluates the safety and efficacy of medicinal herbs, has approved it for laryngitis and other bronchial problems. The suggested dose is 2 teaspoons of dried herb per cup of boiling water for tea. I recommend adding lemon, licorice, and stevia to the tea.

Licorice (*Glycyrrhiza glabra*) Licorice soothes a sore throat and helps remove mucus. People in Europe and China have been using it for centuries. In his book *Chinese Healing Foods and Herbs,* Albert Leung, PhD, a distinguished pharmacist and pharmacognocist (natural product pharmacist), notes scientific documentation of the use of licorice for asthma and its folkloric use for sore throat. He advises adding 5 to 7 teaspoons of licorice root pieces to 3 cups of water and bringing it to a boil. Simmer until half the water has boiled away

Licorice tea may bring relief, but be careful not to drink too much. Long-term use—that is, more than 6 weeks—can cause or aggravate high blood pressure, among other side effects. Besides, if you have a sore throat for that length of time, you should see your doctor!

Sunburn

DURING MY GRADE SCHOOL AND HIGH SCHOOL YEARS, I was one of those sun-worshiping kids who spent every June, July, and August lying at poolside, soaking up the rays and turning bright crimson while trying to turn brown. In college, I again spent my summer evenings playing jazz bass at beach clubs and my days playing in the sun and surf—sometimes soaked with oil, sometimes not. Now, I believe that my sun exposure, like my former habit of smoking three packs of cigarettes a day, has seriously amplified my chances of developing skin and lung cancer. I've already had one squamous cell carcinoma burned off.

I've learned my lesson. As much as I hate them, I now occasionally use sunscreens. I also nearly always wear long-sleeved shirts and sometimes even lightweight gloves and a broad-brimmed hat—especially when I'm traveling by open boat in the tropics. Even then, the sunbeams bouncing off the Amazon sometimes burn me badly, increasing the odds that I'll need to have more cancerous lesions removed.

Healing Foods for Sunburn

So what exactly are we talking about when we talk about sunburn? Why is it different from other types of burns? Sunshine contains not only the visible light that brightens our daytime world but also invisible ultraviolet (UV) rays. These not only cause burns and inflammation but also bring about changes, called mutations, in the molecules that make up the genes in our skin cells. These mutations in turn can incite cells to reproduce uncontrollably and compound into cancerous tumors. Although sunburns are more common in fair-skinned people, they can strike those with darker skin as well, especially in the absence of sunscreen and protective clothing.

Your best defense is the simplest: Avoid the sun when you can and cover up when you can't. But a number of food remedies can also help prevent sunburn and ease the sting if a burn occurs.

★★**Cucumbers** Albert Leung, PhD, a distinguished pharmacist and pharmacognocist (natural product pharmacist), recommends cool cucumbers for soothing burns. These vegetables are a bit cheaper in the summer, and they're probably more useful than many of the over-the-counter remedies you buy at the drugstore. Dian Dincin Buchman, PhD, author of *The Complete Herbal Guide to Natural Health and Beauty,* suggests peeling and chopping cucumbers, then squeezing out the juice and mixing it with glycerin and rosewater for protection from the sun. If you already have a sunburn, I recommend cooling it with mashed cucumber.

★★**Eggplant** This solanum species has a folk reputation for treating sunburn, and more important, it contains compounds used in sunny Australia for the treatment of skin cancers. If I were marooned in the desert without any sunscreen, I might apply the fruit or leaf pulp of any of the several species of solanum.

★★**Olive oil** Dr. Buchanan suggests that polyunsaturated fatty acids (PUFAs) can penetrate and soften skin. Although it contains more monounsaturated fatty acids

(MUFAs) than PUFAs, olive oil is what I used—unfortunately, too rarely—as a beachcombing youth. Some people recommend olive oil with vinegar, others with glycerin and witch hazel. Today, I think I'd try mixing it well with PABA and alpha-tocopherol (vitamin E) and apply the mixture as both a preventive and a palliative.

★★**Potatoes** It turns out the potato is a "comfort food" in more ways than one. In addition to serving up a hefty dose of calming carbohydrates, potatoes can soothe the sting of a sunburn. Simply rub a slice of raw potato on your extra-painful sunburned spots or grate a cold raw potato and apply it to your skin as a poultice. The starch in the potato will both cool the heat and ease the pain.

★★**Sesame oil** Another source of PUFAs, sesame oil "is the one that most fully absorbs the ultraviolet rays of the sun. It is therefore a wonderful natural tanning aid," Dr. Buchanan says. She suggests just sesame oil for swimmers but a mixture of ¼ cup of sesame oil, ¼ cup of anhydrous lanolin, and ¾ cup of water for tanning. Sesame oil ain't cheap, though. There are better and cheaper products, like olive oil (see above) that will do the trick.

★★**Sunflower oil** Sunflower is high in arginine and may help support collagen construction, which is important in repairing burns and sunburned tissue. Sunflower oil also contains the second-highest concentrations of PUFAs recorded in the database and comes in seventh for alpha-tocopherol. Armed with that data, I'd mash milky sunflower seeds in my blender and use them for prevention and treatment of sunburn.

★★**Tea** Tea—particularly green tea—appears to both protect skin from sunburn and soothe it when the damage has already been done. Green tea catechins have proven effective against both chemical and radiation-induced skin cancers, the latter often provoked by sunburn. In one Turkish study, laboratory animals that drank the equivalent of two cups of green tea a day had even greater protection against UV damage than a topical application gave them.

John Boik, PhD, an acupuncturist and author of the power-packed book *Cancer and Natural Medicine*, says that flavonoids—of which tea contains many—may stabilize collagen. To prevent sunburn, you could make iced green tea and drink it regularly whenever you're spending a lot of time outdoors. You could also try applying it topically to a blossoming sunburn. Soak a clean cloth in the tea and apply it to burned areas as a compress or just dab it on with some spent teabags.

★**Flaxseed oil** In addition to providing a healthy dose of omega-3 and omega-6 fatty acids to your body, flaxseed oil is also quite nourishing for skin, particularly

Dr. Duke's Herbal Sunscreen

My herbal sunscreen may be more effective than commercial products, but you'll have to take the time to make it yourself. I'd try avocado and/or carrot, cucumber, or eggplant, or maybe even tomato pulp if I'm in a rush, and ground sesame and sunflower seeds if my blender were handy. After getting sunburned, I might use some of those same things.

skin that has been sunburned. The omegas in the oil help nourish skin membranes, and the omega-3's in particular help the skin produce anti-inflammatory prostaglandins, which promote healing. When applied topically, flaxseed oil helps seal in the skin's moisture, and it acts as a soothing lubricant for sunburn.

★**Guavas** Eating a diet rich in antioxidants can help protect you before you even step outside, and the exotic guava fruit provides nearly five times as much of the skin-healing antioxidant vitamin C as a medium orange (377 milligrams versus 83 milligrams). Other good sources of vitamin C include bell peppers, broccoli, oranges, strawberries, and papayas. In addition to C, other antioxidants that help counteract the free radicals generated by the sun's UV rays, which contribute to sunburn, wrinkles, and skin cancer, include vitamin E, beta-carotene, lycopene, and selenium. Mangoes, blackberries, and apples all provide some vitamin E; cantaloupe, mangoes, and pumpkin all serve up a nice dose of beta-carotene; tomatoes, pink grapefruit, and watermelon are good sources of lycopene; and Brazil nuts are an excellent source of selenium. These antioxidants also improve the production of collagen. Natural and/or nutritional practitioners suggest taking vitamins A, C, and E, plus 100 milligrams of potassium, each day for 2 weeks to take the edge off a sunburn.

In addition to eating foods rich in antioxidants, you may want to try rubbing them on your skin. A study published in the *Journal of Cosmetic Dermatology* found two advantages to using antioxidants topically. First, the skin reaches much higher antioxidant levels in response to topical application than to ingestion (for example, the level of vitamin C after topical application is 20 to 40 times higher than that achieved with oral vitamin C). Second, protective antioxidants won't wash off for several days. The best, most reliable antioxidant creams are available by prescription. Ask your dermatologist what she recommends.

★**Lemon** Lemon juice is often applied to sunburn, but in fact, it may contain some psoralens that at once act as a sunscreen and instigate photodermatitis, an allergy-like inflammation resulting from exposure to sunlight. I have gotten sun-burned lips from sucking an orange in the sun. However, a study done at the Arizona Cancer Center showed that regularly adding some lemon slices to your black tea may cut your lifetime risk of squamous cell skin cancer by up to 70 percent. This may be due to d-limonene, an antioxidant in lemon peel that has been found to kill cancer cells.

★**Oatmeal** If your whole body is burning from sun exposure, add oatmeal to a cool bath and take a soak. I would grind a full cup of oatmeal in a food processor before adding it.

★**Strawberries** Some people make a strawberry wash and bathe their sunburn with it. Tannins in these plants—and, many other members of the rose family—may be beneficial, according to Robert D. Willix, MD, a cardiac surgery and sports medicine specialist. He suggests cutting a berry open and applying the juice topically.

★**Tomatoes** Studies from the medical schools at both Tufts and Boston universities suggest that lycopene, a compound found in tomatoes—as well as in pink grapefruit, calendula, guavas, watermelon, and, to a lesser extent, papayas and apricots—may be superior at quenching skin-damaging free radicals. Research also suggests that fat enhances the absorption of lycopene, so fresh tomatoes sautéed in olive oil, for example, would make a healthful treat for your skin. And a German study showed that people who took 16 milligrams of lycopene a day for 10 weeks had 40 percent less UV damage than those who took a placebo. The researchers concluded that the lycopene fortified skin against damage from the sun.

From the Herbal Medicine Chest

Some of the best treatments for sunburn fall more into the herbal than the food category. Here are some herbs that may help prevent and/or reduce the sting of a sunburn.

Aloe (Aloe vera) For sunburn, alternative practitioners suggest generous application of aloe gel. Cardiac and sports medicine specialist Robert D. Willix, MD, suggests applying the pure aloe gel after a shower and again a few more times during the day. Usually, he says, the redness disappears and the skin does not peel. James F. Balch, MD, a urologist, and Phyllis A. Balch, a certified nutritional consultant, teamed up to prepare the useful book *Prescription for Natural Healing,* in which they recommend three or four applications a day—or even every hour—after healing has started, to reduce pain and scarring.

In Kenya, a local guide taught me something I hadn't known—that aloe gel works as well for preventing a sunburn as for treating one. Wearing a short-sleeved shirt, I applied the gel to one arm and not the other. The difference was obvious—the untreated arm turned red and remained that way for a few days even though we were not in the full Kenyan sun for an entire hour. The treated arm showed far less inflammation and returned quickly to normal.

Calendula (*Calendula officinalis*) Calendula is wonderfully soothing to the skin and a good anti-inflammatory for burns, sunburn, and even radiation burns. According to Aubrey Hampton, author of *Natural Organic Hair and Skin Care*, a poultice of calendula blossoms has been proven helpful in treating abrasions, bedsores, burns, chafing, cuts, eczema, inflammation, and sunburn. Research shows it accelerates wound closing, reduces inflammation, and renews healing tissue in cases of serious burns.

Tinnitus

A SIMPLE WORD THAT COVERS A RANGE OF CONDITIONS and encompasses a multitude of causes, tinnitus affects up to 50 million Americans according to the American Tinnitus Association (ATA), with 12 million of those cases severe enough that sufferers seek medical assistance.

As described by my friend Dr. Alan Tilotson, tinnitus is a condition in which a person hears a sound—whether buzzing, hissing, whistling, roaring, chirping, or ringing—without anything actually making the noise. If you've ever walked out of a rock concert or sports event with a "ringing in your ears," then you have had a (hopefully temporary) first-hand experience with tinnitus.

Note that the sound associated with tinnitus varies from patient to patient. The sound might come and go or it might be constant; it can be a subtle background noise that you notice only in quiet surroundings, or it can be so intrusive that you can't think. Roughly two million people fall into this category, according to the ATA, and the constant clamor in their head makes it difficult to function on a day-to-day basis.

There are multiple possible causes for tinnitus, such as noise-induced hearing loss (from all those concerts), obstruction of the ear canal by wax, infections, inflammation, Ménière's disease (a disorder of the inner ear), otosclerosis (the growth of bone in the inner ear), jaw misalignment, hypertension, arteriosclerosis, or certain medications. Aspirin, sedatives, and antibiotics can also cause tinnitus.

In some cases you can treat the cause—removing the wax, for example, or treating the infection—and the tinnitus will lessen or perhaps vanish. In the case of medications, you can contact the ATA at 800-634-8978, extension 219, and ask for a copy of the "Physicians Desk Reference Guide to Drug Interactions, Side Effects, And Indications for Tinnitus." Loud noises, on the other hand, damage or destroy cilia, sensitive hairs inside the inner ear, and the resulting hearing loss is permanent—as is the tinnitus associated with it.

What can you do to prevent tinnitus, aside from wearing earplugs from dawn 'til dusk? Let's scan the menu and see what stands out.

Healing Foods for Tinnitus

★★**Cashews, pecans, almonds, and other nuts** In addition to being good sources of zinc—a cup of chopped pecans, whole almonds, or raw peanuts has nearly 5 milligrams, while a cup of roasted cashews has more than 7.5 milligrams—nuts and legumes also provide massive amounts of magnesium, which has a DV of 400 milligrams. That same cup of cashews? Packed with a near day's worth at 356 milligrams. The almonds feature 383 milligrams of magnesium while the peanuts have 245 milligrams and the pecans have 132 milligrams.

Why should you care about magnesium? Research has shown that taking additional magnesium could lower the amount of hearing loss caused by exposure to noise, which in turn could affect your chances of developing tinnitus.

★★**Clams** A body doesn't need much vitamin B_{12}—only 6 micrograms according to the FDA—but that doesn't mean that everyone gets enough, and a B_{12} deficiency is connected to chronic tinnitus and noise-induced hearing loss. One study showed that nearly half of the participants who had tinnitus or noise-induced hearing loss were deficient in vitamin B_{12}. Clams are bursting with B_{12}, with 3 ounces containing 42 micrograms—that's seven times the daily recommendation. Oysters, being mollusks as well, also have a healthy supply of B_{12}, with nearly 14 micrograms in 3 ounces. Once again, plants do not manufacture B_{12}, though if you are eating unwashed veggies right out of the garden, you'll get some from the insects still residing there and their unwashed frass.

★★**Oysters, red meat, seafood** Yep, I'd much rather go the fried oyster route (can't stomach the healthier, if clean [i.e., raw] oysters). Wonder how much omega-

3 fatty acids they contain. Research by Japanese scientists in 2003 discovered that low zinc levels are associated with tinnitus not caused by hearing loss. The Daily Value (DV) set by the FDA for zinc is 15 milligrams per day, and you can easily reach that total if your diet includes oysters (32 milligrams in a raw 3-ounce serving).

While other meats aren't quite the zinc powerhouses that oysters are, they can still boost you towards the Recommended Daily Allowance; hamburger, for example, contains 4 milligrams of zinc in a 3-ounce serving, while 100 grams of steamed scallops or lobster contains 3 milligrams. Vegetarians can turn to baked beans as a cup boasts 3.5 milligrams of zinc, but we are talking about large amounts—a pound to get the RV. I think I'd rather take a properly prepared zinc supplement or fried oysters than a pound of beans, or prunes or spinach.

★★**Spinach, leafy veggies, and beans** Research by Japanese scientists in 2003 discovered that low zinc levels are associated with tinnitus not caused by hearing loss. Vegetarians will have to work harder than seafood lovers to get the FDA's assigned daily value of 15 milligrams.

Toothaches

THE CHOCO INDIANS ARE A DISAPPEARING FOREST TRIBE, largely confined to eastern Panama and adjacent Colombia. I have worked more closely with them than with any other Indian group. I mention them here because as early as 1966, a Choco friend of mine told me about a plant, called the Piper, a relative of black pepper, that works as a toothache remedy. In fact, my Indian guide pulled up the root of a Piper plant, scraped off the dirt, and invited me to bite into the inner root bark. When I did, it numbed my mouth. So yes, the people of the jungles do have effective tooth-ache remedies in their natural pharmacopoeia.

Clearly, in the middle of a tropical jungle, plants and roots are your best bet until you can get back to the asphalt jungle of urban America. If you have easy access to a dentist, however, that's where you should go if you have a toothache. Persistent toothaches are sometimes a sign of something more serious, such an active or impending infection. While the following remedies are great for a quick fix, they are no substitute for a professional diagnosis and treatment.

Healing Foods for Toothaches

If you're in the throes of tooth pain, you can take comfort in knowing that you aren't alone. An estimated 98 percent of the population will have a toothache at some point in their lives. You can also take comfort in the following remedies.

★★★**Cloves** Many modern dentists apply eugenol, a main ingredient in true cloves, as a dental anesthetic and analgesic. And clove oil is what Momma gave me for toothaches 70 years ago. Jeffrey Gross, DDS, a staff member at the Case Western Reserve School of Dental Medicine in Ohio, suggests cloves for a quick and easy solution to calm a toothache. The late pharmacognoscist Varro Tyler, PhD, lists clove oil first for treating toothache pain and notes that it is approved by Commission E, the German government agency that evaluates the safety and efficacy of medicinal herbs, as a local anesthetic and antiseptic. Even a scientific committee reporting to our FDA commented that oil of cloves was the only one of 12 commonly found toothache preparations that was "safe and effective for temporary use on a tooth with throbbing pain." In general, cloves are 5 to 20 times richer in eugenol than other eugenol sources in my database. You can rub oil of clove (available at some drugstores and most health food stores) directly on an aching tooth, or, if you don't have oil of clove, you can do it jungle-style: wiggle a whole clove next to the tooth, pointed end down.

★★**Chile peppers** The next time you have tooth pain, you can make good use of Columbus's discovery of the hot pepper by cautiously experimenting with it to get relief. Topically applied, the hot ingredient, capsaicin, burns for a while but depletes the area of substance P, a pain transmitter.

At the Sandoz Institute for Medical Research in London, scientists hope to take the sting out of capsaicin, leaving only its anodyne (painkilling) properties. Studies at the Monell Chemical Senses Center in Philadelphia (where capsaicin is also being studied, along with other pungent compounds, as a bird repellent) can teach us how to cheat in a hot chile–eating contest. Researchers found that capsaicin-laced filter papers placed on the tip of the tongue for a few seconds several times over a 15-minute period temporarily burn, but that sensation is followed by a 2- to 3-hour period of desensitization to the pungency.

Hot peppers, ingested or applied topically, may alleviate toothache pain in a few ways—by stimulating the production of the internal painkillers known as endorphins, and by interfering with substance P, for example. They also contain some natural salicylates, painkilling substances related to aspirin. To use hot pepper for an aching tooth, mix powdered cayenne pepper with enough water to form a paste and apply it directly to the tooth with a cotton ball.

★★Figs The ficin in figs is an analgesic and anti-irritant substance that can destroy the tooth's nerve and/or the surrounding periodontal ligaments. So it's no surprise that around the world, members of the fig family are used to treat cavities and toothache, as well as when extracting teeth. For example, in Madagascar, the country folk prefer the herbal approach to the dental clinic. For 3 days, they insert powdered root of *Pysena sessiflora* into cavities (this doesn't relieve toothache; it's simply preparatory). Next they place a poultice of the bark of a fig relative into the cavity. Two days later, after the tooth's nerves and periodontal ligaments seem to have been destroyed, the healer can use his fingers to extract the tooth with only minor discomfort and virtually no loss of blood.

I mention the fig here since it is available at the supermarket, but it may not be as powerful as the species in Madagascar. A fresh fruit will ooze a little white milky latex if cut properly, and that latex contains the ficin.

★★Ginger Hot in both senses of the word, compresses of hot ginger seem to help alleviate the pain of a toothache. They act as counterirritants, which, as some people correctly suggest, take your mind off the malady. I'd add more heat in the form of hot pepper to such compresses myself. Both ginger and hot pepper (and maybe even horseradish and wasabi) seem to work like the old mustard plasters. Any one or all three might be tried cautiously as hot compresses. Or you can try making a paste of powdered ginger and cayenne pepper by mixing them with a drop or two of water. Then saturate a cotton ball with it and place it on your aching tooth.

★★Oregano Like its relative peppermint, oregano is loaded with two dozen or so analgesic phytochemicals. And even though I find no clinical evidence for its use for toothache, there's plenty of folklore. The British used to dab oregano or its essential oil onto cavities for its analgesic effect. Maybe just biting into the weed would help.

FOODS TO WATCH

Sugary foods not only cause the cavities that lead to toothache, they can worsen the pain once it strikes. Sugar makes it possible for large amounts of bacteria to flourish in your mouth, and over time, these bacteria eat away at the surfaces of your teeth. Fruit juices, which are sometimes recommended as good alternatives to soda, can actually be worse. One Swiss study showed that grapefruit and apple juice actually did more damage to teeth than cola.

★**Peppermint** In addition to its pleasant, refreshing flavor, peppermint has the power to ease the pain of an aching tooth. Try making a peppermint tea by mixing 1 teaspoon of dried leaves with 1 cup boiling water and steeping for 20 minutes. After the tea cools, swish it around in your mouth like mouthwash, repeating as needed. On the trail, I wouldn't hesitate to wad up the leaves of some of the wild mint species, knowing that both wild and domesticated mints are loaded with various painkilling chemicals.

★**Rhubarb** Under the name da-huang, rhubarb root is used in China for toothache, which makes sense since it contains at least six pain-relieving compounds. People in China fry the root, then macerate it in alcohol. The resulting tincture is then applied with a cotton ball to the sore tooth for 5 minutes. If I couldn't find the better foods mentioned elsewhere in this chapter, I might try rhubarb, but it certainly wouldn't be my first choice.

★**Sesame seed** Sesame seeds contain at least seven compounds that relieve pain. If you have a toothache, try boiling 1 part sesame seed in 3 parts water until the liquid is reduced by half, let it cool, and apply the brew to your tooth. You can make it more powerful by adding some cayenne and peppermint.

★**Tarragon** We have tarragon in the Green Farmacy Garden. Michael Castleman, a popular health science writer and author of the bestselling *The Healing Herbs,* suggests chewing the fresh leaves of tarragon as needed for temporary relief of oral pain. He cautions, however, about the remote possibility of a carcinogenic effect due to estragole, which is present in several other spices as well, including sweet basil, sweet fennel, anis vert, and anis star.

From the Herbal Medicine Chest

In addition to the some of the remedies mentioned in this chapter, here are a couple of herbals you might try.

Toothache tree (*Zanthoxylum clava-herculis*) Alabama herbalist Tommie Bass recommends chewing the bark of the toothache tree (which is also called prickly ash, devil's walking stick, and angelica) or making a tea from the bark or berries for either rheumatism or toothache. And in their book *Herbal Medicine—Past and Present*, John Crellin and Jane Philpott recount 19th-century studies that suggest tinctures of toothache tree for the similar ailments.

Willow (*Salix alba*) I have had many dental cavities and frequent toothaches, and I have often resorted to pushing a wad of masticated willow bark into the cavity to temporarily alleviate the pain. To my surprise, in my senior years, I seem to have fewer new caries and tooth-aches, maybe due to a better diet or maybe simply to my age. All poplars and willows contain salicylates, which have an effect similar to that of aspirin.

Ulcers

IN THE 1970S, PEPTIC ULCERS were treated with a bland diet, which didn't help. By the 1980s, doctors were prescribing powerful acid-blocking drugs in attempts at a cure. This, too, didn't work, because even though the ulcers healed, they'd almost always come back—50 to 80 percent of ulcers recurred within a year. All of this effort stemmed from scientists believing that stress and spicy foods were behind these painful stomach lesions. We now know that the real culprit is often an infection caused by *Helicobacter pylori*, a corkscrew-shaped bacterium that settles in the mucous layer that protects the tissue lining the stomach and intestine. This little ulcer-causing bug is now successfully treated with antibiotics.

Yet simply having *H. pylori* in your system doesn't mean you'll get an ulcer. One in five Americans under age 30 and half of those over 60 play host to *H. pylori*. It's a common gastrointestinal infection around the world and often has no symptoms. And not everyone who has an ulcer has *H. pylori*.

The use of certain pain medications called nonsteroidal anti-inflammatory drugs (NSAIDs)—such as aspirin, ibuprofen (Advil, Motrin), and naproxen (Aleve)—can also disrupt the naturally protective lining of the stomach and cause ulcers. Smoking and drinking too much alcohol is linked to them, too.

Technically speaking, an ulcer is a sore in the lining of the esophagus, stomach, or duodenum (the gateway to the small intestine just downstream from the stomach). These kinds of ulcers are called "peptic" ulcers because they occur in areas that are exposed to the digestive enzyme pepsin.

Healing Foods for Ulcers

Ulcers caused by *H. pylori* are generally treated with a combination of antibiotics and bismuth (Pepto-Bismol) or similar stomach-soothing drugs. You might want to try a number of natural anti-ulcer approaches as well.

★★★Bananas These fruits are an old folk remedy for many gastrointestinal problems because they soothe the digestive tract. Research shows that they have an anti-ulcer effect. In particular, plantains—cousins of the banana—contain an enzyme that stimulates mucus production in the lining of the stomach, strengthening its natural defenses against culprits such as *H. pylori*. Plantains that are green and not quite ripe are best because they're believed to contain more of the healing enzyme.

★★★Bilberries and blueberries Both of these berries contain compounds known as anthocyanosides, which have proven to offer significant protection against ulcers. These compounds help stimulate the production of mucus that protects the stomach lining from digestive acids. Researchers have also found that blueberries contain a specific compound that may reduce the risk of colon cancer.

★★★Cabbage Cabbage is one of the oldest folk remedies for ulcers. It contains glutamine, an amino acid that increases blood flow to the stomach and helps strengthen its protective lining. Michael Murray, ND, a naturopathic doctor and author of *Natural Alternatives to Over-the-Counter and Prescription Drugs,* hails cabbage as an extremely effective ulcer treatment, saying that healing usually happens in less than a week. In studies of glutamine, daily doses of 1,600 milligrams proved as effective as conventional antacids in treating ulcers.

Cabbage is also a good source of fiber, which can help and even heal ulcers. This is because foods that contain lots of fiber encourage the growth of the stomach's protective layer.

The folk recommendation for treating ulcers with cabbage is to drink 1 quart of raw cabbage juice a day. That may be hard to swallow, so I suggest concocting a tasty cabbage soup or stew with some of the other goodies mentioned in this chapter thrown in for good measure.

★★★Chile peppers Despite popular belief, hot spices don't cause ulcers. In fact, they may even protect the stomach against them. Capsaicin, the compound that

Anti-Ulcer Chewing Gum

The leaves of the mastic tree, a native of the Mediterranean region, contain a resin that can kill *Helicobacter pylori* bacteria. It's believed that chewing mastic gum may help reduce the risk of ulcers. You can buy it online and from select health food stores, too.

makes chiles hot, has been shown to prevent ulcers. In addition, recent studies have reported that carotenoids, the natural pigments that give many fruits and vegetables their bright red, orange, or yellow color, seem to protect the lining of the stomach. Eating plenty of hot peppers and cayenne can give you triple protection against ulcers.

Medicinal herb expert Andrew Weil, MD, professor at the University of Arizona College of Medicine in Tucson, suggests sipping red pepper tea to calm an ulcer. Just steep ¼ teaspoon of cayenne in a cup of hot water.

★★★**Yogurt** It's a fight among the microbes: The live bacteria in yogurt have no fear of taking on *H. pylori* in full-force combat—and they're strong enough to win. When the fight is over, a natural sugar in yogurt called lactose breaks down during digestion and helps restore a healthy acid balance in your intestines. Yogurt, in short, is your ally in your defense against ulcers.

If you try this approach to taming an ulcer, be sure to buy yogurt that has "live, active cultures" listed on the label. You can eat a cup three or four times a day to help get your stomach back in order.

★★**Chamomile** Rudolf Fritz Weiss, MD, a German medical herbalist and author of *Herbal Medicine*, says that chamomile is the remedy of choice for stomach ulcers. Widely used as a digestive aid in Europe, this herb is uniquely suited to treating stomach ailments, including ulcers because it combines anti-inflammatory, antiseptic, antispasmodic, and stomach-soothing properties. If I had an ulcer, I'd drink chamomile tea with licorice.

★★**Garlic** In preliminary studies, scientists were able to kill *H. pylori* bacteria using garlic extract. Other studies have shown garlic to be toxic to many "bad" bacterial strains, even some that resist antibiotics. Researchers in India have found that garlic may actually enhance the "good" bacteria in the intestine.

If you want to try a course of garlic therapy, eat nine cloves a day. You can chop each dose of garlic with one carrot and some celery and eat it raw, or you can cook or pickle it. You might also try whipping up an anti-ulcer gazpacho that's heavy on the garlic and red pepper (another anti-ulcer food).

★★**Ginger** Long known for its many healing properties, ginger contains 11 compounds that have shown anti-ulcer effects. That's a lot of anti-ulcer chemistry concentrated in a single humble spice. Ginger is a proven anti-inflammatory and also has antibacterial properties.

Eating candied ginger is a tasty treatment for ulcers, and the combination of ginger and honey (another antibacterial) is particularly effective, working synergistically to clean up *H. pylori* in your stomach.

FOODS TO WATCH

Some foods are great for soothing an ulcer, but others, not so much. Here are three to avoid.

Alcohol. Drinking alcohol increases the amount of acid that your stomach produces, which can irritate and break down the stomach lining. If you have an ulcer (or are trying to avoid one), refrain from alcoholic beverages.

Coffee. The caffeine in coffee can make you more susceptible to developing an ulcer, and if you already have one, drinking coffee can make it worse.

Milk. Once thought to help prevent ulcers, milk is no longer believed to be a good choice. It increases acid production in your stomach, which can irritate an ulcer. In addition, food allergies may cause ulcers, so people allergic to milk are at higher risk.

★★**Honey** Raw, unprocessed honey has been shown to strengthen the lining of the stomach. A study at the University of Waikato in New Zealand found that honey made from the nectar of the manuka flower completely stopped the growth of ulcer-causing bacteria.

If you want to try honey to prevent and treat ulcers, I suggest consuming it raw and unprocessed, because the heat-processed product doesn't contain any of the beneficial substances. Take 1 tablespoon on an empty stomach at bedtime. Doing this every day can help an ulcer heal and prevent recurrence.

★★**Peppermint** Herbalists have a special regard for peppermint's ability to soothe the lining of the stomach, and it has been used for centuries to treat a wide range of digestive ailments.

If you have a nagging ulcer, I suggest drinking a mix of peppermint and chamomile tea, as both have a soothing effect on the stomach. You can also use fresh or chopped peppermint leaves in a variety of drinks and dishes. Fresh peppermint is now available in many supermarkets.

★★**Pineapple** Like cabbage, pineapple has a fair amount of glutamine, a compound that helps protect the stomach lining. Pineapple also contains bromelain, a natural anti-inflammatory that may help reduce the painful swelling and inflammation of ulcers.

★★**Rhubarb** Eating rhubarb has been shown to help reduce the effects of ulcers within a few days. However, eat only the stalks; rhubarb leaves contain high levels of toxins called oxalates that can cause stomach irritation and kidney problems. Rhubarb also has powerful natural laxative action, so watch out for diarrhea. If you experience problems, cut back on the amount you're using or discontinue it altogether.

★★**Turmeric** This culinary herb, the main ingredient in Asian and Indian curry dishes, is a powerful anti-inflammatory that's been used as a natural medicine for thousands of years. India's traditional Ayurvedic doctors used it for all kinds of swelling, and it's believed to have a number of gastrointestinal benefits.

Turmeric has been called the poor person's ulcer treatment. Physician researchers in Thailand found that it relieved ulcer pain only about half as well as over-the-counter antacids after 6 weeks. However, antacids are about eight times more expensive than turmeric, so if your budget is tight, this herb may be for you.

★**Nutmeg** Researchers at the University of Chicago found nutmeg to be a potent anti-ulcer herb. In other recent studies, nutmeg oil has shown considerable activity against 25 different types of bacteria. Although more research is needed to confirm nutmeg's true anti-ulcer effects, this research supports its long-time use as an antiseptic.

From the Herbal Medicine Chest

In addition to the ulcer-fighting foods mentioned in this chapter, there are some great herbal remedies as well. Here are some to try.

Aloe (*Aloe vera*) This plant contains enzymes that relieve pain, reduce inflammation, and decrease swelling. It also has antibacterial properties, which can prevent sores from becoming infected. Aloe can help heal ulcers, so Andrew Weil, MD, professor at the University of Arizona College of Medicine in Tuscon, suggests taking a teaspoon of aloe juice after each meal. But buy the juice; don't make your own. The unprocessed gel taken directly from the plant has extremely powerful laxative properties that can damage your intestine.

Calendula (*Calendula officinalis*) Herbalists say that calendula is a remedy for sores in the mouth; inflammations of the mouth, throat, and nose; and digestive disorders such as peptic and duodenal ulcers. Clinical trials in Europe suggest that extracts may also be useful for duodenal ulcers.

Licorice (Glycyrrhiza glabra) Licorice contains several anti-ulcer compounds that help protect the lining of your stomach and intestine. Deglycyrrhizinated licorice (DGL) is a processed form of the herb and the preferred type for ulcers. Add ½ teaspoon of DGL powder to your favorite herbal tea or use it by itself to make a sweet, pleasant-tasting tea.

Slippery elm (Ulmus rubra) The demulcent nature of the inner bark of slippery elm makes an effective stomach coating to help soothe and perhaps even prevent ulcers. You can chew on slippery elm bark or dry and grind it to make a satisfying tea.

Vaginitis

THE VAGINA NORMALLY CONTAINS lots of friendly bacteria called lactobacilli, plus a few other types of bacteria called anaerobes. Too many anaerobes can cause bacterial vaginosis (BV), the most common of three vaginal infections that fall under the category known as vaginitis. BV was called different names in the past, including nonspecific vaginitis and *Gardnerella vaginalis* vaginitis. The other two infections are trichomoniasis, a sexually transmitted disease, and the fungal infection commonly known as a yeast infection (see page 372).

BV disrupts the vaginal ecosystem. Some women infected with BV have up to 1,000 times more anaerobic bacteria (bacteria that require no oxygen to live) than uninfected women. Once this imbalance occurs, the body has difficulty getting back to normal.

The most common symptom of BV is a vaginal discharge similar in consistency and appearance to skim milk. The discharge caused by the infection often has a strong fishy odor that may become worse after sex because semen changes the acidic level of vaginal fluids. BV also may cause vaginal itching and irritation. BV is often mistaken for a common yeast infection or other vaginal infection because the symptoms are similar. But about 50 to 75 percent of all women with BV experience no symptoms.

Despite adequate treatment, BV recurs within 3 months in about 30 percent of women. One cause of recurrent BV may be that even after the harmful bacteria are reduced, the good bacteria have trouble growing back in the vagina. Scientists are not sure what makes some women more prone to recurrent BV. But the greatest risk factors are having a new sex partner or having multiple sex partners. Commercial douches also appear to increase the risk of developing it.

FOODS TO WATCH

You need fats in your diet to give you energy, keep your body warm, protect your organs, support cell grow, and a host of other reasons—just don't overdo it.

A diet too high in fat increases your risk of developing BV, and the more total fat you consume, the higher your risk of developing severe BV, according to the University of Alabama, Department of Human Nutrition, study that evaluated the association between diet and BV in 1,521 women.

The recommended Daily Value for fat, based on a 2,000-calorie diet, is 65 grams.

Another reason BV so often recurs may be that the drugs used to treat the condition are not getting the job done. One recent study published in the *Journal of Infectious Diseases* concluded that the current recommended treatment (oral metronidazole therapy) is not preventing the recurrence of BV or abnormal vaginal flora in the majority of women. Another recent study concluded that 45 percent of over-the-counter products available to women in the feminine hygiene section of the stores surveyed could not be confirmed to be effective for treating infectious vaginitis.

BV is the least understood and most often ignored or misdiagnosed vaginal condition. However, it's gaining more attention as more research shows that untreated BV can lead to significant health complications, including premature delivery, postpartum infections, clinically apparent and subclinical pelvic inflammatory disease (PID), postsurgical complications (after abortion, hysterectomy, cesarean section, and other reproductive procedures), increased vulnerability to HIV infection and, possibly, infertility.

With so many negative outcomes now linked to BV, it's important that women get tested and treated. And to help keep infections from returning, you might try a few of these food remedies.

Healing Foods for Vaginitis

★★**Beans, peas, and cowpeas** The University of Alabama study also found that folate (folic acid) may decrease the risk of getting severe BV. Beans and peas are ideal foods to fulfill your recommended folate requirements (400 micrograms daily for adults). A ½ cup of cooked cowpeas (blackeyes) provides 105 micrograms (25 percent

Daily Value [DV]); a $\frac{1}{2}$ cup of Great Northern beans provides 90 micrograms (20 percent DV); and the same quantity of green peas provides 50 micrograms (15 percent DV).

★★**Low-fat yogurt** Early studies suggested that eating yogurt with live *Lactobacillus acidophilus* cultures increases the good bacteria in the vagina and may reduce episodes of BV. But eating yogurt may not be the only way live cultures can help.

In a recent study, scientists at the University of Milan, Italy, treated 40 BV patients with a *L. acidophilus* douche. Vaginal smears were collected when the women were diagnosed, after the 6-day treatment, and 20 days after treatment. At the end of the study, the researchers concluded that this regimen helped restore the women's normal vaginal microflora.

The high calcium content of low-fat yogurt may provide yet another reason to add this food to your grocery list. After evaluating the association between diet and the presence of BV in a subset of 1,521 women (86 percent African American) from a larger study of vaginal flora, researchers at the University of Alabama, Department of Human Nutrition, concluded that increased intake of calcium decreased the risk of developing severe BV.

Self-Care Strategies

Here are some tips for decreasing your risk of BV or recurrent BV:

- Avoid commercial douches.
- Wipe from front to back after urination.
- Avoid sexual contact with someone who has a sexually transmitted disease; use condoms if you're uncertain.
- Use condoms to reduce semen exposure, which can affect the vaginal bacteria balance.
- Avoid local irritants, such as bubble baths, harsh soaps, feminine hygiene sprays, and deodorant tampons, which can affect the normal pH of the vagina.
- Try a vaginal moisturizer after sexual intercourse or after your period.
- Don't smoke.
- After a few weeks of therapy for BV, ask your health care professional to retest you for the infection.

An 8-ounce serving of plain, low-fat yogurt contains 415 milligrams of calcium; that's 42 percent of the recommended DV. Eat it cold right out of the fridge to retain the highest level of live cultures.

★★**Spinach** Spinach not only gets high points for containing folate (a cooked ½ cup serving provides 100 micrograms, 25 percent DV), it also provides you with 230 percent DV for vitamin A, another nutrient found to lower the risk of getting severe BV in the University of Alabama study.

You can tuck fresh, chopped spinach into any number of favorite recipes, from pizza to pasta to soup. Or simply steam a bunch of the fresh greens and top with minced garlic and olive oil.

★**Apple cider vinegar** An apple cider vinegar soak is an old folk remedy that many physicians also recommend for several types of vaginitis. My friend Jeanne Rose, distinguished California herbalist and prolific author of several herbal books, including *Herbs & Aromatherapy for the Reproductive System*, suggests that vinegar baths and douches help restore normal vaginal acidity. Normal acidity helps banish candida, trichomonas, and gardnerella.

To try this approach, add 3 cups of apple cider vinegar to a hot bath and soak in the tub for at least 20 minutes, spreading your legs to allow water to flow into the vagina.

From the Herbal Medicine Chest

Jeanne Rose, author of *Herbs & Aromatherapy for the Reproductive System*, finds that most types of vaginal infection, including pelvic inflammatory disease (PID), respond to two types of herbal treatments: herbal capsules taken orally, and herbal suppositories inserted in the vagina.

For the capsules, she suggests what she calls the Yegg formula: 1 ounce yellowdock root to cleanse the blood; 2 ounce echinacea root to boost the immune system to fight infection; 1 ounce goldenseal root to counter bacteria and viruses; and 1 ounce ginseng root to improve health of the lymphatic system.

For the suppository, she adds the following to the Yegg herbs: comfrey root, marshmallow root, and slippery elm bark (and sometimes chickweed and squawvine). Then she mixes the herbs with melted cocoa butter for easier insertion high into the vagina. The concoction can be held in place with a tampon for 36 hours. Then douche it out with a mixture of water, comfrey, goldenseal, and yellowdock.

Varicose Veins

IT'S PROBABLY NOT MUCH CONSOLATION, but if you're bothered by large, unsightly veins, especially in your legs, you have lots of company. According to the American College of Phlebology (the field of medicine that deals with vein diseases), more than 80 million Americans have varicose veins or their mini-versions, spider veins. Women are four times more likely to develop them than men are, with up to half of American women affected. Hormonal factors are likely triggers—puberty, pregnancy, menopause, and taking birth control pills can all activate the disease. Spending long hours standing or sitting with crossed legs raises your risk as well.

If you're looking for a root cause, however, this is one time you'd be right to point your finger at Mom. Heredity is the number one risk factor for the condition—probably an inherited weakness in the veins' walls or valves.

Put a genetic predisposition together with a trigger, and voilà: varicose veins. Here's how they develop. Your arteries work like a plumbing system, carrying oxygen-rich blood pumped from your heart to your extremities. From there, the blood has to make the round trip for cleaning and recirculating, but it doesn't have a pump to help it along. So your veins, which carry the oxygen-depleted blood back to your heart, have one-way valves to keep it flowing in the right direction. If the valves don't function well, the blood doesn't flow efficiently. The veins first become congested and then enlarged. They may end up looking blue, swollen, stretched out, kinked, or twisted. They can also leak blood and fluid into surrounding tissue, which causes swelling.

This happens most frequently in the legs, but it can occur elsewhere, too. When varicose veins occur in and around the anus, they're called hemorrhoids; in the scrotum, they're varicoceles. Both of these conditions are usually harmless. However, in the esophagus, they're known as varices, and if left untreated, they can rupture and bleed uncontrollably.

Besides being unsightly, varicose veins of the legs can cause pain that ranges from dull throbbing to acute burning. Sometimes they cause a feeling of pressure or heaviness in the legs, make your feet and ankles swell, or cause surrounding skin to itch.

Modern medicine can treat them with laser therapy, sclerotherapy (injection of a special solution), or surgery. Now brace yourself for the bad news: Treatments aren't always covered by insurance, and even if they are, they may not work the way you would like. Sclerotherapy isn't always permanent, and surgery leaves scars (and can't prevent new varicose veins from developing).

Now here's the good news: Dietary changes can help. For example, you can eat more fiber. Promoting regularity eases the pressure on veins in the legs. Some of the best sources of fiber are in your supermarket's bean aisle: navy beans, split peas, lentils, and pinto beans, to name a few. Whip up a mixed-bean VaricoSoup, and include a few of the better anti-varicose spices, such as basil, bay, chili powder, garlic, ginger, onion, oregano, rosemary, sage, and turmeric. You'll get more than a dozen COX-2-inhibiting compounds (which help with pain) in the process.

Healing Foods for Varicose Veins

Besides fiber, other food remedies, such as those I've listed below, may be helpful for preventing or treating spider veins and varicose veins.

★★★**Buckwheat and other sources of rutin** Certified lactation consultant Sheila Humphrey, RN, notes that buckwheat is noteworthy for strengthening capillaries. Science bears this out: Buckwheat contains a compound called rutin. Researchers in Germany found that when pregnant women were given hydroxyethylrutosides, a type of flavonoid derived from rutin, their varicose veins improved.

In a 2003 article titled "From Medical Herbalism to Phytotherapy in Dermatology: Back to the Future," A.M. Dattner, MD, mentions buckwheat bioflavonoids as a first-line defense against varicose veins. Further, he states that plant-based therapeutic preparations serve as "therapeutic alternatives, safer choices, or in some cases, the only effective treatment."

Medical texts say that taking 20 to 100 milligrams of rutin each day can significantly strengthen capillaries. A ½ cup of buckwheat contains a lot of rutin, more than you'd need to shore up your capillaries. Try eating buckwheat pancakes or kasha, which is a cereal-like product that is made from buckwheat groats and is widely available in supermarkets.

Some people are allergic to buckwheat. If you develop hives or hay fever–like symptoms, try another remedy instead.

Not big on buckwheat? Parsley is the next richest source of rutin in my database, and it's readily available. At restaurants, most people leave the parsley on their plates, failing to recognize that this dark green nutritious herb may prevent those purple spiders. Don't throw your parsley away! A single ounce could contain 180 milligrams of rutin.

★★**Blueberries, bilberries, and grapes** These sweet, tart, tangy berries are nutritional powerhouses. They contain antioxidant phytonutrients called anthocyanidins, which strengthen capillaries and may also decrease the swelling of varicose veins. These high-fiber berries will also help prevent constipation, which is often a trigger for hemorrhoids.

A small, preliminary study done in the 1980s found that supplementing each day with 150 milligrams of proanthocyanidins improved the function of leg veins after just one dose. More studies are needed, but in the meantime, eating more blueberries and related foods couldn't hurt. Some scientists add that frozen blueberries are as good medicinally as fresh. There are also several blueberry capsules containing concentrated active compounds. Other sources of anthocyanidins include black beans, black currants, blackberries, cherries, grapes, and tea.

★★**Grapes and chocolate** These two foods are high in compounds called flavonoids, which are responsible for many of the brilliant colors in plants. One of the many benefits of high-flavonoid foods is protection against varicose veins by reducing the permeability of blood vessels, especially the capillaries.

By the way, before you tear open a caramel-coated, marshmallow-topped, peanut butter–filled candy bar, keep in mind that the more chocolate is processed, the more its flavonoids are lost. Choose dark chocolate over milk chocolate and, if possible, buy brands that give the cocoa content on the label.

★**Bay leaves and olive oil** Here's an old-time folk remedy you could try. Place three bay leaves and 4 teaspoons of olive oil in a pan and warm over low heat. Let the mixture cool, then strain it and apply it to your varicose veins with a clean, soft cloth.

From the Herbal Medicine Chest

The horse chestnut tree, which is native to Greece and Bulgaria, gets its name from horseshoe markings that appear on the branches—actually scars from where leaves previously grew.

According to Linda White, MD, coauthor of *The Herbal Drugstore,* horse chestnut seed is the most popular treatment for varicose veins in Germany. It's commonly recommended by herbalists in the United States as well.

Researchers in Switzerland recently reviewed five studies that had been conducted on horse chestnut and varicose veins. They used a product called Aesculaforce, which is an extract made from horse chestnut seeds (available on the Internet). The researchers found that the product was effective at reducing lower-leg swelling and alleviating leg pain, heaviness, and itching in people with varicose veins and a related condition called chronic venous insufficiency.

Preliminary evidence suggests that horse chestnut may be as effective as compression stockings—which people who've tried them tell me are expensive and annoying.

Horse chestnut has a long history of use for varicose veins and hemorrhoids in traditional herbal medicine. Botanists have isolated the most active compound, aescin, and learned that it helps strengthen capillary cells and reduce fluid leakage.

If you're going to use horse chestnut, you must buy a standardized extract and follow the package directions carefully. If you have diabetes, be especially cautious if you try this remedy because it causes an increased risk of low blood sugar.

Commission E, Germany's official agency charged with evaluating herbal medicines, approves witch hazel to treat venous conditions. Witch hazel is primarily known for treating hemorrhoids, and in fact it's the ingredient in over-the-counter remedies such as Tucks medicated pads. But it may also be useful for treating varicose veins.

Dip a cotton ball in witch hazel extract and apply it to your varicose veins three or more times a day. If you try this remedy, be patient; you'll have to use it for 2 or more weeks before you can expect to see results.

Warts

WARTS MAY NOT SEEM LIKE A BIG DEAL—unless you have them. Researchers in Australia found that the vast majority of people with warts are moderately to extremely embarrassed by them, and more than half said their warts cause them some level of discomfort.

Common warts plague 7 to 10 percent of all people, and ironically, most of them are in the hyper-image-conscious preteen years. For some unknown reason, some people tend to be more prone to warts than others, so if you've had them, you're more likely to get them again.

Despite the legend that warts are caused by toads, they're actually a result of a virus called human papillomavirus (HPV). They appear most commonly on the hands (usually called common warts), feet (plantar warts), and genitals (genital warts). While you can't catch a wart from a toad, you can catch one from a person—either from direct contact or from unclean surfaces in areas such as bathrooms and swimming pools. That said, the risk of catching a wart from another person is really quite small unless you have a weakened immune system.

Most of my food farmacy items for warts are applied topically, not eaten, in hopes of making the warts disappear, but immunity boosters may help you avoid them in the first place.

Number one among my immunity-stimulating foods is garlic, but bilberry, burdock, calendula, camu-camu, cantaloupe, chamomile, chickpeas, cinnamon, dandelion, fenugreek, ginger, ginseng, grapes, jujube, marshmallow, oats, pepper, shitake, spinach, sweet potato, thyme, and turmeric also come to mind. The inulin-bearing herbs (artichoke, burdock, chicory, dandelion, elecampane, Jerusalem artichoke, and salsify) act as prebiotics and also boost the immune system. Because stress weakens the immune system, I think of the stress-reducing herbs hops, kava, St. John's wort, skullcap, and valerian, but they aren't exactly foods. Some stress-reducing foods include celery, chamomile, lavender, lemon balm, licorice, passion-flowers, and of course poppy.

Doctors have several treatments for warts at their disposal, including lasers, injections, and cryotherapy (freezing). At the opposite end of the spectrum, folklore treatments for warts abound. The good news is that between these two extremes, you'll find the following food remedies, which are worth a try. The *best* news is that some warts just disappear on their own!

Healing Foods for Warts

★★★**Garlic** Garlic provides a one-two punch against warts. First, it kills viruses. Second, it keeps virally infected cells from multiplying. Garlic showed more phyto-chemical evidence than any of the others I checked with my Multiple Activities Menu query, but better evidence comes to us from Iran. Researchers there treated 23 people who had between 2 and 96 warts with an extract of garlic. Every single one of their warts disappeared within 1 to 2 weeks.

If you want to try this remedy, crush or slice fresh garlic cloves and apply them directly to the wart, avoiding the surrounding skin. Cover the garlic with a bandage, leave it in place overnight, and wash it off in the morning. Blisters may form (I didn't blister when I applied a split garlic clove for an ear infection), but repeat the treatment a few times until the wart disappears.

Never apply raw garlic to an infant or child's delicate skin because it can cause serious burns.

★★**Figs** If the only association you've ever had with a fig involved the word *Newtons*, you've been missing out. There is nothing like the unique taste and texture of fresh figs. To get rid of a wart, though, you're not going to eat them.

In rural Iran, they traditionally use fig latex applied topically. Researchers there

Kissing a toad may not give you warts, but other things that you put to your mouth just might. Here are some foods and beverages to avoid.

Alcohol. Researchers think there's a link between drinking alcohol and genital warts, which are caused by the same virus as common warts. Researchers in Seattle found that drinking two to four alcoholic drinks a week was associated with an almost doubled risk of genital warts. Consuming five or more alcoholic drinks a week increased the risk even more. Researchers aren't sure why, but they suspect it's because of alcohol's effect on immunity.

Pork. In a study in West Germany, researchers found that a young man's genital warts regressed when he stopped eating fried pork, at the same time he was being treated with interferon gamma, an antiviral drug. The researchers believe that eating pork may be involved in developing diseases related to the human papillomavirus.

wanted to confirm its effectiveness, so they recruited 25 HPV-infected people and asked them to apply fig tree latex to warts on one side of their bodies. The warts on the other side of their bodies were treated with cryotherapy. The fig treatment was only marginally less effective than the cryotherapy. The researchers aren't sure why fig works, but they think it's because of the protein-digesting activity of the latex enzymes.

If you'd like to give this treatment a try, apply the milk from fresh figs to your warts once a day for 5 to 7 days.

★★**Sesame oil** This fragrant oil, which of course comes from sesame seeds, is especially popular in India and the Orient. My database and synergy scores gave sesame good ratings for effectiveness against warts.

In an interesting twist, researchers in the 1980s conducted a study to test the effectiveness of a medication called bleomycin when it was directly injected into warts. They used sesame oil as a placebo (sham treatment) for comparison. Ironically, 46 percent of the people who got the sesame oil saw improvement in the number of warts cured compared with only 18 percent who got the drug.

★★**Turmeric** Curcumin, the major active compound in the spice turmeric, has proved active against papillomavirus, and turmeric contains at least 10 other antiviral compounds. It's a popular home remedy for warts.

I don't remember having any warts since childhood. But if one suddenly appeared, I might apply some of the turmeric growing in my garden, though the treatment is messy and can stain clothing.

★**Banana peel** Rubbing a wart with the inside of a banana peel is another popular food remedy. You might give it a try two to four times a day for 5 to 7 days. A study published in the *Journal of Reconstructive Surgery* in the 1980s suggested that this might work.

★**Lemon juice** There isn't a lot of scientific evidence for lemon juice, but I'm lucky enough to have the compilation of all 11 parts of Jonathan Hartwell's *Plants Used against Cancer,* a compendium of more than 3,000 plants with histories as folk remedies. I'll wager there are hundreds of references therein to plants used against warts. Lemon juice, for example, appears in the traditional folk medicines of Australia, and in the United States, of Illinois and Kentucky.

In the spirit of "it won't hurt, so why not give it a shot," you may want to try this home remedy: Dab lemon juice straight onto your warts, repeating for several days until the acids in the juice dissolve the growths. It's not nearly as messy as the turmeric.

★**Spinach and other foods high in zinc** This we know: People with weakened immune systems are more likely to get warts, and zinc can profoundly affect the immune system. It has been used to treat a host of skin disorders.

To this we can add some hard science: Researchers in Iraq conducted a study in which 9 out of 10 people taking daily zinc (10 milligrams per kilogram of body weight) reported that their warts completely disappeared within 2 months.

If I had a stubborn wart, I'd add more spinach, parsley, collards, Brussels sprouts, and cucumbers, which are all high in zinc, to my diet.

From the Herbal Medicine Chest

The small yellow flowers and leaves of greater celandine have been used in herbal remedies. This plant grows primarily in Europe and Asia, but it has been introduced in North America. Although the results haven't been confirmed by double-blind clinical trials, preliminary reports from Russia and China have indicated that a tincture of greater celandine applied topically was useful for getting rid of warts.

To give this herb a try, make a strong tea with the dried herb and apply it to your warts. If you have access to the fresh plant, squeeze some juice from the stems and apply it once or twice a day for 5 to 7 days.

From the Herbal Medicine Chest

I was surprised to read (in the *PDR for Herbal Medicines*, 2nd edition) that the German Commission E, a government agency that evaluates the safety and efficacy of medicinal herbs, had approved oat straw for warts—especially since it doesn't indicate either how the oat straw was used or the rationale for its use. In general, I consider Commission E's opinions worthwhile, though they are unreferenced. My referenced Multiple Activities Menus list seven antiviral compounds in oat straw, which certainly suggests it could battle the human papillomavirus.

Wrinkles

WHEN I TOUR THE GREEN FARMACY GARDEN, I hide my wrinkles under a broad-rimmed sombrero since it's too late for me to avoid them. I should have worn that big sombrero when I was a sun-worshiping kid.

Like most young people, in those days, I wasn't worried about worry lines or wrinkles. I was living for today, not tomorrow. Now moderately wrinkled at age 79, I'm a worry wart, worrying more about tomorrow than today.

In general, I rarely offer prescriptions, but I feel safe with this one: Don't you do that. Worrying is unhealthy. Take up stress relief—or else. Time has a funny way of catching up with you, and wrinkles are one of its calling cards. The more you fret and worry, the more you'll wrinkle.

As we age, four main factors conspire to etch lines and furrows into our skin. First, as you get older, the process of cell turnover slows down. New young cells aren't produced as quickly, and old ones hang on longer. Second, your body is assaulted by free radicals—unstable oxygen molecules from pollution, stress, and the sun—that cause cell irregularities and discoloration. Third, your body slows down its production of collagen, the protein that helps keep your skin plump and elastic. And fourth, your skin loses moisture and dries out.

That's a lot to deal with, I know. But before you throw in the towel along with your moisturizer, take heart from the fact that certain nutrients can help minimize the appearance of—or even prevent—wrinkles and enhance your skin's natural beauty. Below are some food remedies to try—but take it from me, wearing a big ol' sombrero won't hurt either.

Healing Foods for Wrinkles

★★★**Soy foods** Researchers in Japan conducted a double-blind, placebo-controlled study to determine the effect of the soy isoflavone aglycone on the skin of women in their late thirties and early forties.

Twenty-six women were divided into two groups. The women in one group ate foods containing 40 milligrams of aglycone each day for 12 weeks, and the women in the other group ate foods with no known anti-wrinkle effect. As the researchers evaluated the women's wrinkles along the way, they found that the women who ate the soy showed a statistically significant improvement in skin elasticity after 8 weeks and an improvement in fine lines after 12 weeks compared with the control group.

You can get soy isoflavones in many soy-based foods. For example, ½ cup of miso contains 59 milligrams, 1 cup of soy milk has 30 milligrams, and ½ cup of boiled edamame (green soybeans) offers 12 milligrams.

If soy isoflavones can help wrinkles as this study suggests, then so can most bean isoflavones. As a matter of fact, you can get "soy" isoflavones in almost all edible beans. Soy is good, but it isn't necessarily better. Researchers analyzed 75 varieties of beans and found that many of them had more of the isoflavones genistein and/or daidzein than some varieties of soybeans. Other terrific beans to add to your diet include yellow split peas, black turtle beans, baby limas, anasazi beans, and red kidney beans, all of which, according to the study, contain more genistein than soy beans do!

★★**Carrots** I'll spare you any jokes about Bugs Bunny not having any wrinkles even though he's in his seventies. Carrots are high in beta-carotene, the vegetarian precursor of vitamin A, as well as the vitamin itself, offering you double the wrinkle protection.

Researchers at the University of Michigan Medical School conducted a study to determine how well vitamin A applied topically improved the look of aged skin. Thirty-seven senior citizens applied a lotion containing vitamin A to one arm three times a week and applied a lotion without vitamin A to the other arm. Neither the researchers nor the volunteers knew which arm got which lotion.

After 24 weeks, there were significant differences in wrinkling between the two arms. The researchers think that vitamin A protects the skin from injury and improves its appearance in general.

Want to try this at home? Buy carrot oil, which is high in vitamin A, and apply it to your skin. I've never tried the oil, but I have mashed carrots in a blender and applied them to my face as a mask. If you try it, wash the mask off after 15 to 30 minutes.

★★**Chocolate** I'll pause while you cheer. Yes, it's true: Not only does chocolate *not* cause acne, it's actually good for your skin. If free radicals are one of your skin's worst enemies, then antioxidants, which combat the cellular damage they cause, are among your skin's best friends. And just 0.5 ounce of dark chocolate contains more antioxidants than a glass of orange juice.

★★**Fish** Fatty fish contain essential fatty acids called omega-3's. Researchers from the University of California, Davis, found that the anti-inflammatory properties of omega-3's may extend to the skin, helping to reduce puffiness.

Omega-3's make up an integral part of the membranes that surround our skin cells, and they're key components of the lubricating layer that keeps skin supple. Eicosapentaenoic acid (EPA) from fish oil is a COX-2 inhibitor, increases collagen and elastic fibers, and even has potential as an anti–skin-aging agent. But your body can't make omega-3's, so you have to get them from food or supplements.

Experts recommend eating fatty cold-water fish such as salmon, mackerel, or albacore tuna twice a week.

★★**Green tea** Researchers at Dartmouth Medical School found that people who drink green tea regularly have less sun-related skin damage than people who don't drink tea. They think it's due to a powerful antioxidant in the tea called EGCG.

This is great news for regular green tea drinkers, but the truth of the matter is that I drink green tea only on social occasions. For some conditions, experts may suggest drinking as much as five cups of green tea a day, but I wouldn't recommend more than three, for the stress busting more than the anti-wrinkle effect.

★★**Pineapple** This tropical fruit has been known as a symbol of welcome, but besides being a great welcome gift, it's great for your skin and health. Pineapple is a good source of alpha-hydroxy acids (AHAs), which are used in a great many skin care products.

Researchers in the land of the rising sun suggest that AHAs help the outer layer of skin shed old skin cells and grow new ones, so they are useful for rejuvenating sun-damaged skin.

In a study, people applied a lotion containing AHAs to one arm and a placebo lotion to the other. After about 6 months, the skin on the arm that received the AHAs had increased its thickness by 25 percent. It was also more elastic and

FOODS TO WATCH

Pass up foods containing white flour and white sugar. A diet high in these two ingredients can create chemical reactions between molecules in your skin that sap its collagen and make it less elastic, leaving your skin looking much older.

contained more collagen. All of this led the researchers to conclude that the AHAs significantly reduced the effects of photo-aging.

If I should ever decide to do something about my wrinkles, I'll start by liquefying the peel and core of a whole pineapple in my blender and applying the mash to my face to help remove the surface layer of dead skin cells. Then I'll put my feet up and relax with a good book for 15 to 30 minutes before rinsing it off.

Bear in mind that some people are allergic to pineapple. If you develop itching or a rash when trying this remedy, stop using it immediately.

Not in love with pineapple? Other good sources of citric acid include lemon, tamarind, and black currant.

★★**Pomegranate** Can a bite of the "apple" of the Garden of Eden have an anti-aging effect? I believe that the pomegranate was *that* apple, and I know that it contains three reportedly anti-aging phytochemicals: apigenin, caffeic acid, and quercetin. It's true that these chemicals are more abundant in many other herbs, but pomegranate is uniquely rich in phytoestrogens. Clinical trials involving a type of phytoestrogen from pomegranate concluded that 7 months of hormone replacement therapy can help the skin in several ways. Skin elasticity, skin hydration, and skin thickness were all measurably improved. The authors concluded, "While skin aging is no indication for systemic hormone supplementation, a positive effect on aging skin can be observed."

Candidly, I think that both eating pomegranate and putting it on your skin can help. If I wanted to whip up a facial peel for wrinkles, I'd add lemon, pineapple, roselle, and tamarind to meld with those dozen or so reported estrogenic compounds in pomegranate.

★★**Red bell peppers** If you take a stroll around a department store's cosmetics department, carefully dodging those women wielding perfume atomizers, you'll see many products containing vitamin C. That's for good reason. Your body needs this vitamin to produce collagen, which is a building block of healthy skin. Research has shown that when lab animals eat vitamin C–fortified food, their skin becomes more resistant to wrinkling and discoloration.

Before you reach for a carton of orange juice, though, consider this: Red bell peppers contain more C, cup for cup, than oranges. For skin health, experts suggest eating at least 500 milligrams of vitamin C each day; one bell pepper contains nearly 285 milligrams. Other great sources include camu-camu, bitter melon, and guava.

★★**Sunflower seeds** Here's a little bit of irony: The seeds from a flower named for the sun can help protect you against it! Sunflower seeds are one of the better sources of vitamin E, which, besides protecting you against heart disease, colds, flu, and skin cancer, can prevent wrinkles. Researchers in Korea discovered that mice that ate vitamin E (along with a cocktail of other antioxidants) were less likely to get wrinkles.

If you don't like sunflower seeds, you can get a healthy vitamin E boost from buckwheat, purslane, wheat grains, and corn.

★★**Tomatoes** Red and orange foods are rich in two carotenoids—beta-carotene and lycopene—that protect your skin. These antioxidants actually protect the plants from sunlight, and that protection then extends to you when you eat their fruit.

Beta-carotene and lycopene settle into the outer layer of your skin, where their antioxidant action helps repair cells damaged by sunlight. Researchers in Germany found that eating foods rich in carotenoids may contribute to lifelong protection against harmful ultraviolet radiation. While many fruits and vegetables contain beta-carotene and lycopene, tomatoes are a source of *both*.

My granddaughter Cena would turn orange just from eating some baby food squash or sweet potato, and I'd have thought they were the richest beta-carotene sources around. Now, more than a decade later, I go to my phytochemcial database and find that those two vegetables by no means tops on the beta-carotene hit parade. Other things being equal, I think Cena could have turned more colorful had she eaten the same amount of carrots, spinach, watercress, or nasturtium flowers, each of which contains more beta-carotene than sweet potatoes, most squashes, and pumpkins.

★**Honey** The average woman begins to notice lip lines at age 35. Eating honey, however, could help keep those lines at bay. Honey contains natural sugars that tend to stick to your lips, increasing their ability to attract and maintain moisture—and look younger longer. Get two food remedies for the price of one by sweetening your green tea with a bit of honey.

★**Shortening** Folklore suggests that Crisco is an excellent skin moisturizer. Use it on your face every night before bed.

From the Herbal Medicine Chest

A few plants in the Green Farmacy Garden can offer some help with those pesky worry lines.

Aloe (*Aloe vera*) I have had good experience with an alpha-hydroxy facial cleanser smoothing out my wrinkles a bit. The first ingredient listed on its label is aloe.

Cleopatra is said to have massaged aloe gel into her face daily. It probably can't hurt to give it a try. Simply break open a leaf and smooth the gel on your skin each night before bed.

Echinacea (*Echinacea* spp.) New studies suggest that antioxidant protection against sun damage to collagen may also be a good sunburn preventive, which in turn may protect against wrinkles. Several compounds in echinacea diminish destruction of collagen.

Yeast Infection

MANY PEOPLE THINK YEAST INFECTIONS, also known as candidiasis, occur only in women. While vaginal yeast infections are common in most women, men can also develop candidiasis, especially if they're uncircumcised. A man with yeast typically shows no symptoms, but each time his partner is treated and gets rid of her infection, he infects her again. Yeast infections are easily treated. But if you're a woman troubled by recurrent yeast infections, your partner should get checked, too.

A group of yeastlike fungi called candida causes candidiasis. *Candida albicans* is the most common culprit, but it's not the only one. Everyone has a certain amount of candida living on them and in them, but not everyone develops candidiasis. Yeast live in the lining of the mouth, in the vagina, and on other moist areas of the body. Only when they overgrow do they cause problems. When it overgrows in the vagina, it causes uncomfortable symptoms, such as vaginal itching, burning, and discharge. In the mouth, a yeast infection is known as thrush; in the respiratory tract, it's known as bronchocandidiasis; and on the skin, it's known as dermatocandidiasis.

Most women—as many as 75 percent—will have at least one diagnosis of vaginal yeast infection during their lifetime. Yeast infections are more common during pregnancy, perhaps because of a chemical change in the vaginal environment—essentially there is more sugar in the vaginal secretions that nourishes the fungus. For the same reason, people with diabetes also get yeast infections more frequently.

In modern times, yeast infections have become more common, most likely because several modern drugs spur yeast overgrowth, particularly antibiotics, steroids, and birth control pills. The contraceptive sponge, diaphragm, and spermicidal cream can also produce yeast overgrowth.

Doctors treat yeast infections with antifungal medications that used to be available only by prescription. But several have become available over the counter, and they are advertised extensively, such as nystatin (Mycostatin) and miconazole (Monistat). If you have symptoms, speak with your health care practitioner.

There's more than one way to address the problem, however. Her are some food remedies that might help.

Healing Foods for Yeast Infection

★★★**Garlic** Garlic is a well-known antibacterial antibiotic, but since it also inhibits fungi quite well, some people use it to treat both vaginal candidiasis and thrush. The typical oral dose may range up to a dozen raw, chopped cloves taken two or three times a day in juice. You have to like the taste of garlic to live with this particular treatment, but it's worth a try, as garlic does pack a powerful anti-yeast wallop. Onions have a similar but less potent effect.

Garlic contains dozens of chemical compounds, among them ajoene, allicin-alliin, and diallyl sulfide, which have been proven powerful against fungal infections. In a laboratory study at Loma Linda University in California, animals with yeast infections were given either a placebo (inactive) saline solution or a solution made with aged garlic extract. (This is much lower than 12 cloves, I'll wager; I take New Chapter's product [one capsule supposedly equals one clove; I rarely take more than four a day]). Two days later, animals in the saline group were still infected. Those in the garlic group, however, were completely free of the fungus.

FOODS TO WATCH

Yeast thrives on sugar, so if you have chronic yeast infections, you may find that cutting down on sugar, refined carbohydrates, and alcohol helps. If you have chronic yeast infections and diabetes, it's especially important to control your blood sugar.

If you're fighting boomerang yeast infections with yogurt, choose plain rather than sweetened yogurt. In a surprising study, researcher Betsy Foxman, PhD, of the University of Michigan's School of Public Health, found that women who ate acidophilus-rich products had a higher risk for another yeast infection. She suspects that the sugars in sweetened yogurt may provide food for the yeast you're trying to discourage—and may overpower the "good" yeast-fighting acidophilus bacteria.

Fresh garlic is available all the year round. Other than juicing, you can chop or purée garlic to season your favorite recipes, from salads, to soups, to sides, to main courses. To use garlic, break a clove or two or three away from the bulb. To remove the skin, pound the clove once or twice with the side of a large knife. Then crush, chop, mince, or mash. In recipes that call for whole garlic cloves, simply break the cloves from the bulb, peel, and add to dish.

★★★**Yogurt** A cup of acidophilus yogurt a day may actually prevent recurrent yeast infections (provided it's sugar-free or plain), according to Eileen Hilton, MD, an infectious disease specialist and president of Biomedical Research Alliance of New York.

A study at Long Island Jewish Medical Center suggests that eating live-culture yogurt, especially yogurt containing bacteria called *Lactobacillus acidophilus*, may help keep fungus under control. In the study, women who frequently had vaginal yeast infections were asked to eat 8 ounces of yogurt a day for 6 months. At the end of the study, the rate of yeast infections had dropped significantly. The women were so satisfied, in fact, that when researchers asked them to stop eating yogurt, many of them refused to give it up.

Candidicidal Soup

If you're plagued by recurring yeast infections and enjoy the taste of garlic and onions, here's a tasty soup that might help.

Ingredients:

4 cups water

2 onions, finely chopped

4 cloves garlic, minced

Sage

Thyme

Ground cloves

Salt

Ground black pepper

Acidophilus yogurt

Place the water, garlic, and onions in a medium saucepan. Bring to a boil over high heat. Then reduce the heat, cover, and simmer for 5 minutes, or until the vegetables are tender. Season to taste with sage, thyme, cloves, salt, and pepper, but use the spices somewhat sparingly. Top each serving with a dollop of yogurt.

Makes 4 servings

The Long Island researchers speculate that eating yogurt helps keep the vagina's natural bacterial environment in balance, making it harder for the yeast fungus to thrive. Additional studies need to be done, Dr. Hilton says, but in the meantime, women who are trying to prevent yeast infections may want to try eating 1 cup of yogurt a day—the same amount that was used in the study.

Yogurt makes a delicious snack, and also serves as a healthy substitute for milk with breakfast cereal, or sour cream in recipes. It's important, however, to eat yogurt that contains live cultures, Dr. Hilton says. Yogurt that has been heat-treated doesn't contain bacteria and probably won't be effective. Read the label to find out if your brand has been heat-treated. Cooking also destroys yogurt's friendly bacteria, so it's better to add it to recipes just before serving.

★★**Brazil nuts** Brazil nuts, seeds of the Brazil nut tree, are one of the most widely used tropical nuts. They are harvested almost entirely from wild trees during rainy seasons in various parts of the Amazon, not just Brazil. Brazil nuts are a top-notch source of the mineral selenium; they also contain vitamin E (tocopherols and tocotrienols) as well as trace amounts of vitamins A (beta-carotene) and C (ascorbic acid). Collectively these nutrients may bolster immunity. Stephen Levine, PhD, a candida victim himself, took 400 micrograms of selenium a day, about what one would get in five or six Brazil nuts. Eat them whole, or grind them into creamy nut butter.

★★**Purslane** Vitamins A (and beta-carotene), C, and E are my personal "ACE in the hole" for supporting the immune system. And this ubiquitous weedy herb, not in many supermarkets but in a few farmers markets, packages all of these up together. Although the research is still preliminary, evidence suggests that eating more foods containing these vitamins can help prevent yeast infections. Researchers at Albert Einstein College of Medicine in the Bronx, New York, found that women with yeast infections had significantly less beta-carotene in their vaginal cells than women without infections. The researchers speculate that women with higher levels of beta-carotene may be more resistant to the fungus.

You definitely want to give the immune system help when it's fighting a yeast infection of any kind. Purslane is the best food source of all of these nutrients. I suggest enjoying young shoots of this tasty vegetable in a salad or steaming the leaves as you would spinach.

★**Apple cider** In their book, *Prescriptions for Nutritional Healing,* James F. Balch, Jr., MD, and Phyllis A. Balch also recommend adding 3 cups of pure cider vinegar to the bath water and soaking in the tub for 20 minutes, allowing the water to flow into the vagina. They also say that apple cider vinegar is preferable to over-the-counter douching products. Some would argue that since yeasts make vinegar, vinegar cannot be especially toxic to candida. My friend Jeanne Rose, distinguished California herbalist and prolific author of herbal books, including *Herbs & Aromatherapy for the Reproductive System*, suggests that vinegar douches can restore normal vaginal acidity and are useful for candidiasis.

★**Cranberry** These colorful berries are not just for Thanksgiving. Arbutin, a compound found in cranberries (and bearberries and blueberries), may help treat candida infections, according to naturopaths Joseph Pizzorno, ND, president of Bastyr University in Seattle, and Michael Murray, ND, authors of *Textbook of Natural Medicine*. If you like drinking cranberry juice or eating cranberry sauce, look for plain, unsweetened varieties.

From the Herbal Medicine Chest

You might consider using echinacea in addition to whatever your doctor prescribes for your yeast infection. In studies using laboratory animals, treatment with echinacea protected mice from *Candida albicans* infections. It works by stimulating the white blood cells to gobble up yeast organisms, a process known as phagocytosis.

In an impressive German study, women with recurrent vaginal yeast infections were either given a standard antifungal medication or the antifungal plus an echinacea extract. Among those taking just the antifungal, 60 percent suffered recurrences. But among the women taking the drug plus echinacea, only about 10 percent experienced recurrences. That sounds to me like a good rationale for giving echinacea a try.

Index

Underscored page references indicate boxed text.

Aniseed *(cont.)*
  for laryngitis, 339
  for sore throat, 339
Anthocyanins, 36, 45, <u>228</u>
Apple cider vinegar
  for dandruff, 136
  for insect bites and stings, 249
  for psoriasis, 319
  for vaginitis, 359
  for yeast infection, 375–76
Apples
  for burns, 86
  for cold sores, 115
  for constipation, 118, 258
  for diarrhea, 152, 260
  for diverticulitis, 155
  for food allergies, 180
  for hemorrhoids, 225
  for irritable bowel syndrome, 258, 260
Apricot kernel oil for psoriasis, 318
Apricots for cold sores, 115
Arachadonic acid, <u>173</u>
Arginine, 29, 114–15
Arthritis, <u>6</u>
Artichoke for gallstones, 186
Artificial sweeteners, <u>98</u>, <u>153</u>, <u>259</u>
Aspartame, <u>98</u>. *See also* Artificial
  sweeteners
Asthma, 46–48, <u>49</u>, 50–53, <u>53</u>
Astragalus for colds and flu, <u>112</u>
Athlete's foot, 54–56, <u>56</u>
Atkins Diet, 11
Atopic dermatitis, 333
ATP, <u>174</u>
Avocados
  for angina, 44–45
  for carpal tunnel syndrome, 99
  for dry and itchy skin, 335
  for high cholesterol, 239
  for osteoporosis, 289–90
Ayurveda, 3, 158, 308

B

Backache, 57–61, <u>58</u>, <u>59</u>, <u>61–62</u>
Bacterial vaginosis (BV), 356, <u>358</u>. *See also*
  Vaginitis

Bad breath, 62–66, <u>63</u>, <u>65–66</u>
Baking soda
  for athlete's foot, 55
  for hives, 241
  for insect bites and stings, 249–50
  for poison ivy, oak, and sumac, 310
  for psoriasis, 319
Bananas
  for hangover, 203
  for heartburn, 214
  for high blood pressure, 235
  for ulcers, 352
  for warts, 366
Barley for dandruff, 136
Basil
  for carpal tunnel syndrome, 98
  for indigestion, 243
  for insect bites and stings, 248
  for pneumonia, 306
Bay leaves
  for diabetes, 146–47
  for varicose veins, 362–63
Beans. *See also specific type*
  cooking, <u>176</u>
  effects on
    flatulence, <u>176</u>, <u>177</u>
    irritable bowel syndrome, <u>259</u>
  nutritional overview and eating tips,
    16–17
  in treating and preventing
    cold sores, 114
    constipation, 118
    depression, 140
    diabetes, 147
    erection problems, 164–65
    heart disease, 219
    hemorrhoids, 225–26
    high blood pressure, 236
    high cholesterol, 238
    menopausal symptoms, 271–72
    osteoporosis, 291–92
    overweight, 298
    premenstrual syndrome, 302
    sinusitis, 331–32
    tinnitus, 347
    vaginitis, 357–58
Bearberries for bladder infections, <u>70</u>
Beat-the-Heat Soup, <u>109</u>

Beautyberries for insect bites and stings, 250–51
Bee pollen for cataracts, 104
Beeswax
  for dry and itchy skin, 333
  for psoriasis, 318
Beet greens for gallstones, 185
Beets for psoriasis, 319
Bell peppers
  for gingivitis, 191
  for glaucoma, 193
  for menstrual cramps, 276
  for shingles, 328
  for wrinkles, 370
Benign prostatic hyperplasia (BPH), 311, 314. See also Prostate enlargement
Berries. See also specific type
  for constipation, 119, 258
  for hemorrhoids, 226
  hives and, 242
  for intermittent claudication, 254
  for irritable bowel syndrome, 258
Beta-carotene, 5, 7
Beverages. See Fluid intake; specific type
Bilberries
  for angina, 45
  for diabetes, 149
  for diarrhea, 152, 260
  for gallstones, 186
  for intermittent claudication, 254
  for irritable bowel syndrome, 260
  for ulcers, 352
  for varicose veins, 361–62
Bitter greens for high blood pressure, 235
Blackberries
  for angina, 45
  for hemorrhoids, 228
Black currants
  for glaucoma, 193
  for shingles, 328
Black haw for menstrual cramps, 276
Black pepper
  for colds and flu, 111
  for coughs, 128
  for osteoporosis, 297
  turmeric and, 36–37
Bladder infections, 66–70, 67, 68, 69, 70
Blood-type theory of eating, 12–13

Blueberries
  for angina, 45
  for bladder infections, 69–70
  for bruises, 81
  for diabetes, 149
  for diarrhea, 152, 260
  for gallstones, 186
  for hemorrhoids, 228
  for high cholesterol, 6
  for intermittent claudication, 254
  for irritable bowel syndrome, 260
  for memory loss, 268
  for ulcers, 352
  for varicose veins, 361–62
BMD, 296
Body odor, 71–73, 72, 73
Bok choy for menstrual cramps, 275
Bone fractures, 289
Bone loss, 288–97, 294
Bone mineral density (BMD), 296
Borage seed oil for bronchitis, 79
Boswelia for rheumatoid arthritis, 326
BPH, 311, 314. See also Prostate enlargement
Bran
  for bronchitis, 77
  for diverticulitis, 158
Brazil nuts
  for asthma, 51
  for colds and flu, 110–11
  for prostate enlargement, 313
  selenium in, 7, 51
  for yeast infection, 375
Broccoli
  for asthma, 47–48
  for cataracts, 102–3
  for gingivitis, 191
  for hay fever, 205
  for macular degeneration, 263
  for menstrual cramps, 275
  for overweight, 299–300
  for prostate enlargement, 313
  for shingles, 328
Bromelain, 46, 60. See also Pineapples
Bronchitis, 73–79, 74, 76, 79–80
BronchoBuster Spread, 305
Broths for dry mouth, 161
Bruises, 80–83, 82, 83

Brussels sprouts for gingivitis, 191
Buckwheat
    for diabetes, 149
    for fibromyalgia, 171
    for varicose veins, 361
Bulbs, 17–18. *See also* Garlic; Leeks;
    Onions
Burns, 83–87, <u>87–88</u>, <u>230</u>
Bursitis, 88–93, <u>93</u>
Butcher's broom for hemorrhoids, <u>231</u>
Butterbur
    for hay fever, <u>208</u>
    for headaches, <u>213</u>
BV, 356, <u>358</u>. *See also* Vaginitis
B vitamins and neuropathy, 7

C

Cabbage for ulcers, 352
Caffeinators. *See also* Chocolate; Coffee;
    Tea
    effects on
        colds and flu, <u>106</u>
        fatigue, <u>169</u>
        insomnia, 48, <u>252</u>
        laryngitis, <u>338</u>
        menstrual cramps, <u>275</u>
        osteoporosis, <u>294</u>
        sore throat, <u>338</u>
    nutritional overview and eating tips,
        18–20
    in treating and preventing, asthma,
        48
Caffeine withdrawal, <u>169</u>
Calaguala for psoriasis, <u>319–20</u>
Calcium
    kidney stones and, 184–85
    for osteoporosis, 290–91
Calcium channel blockers, 45
Calendula
    for burns, <u>88</u>
    for cuts and scrapes, <u>135</u>
    for dry and itchy skin, <u>336</u>
    for insect bites and stings, <u>251</u>
    for sunburn, <u>345</u>
    for ulcers, <u>355</u>
Calluses, 124

Camu-camu for bronchitis, 77
Candidicidal Soup, <u>374</u>
Candy and diarrhea, <u>153</u>
Canker sores, 94–95, <u>95–96</u>
Canned foods, 33, 35, <u>234</u>
Cantaloupes
    for angina, 46
    for cold sores, 115
    for shingles, 328–29
Capers for cataracts, 104
Capsaicin. *See also* Chile peppers
    in peppers, 25–26, 58, 99–100
    substance P and, 58, 198, 322
Caraway seeds
    for colds and flu, 111
    for fungal infections, 181
Carbohydrates, 11, 42, <u>211</u>
Cardamom
    for laryngitis, 337
    for sore throat, 337
Carob
    for diarrhea, 152–53
    for heartburn, 214
    for intermittent claudication, 255–56
Carotenoids, 8, 35, 37
Carpal tunnel syndrome (CTS), 96–101,
    98, <u>101</u>
Carrots
    for angina, 45
    for cataracts, 103
    for diarrhea, 154, 261
    for high cholesterol, 239
    for irritable bowel syndrome, 261
    for osteoporosis, 292
    peels of, 36
    for psoriasis, 316
    for wrinkles, 368
Cashews for tinnitus, 346
Castor oil for corns, 125
Cataracts, 101–4
Cauliflower for dry and itchy skin, 335
Cayenne
    for bronchitis, 77–78
    for bruises, <u>83</u>
    for nausea, 279
    for overweight, 298–99
Celecoxib (Celebrex), <u>6</u>, 61, 89, 98,
    322

Celery
  for bad breath, 64
  for bladder infections, 67
  for bursitis, 88–89
  for fungal infections, 181
  for gout, 195
  for hay fever, 206
  for high blood pressure, 232–33
  for indigestion, 243
  for memory loss, 268–69
  for menopausal symptoms, 273
  nutritional overview and eating tips,
    20–21
  for pneumonia, 307
Cepaenes, 48, 50
Cereal for fatigue, 168
CFS, 167. *See also* Fatigue
Chamomile
  for body odor, 71–72
  for bronchitis, 79–80
  for bruises, 82
  for burns, 84–85
  for bursitis, 90
  for canker sores, 95
  for carpal tunnel syndrome, 99
  for coughs, 128
  for diverticulitis, 156
  for food allergies, 180
  for fungal infections, 182
  for gout, 198
  for hay fever, 208
  for heartburn, 214
  for hemorrhoids, 230
  for high blood pressure, 235
  for hives, 241
  for indigestion, 244
  for nausea, 279–80
  for psoriasis, 320
  for ulcers, 353
Charles Bonnet syndrome, 262
Cheese
  for cold sores, 115
  constipation and, 119
  for dry mouth, 160–61
  for gingivitis, 191–92
Cherries
  for angina, 45
  for backache, 60

for gout, 26, 195
  for hemorrhoids, 228
  for insomnia, 252
Chest pain, 43–46, 45
Chewing gum
  for bad breath, 63–64
  diarrhea and, 153
  for ulcers, 352
Chia
  alpha-linolenic acid in, 8
  for menstrual cramps, 274–75
  omega-3 fatty acids in, 23
Chicken pox, 327. *See also* Shingles
Chicken soup
  for colds and flu, 105–6
  for coughs, 126
Chicory for diabetes, 147
Chile peppers
  for backache, 58–59
  for bronchitis, 77–78
  for bursitis, 90–91
  for carpal tunnel syndrome, 99–100
  for cold sores, 114
  for coughs, 128
  for dry and itchy skin, 336
  for dry mouth, 161
  for fibromyalgia, 172
  for gout, 198–99
  for hay fever, 206–7
  for indigestion, 245–46
  for osteoarthritis, 282–84
  for psoriasis, 316, 318
  for rheumatoid arthritis, 322–23
  for shingles, 327–28
  for toothaches, 348
  for ulcers, 352–53
Chiso for menstrual cramps, 274–75
Chocolate. *See also* Caffeinators
  caffeine in, 48
  effects on
    heartburn, 215
    hives, 242
  in treating and preventing
    coughs, 128–29
    depression, 140–41
    high cholesterol, 239
    varicose veins, 362
    wrinkles, 368–69

Cholesterol. *See also* High cholesterol
  dietary fats and, 7–8
  gallstones and, 184
  HDL, 7, 240–41
  LDL, 7, 11, 218, <u>221</u>, 239–41, 256
Cholorophyll, 72–73
Chromium
  for diabetes, 145
  for overweight, 299–300
Chronic fatigue syndrome (CFS), 167. *See also* Fatigue
Cineole, <u>67</u>
Cinnamon
  for bad breath, 63–64
  for diabetes, 145–46
  for fatigue, 167–68
  for fungal infections, 182
  for hangover, 202
  for heartburn, 216
  for indigestion, 244
  for insect bites and stings, 250
  for nausea, 278
  nutritional overview and eating tips, 21–22
  for pneumonia, 307
Ciprofibrate, <u>6</u>
Citrus fruits. *See also specific type*
  for asthma, 47–48, 50–51
  for bruises, 81–82
  for colds and flu, 106–7
  for cuts and scrapes, 133–34
  for fatigue, 169
  for food allergies, 179
  for gingivitis, 190
  for hay fever, 205
  for memory loss, 266–67
  for nausea, 280
  nutritional overview and eating tips, 22–23
  peels of, 36, 50–51
  for pneumonia, 306
  for sinusitis, 330
Clams
  for glaucoma, 194
  for tinnitus, 346–47
Cloves
  for altitude sickness, 41
  for cold sores, 114

for coughs, 127
for cuts and scrapes, 132
for diabetes, 150
for insect bites and stings, <u>251</u>
for toothaches, 348
Cluster headaches, 209. *See also* Headaches
Coca leaf for altitude sickness, 40
Coenzyme Q10 (CoQ10), 44
Coffee. *See also* Caffeinators
  caffeine in, 48
  effects on
    angina, <u>44</u>
    gallstones, <u>187</u>
    heartburn, <u>215</u>
    hemorrhoids, <u>227</u>
    irritable bowel syndrome, <u>259</u>
    menopausal symptoms, <u>270</u>
    ulcers, <u>354</u>
  in treating and preventing
    asthma, 48
    constipation, 123
    gout, 195–97
Cold-fx, 112
Colds and flu, 104–8, <u>106</u>, <u>109</u>, 110–11, <u>111–13</u>
Cold sores, 94, 113–15
Collagen, <u>325</u>
Collard greens
  for cataracts, 103
  for hay fever, 205
  for macular degeneration, 263
  for menstrual cramps, 275
Commission E, 76, 79, 112, 157, 186, 207, 339, <u>340</u>, <u>367</u>
Constipation, 116–25, <u>119</u>, <u>120</u>, <u>121</u>, <u>123</u>, 258–60
Cooking, 35–37, <u>176</u>
CoQ10, 44
Coriander
  for bad breath, 64–65
  for indigestion, <u>245</u>
  for nausea, 279
Corn and irritable bowel syndrome, <u>259</u>
Cornmeal for osteoporosis, 292–93
Corns, 124–25
Corn silk for corns, 124
Cornstarch for hives, 242

Eye problems
    cataracts, 101–4
    glaucoma, 192–94

F

Farmer's markets, 32
Fasting followed by doses of olive oil, <u>188</u>
Fatigue, 167–70, <u>169</u>
Fava beans
    for erection problems, 164–65
    for high blood pressure, 236
Female health problems
    menopause-related, 269–73, <u>270</u>,
        <u>273–74</u>
    menstrual cramps, 274–76, <u>275</u>, <u>276</u>
    premenstrual dysphoric disorder,
        301–2
    premenstrual syndrome, 301–4
Fennel
    for heartburn, 216
    for nausea, 279
Fenugreek
    for diabetes, 147
    for diarrhea, <u>154</u>
    for high cholesterol, <u>240–41</u>
Fever, <u>109</u>
Feverfew for headaches, <u>213</u>
Fiber
    for constipation, 116–18
    for diabetes, 146
    for gallstones, 186
    for hemorrhoids, 225
    for irritable bowel syndrome, 257
    for kidney stones, 188
    for overweight, 298
Fibromyalgia, 170–74, <u>173</u>, <u>174–75</u>
Figs
    for cold sores, 113, 115
    for constipation, 121, 260
    for fibromyalgia, 171
    for irritable bowel syndrome, 260
    for toothaches, 349
    for warts, 364–65
Fish
    effects on
        dry and itchy skin, <u>334</u>
        eczema, <u>334</u>

omega-3 fatty acids in, 8, 51
in treating and preventing
    angina, 44
    asthma, 51–52
    colds and flu, 110–11
    dandruff, 137
    depression, 141
    fatigue, 168
    gallstones, 186, 188
    gingivitis, 191
    high blood pressure, 234
    insomnia, 253
    intermittent claudication, 256
    macular degeneration, 263–64
    rheumatoid arthritis, 321–22
    wrinkles, 369
Fish oil for depression, 139
Flatulence, 175–78, <u>176</u>, <u>177</u>
Flavonoids, <u>6</u>, 8, 17, 48, 229
Flax
    for dry and itchy skin, 335
    for menstrual cramps, 274–75
Flaxseed
    for burns, 86–87
    for bursitis, 92
    for carpal tunnel syndrome, 100
    for constipation, 120, 258
    for diverticulitis, 156
    for hemorrhoids, 226
    for irritable bowel syndrome,
        258
    for menopausal symptoms, 272
    omega-3 fatty acids in, 8
    for premenstrual syndrome, 302
    for prostate enlargement, 315
    for psoriasis, 318
Flaxseed oil for sunburn, 342–43
Floral teas for depression, 142
Flu. *See* Colds and flu
Fluid intake. *See also* Water
    bladder infections and, <u>68</u>
    for fever, <u>109</u>
    for laryngitis, 339
    for sore throat, 339
Folate for memory loss, 265
Food allergies, <u>49</u>, 178–80, <u>179</u>, <u>242</u>,
    <u>309</u>, <u>329</u>
Food diary, keeping, <u>211</u>
Food labels, reading, <u>179</u>

for irritable bowel syndrome, 259,
261
for laryngitis, 337–38
for memory loss, 269
for menstrual cramps, 275–76
for motion sickness, <u>6</u>
for nausea, 277–78
nutritional overview and eating tips,
23–24
for osteoarthritis, 284
for pneumonia, 307
for sore throat, 337–38
for toothaches, 349
for ulcers, 353
Gingivitis, 190–92
Ginkgo
for altitude sickness, <u>43</u>
for asthma, <u>53</u>
for erection problems, <u>166–67</u>
for intermittent claudication, <u>256</u>
for memory loss, <u>269</u>
Ginseng
for colds and flu, <u>111–12</u>
for sinusitis, <u>333</u>
Glaucoma, 192–94
Glycemic index, 11
Goldenseal
for pneumonia, <u>308</u>
for sinusitis, <u>333</u>
Gout, <u>26</u>, 194–200, <u>196</u>, <u>200</u>
Grains for insomnia, 252
Grapefruit
for cold sores, 115
for osteoarthritis, 286
psoriasis and, <u>317</u>
for shingles, 328–29
Grape leaves for colds and flu, 111
Grapes
for memory loss, 267
for varicose veins, 361–62
Gravies for dry mouth, 161
Grazing, 14
Greater celandine for warts, <u>366</u>
Green tea
for food allergies, 180
for high blood pressure, 234
for pneumonia, 307
for prostate enlargement, 313–14

for psoriasis, 319
for rheumatoid arthritis, 324
for wrinkles, 369
Guavas
for bronchitis, 76
for bruises, 81
for glaucoma, 193
for menstrual cramps, 276
for shingles, 328
for sunburn, 343
Gum disease, 190–92

H

Hair problems, 136–37, <u>137</u>, <u>138</u>
Halibut, for insomnia, 253
Halitosis, 62–66, <u>63</u>, <u>65–66</u>
Hangover, 201–3, <u>202</u>, <u>203</u>
Hawthorn for high blood pressure,
<u>236</u>
Hay fever, 204–7, <u>205</u>, <u>207</u>, <u>208–9</u>
Hazelnuts
for cataracts, 103
for glaucoma, 194
HDL, 7, 240–41
Headaches, 209–12, <u>211</u>, <u>213</u>
Health Professionals Follow-Up Study,
196–97
Heartburn, 213–17, <u>215</u>, <u>217</u>
Heart disease, 4, 7, 218–24, <u>221</u>
Hemorrhoids, 224–30, <u>227</u>, <u>228</u>, <u>230</u>,
<u>231–32</u>
Hemp for menstrual cramps, 274–75
Hempseed
for diverticulitis, 156–57
for nausea, 280
omega-3 fatty acids in, 8
Herbal remedies, 2. *See also specific herb*
for constipation, <u>121</u>
for flatulence, 178
for gallstones, <u>189</u>
for gas and cramps, 261
for insomnia, <u>254</u>
for irritable bowel syndrome, 261
for kidney stones, <u>189</u>
for sunburn, <u>343</u>
for vaginitis, <u>359</u>

Herpes zoster, 327–29
High blood pressure, 232–36, <u>233</u>, <u>234</u>, <u>236</u>
High-carbohydrate foods for altitude sickness, 42
High cholesterol, <u>6</u>, 17, 237–40, <u>238</u>, <u>240</u>, <u>240–41</u>
High-fat foods
  bronchitis and, <u>74</u>
  coughs and, <u>127</u>
  heartburn and, <u>215</u>
  heart disease and, <u>221</u>
  pneumonia and, <u>307</u>
  psoriasis and, <u>317</u>
  vaginitis and, <u>357</u>
Hives, 241–42, <u>242</u>
Honey
  for asthma, 52
  for burns, 87
  for colds and flu, 108, 110
  for constipation, 122
  for coughs, 128
  for cuts and scrapes, 134
  for dandruff, 136
  diarrhea and, <u>153</u>
  for dry and itchy skin, 333
  for hemorrhoids, 231
  for laryngitis, 339
  for nausea, 280
  for psoriasis, 318
  for sore throat, 339
  for ulcers, 354
  for wrinkles, 371
HOPE (Heart Outcomes Prevention Evaluation) study, 4
Horehound
  for laryngitis, <u>340</u>
  for sore throat, <u>340</u>
Hormone replacement therapy (HRT), <u>6</u>, 27, 269–70
Horse chestnut tree for varicose veins, <u>362</u>
Horseradish
  for bronchitis, 77–78
  for coughs, 129
  for hay fever, 206–7
  for laryngitis, 339
  for sinusitis, 332
  for sore throat, 339

Hot flashes, 270, <u>270</u>
Hot pepper sauce for hangover, 202
HPV, 363
HRT, <u>6</u>, 27, 269–70
Human papillomavirus (HPV), 363
Hummus for high cholesterol, <u>238</u>
Hydrogenation, 11
Hypertension, 232–36, <u>233</u>, <u>234</u>, <u>236</u>

I

IBS, 257–61, <u>259</u>, <u>262</u>
IC, 254–56, <u>256</u>
Ice
  for insect bites and stings, 250
  for laryngitis, 339
  for sore throat, 339
Ice cream for dry mouth, 161
Inca peanut, research on, 8
Indigestion, 243–46, <u>245</u>, <u>246–47</u>
Infections
  bacterial vaginosis, 356, <u>358</u>
  bladder, 66–70, <u>67</u>, <u>68</u>, <u>69</u>, <u>70</u>
  cystitis, <u>67</u>
  ear, 162
  fungal, 180–83, <u>183</u>
  sinusitis, 329–32, <u>329</u>, <u>332–33</u>
  urinary tract, 66–70, <u>67</u>, <u>68</u>, <u>69</u>, <u>70</u>
  vaginitis, 356–59, <u>357</u>, <u>358</u>, <u>359</u>
  yeast, 372–76, <u>373</u>, <u>374</u>, <u>376</u>
Inflammation
  arthritis, <u>6</u>
  asthma, 46–48, <u>49</u>, 50–53, <u>53</u>
  bronchitis, 73–79, <u>74</u>, <u>76</u>, <u>79–80</u>
  bursitis, 88–93, <u>93</u>
  osteoarthritis, 281–87, <u>283</u>, <u>286</u>, <u>287–88</u>
  processed foods and, <u>90</u>
  rheumatoid arthritis, 320–26, <u>323</u>, <u>325</u>, <u>326</u>
  snack foods and, <u>41</u>
Inhalers, 47
Inositol-rich foods for depression, 142–43
Insect bites and stings, 247–50, <u>248</u>, <u>250–51</u>

Mental problems
  depression, 138–43, <u>143</u>
  memory loss, 264–69, <u>265</u>, <u>269</u>
Menthol
  for backache, 60
  for sinusitis, 331
Metabolic syndrome, <u>151</u>
Micronutrients, 5
Migraines, 209. *See also* Headaches
Milk
  effects on
    eczema, <u>334</u>
    hay fever, <u>207</u>
    hives, <u>242</u>
    irritable bowel syndrome, <u>259</u>
    ulcers, <u>354</u>
  in treating and preventing
    cold sores, 115
    dry and itchy skin, <u>334</u>, 336
    gingivitis, 191–92
    hives, 242
    psoriasis, 318
Minerals, 184–85. *See also specific type*
Mints. *See also* Peppermint
  for backache, 60
  for bronchitis, 78–79
  for bursitis, 91–92
  for gout, 197
  for hay fever, 207
  for headaches, 212
  nutritional overview and eating tips, 24–25
  for sinusitis, 331
Monosodium glutamate (MSG), <u>211</u>
Motion sickness, <u>6</u>, <u>279</u>, 280
Mouthwash, herbal, <u>65–66</u>
MSG, <u>211</u>
Mushrooms. *See also specific type*
  for altitude sickness, 42–43
  for bad breath, 65
  for colds and flu, 111
  for fatigue, 170
  fungal infections and, 180–83, <u>183</u>
Mustard
  for bronchitis, 77–78, <u>78</u>
  for hay fever, 206–7
  for laryngitis, 339
  for sore throat, 339

Mustard Blaster Salad Dressing, <u>78</u>
Mustard greens for fatigue, 168
Myers' Cocktail, <u>175</u>
Myrrh for canker sores, <u>96</u>

N

Nausea, 276–81, <u>279</u>, <u>281</u>
Nerve disorder, 7
Neuropathy, 7
Nonsteroidal anti-inflammatory drugs (NSAIDs), 274, 282, 351
Nonsweetened beverages for dry mouth, 160
NSAIDs, 274, 282, 351
Nutmeg for ulcers, 355
Nutrients. *See also specific type*
  dietary fats, 7–8
  in fruits, decline of, 31
  loss of, in modern diet, 31–32
  maximizing, 31
  new stars, 5, 8–9
  old standbys, 6–7
  peels and, 36
  in potatoes, decline of, 31
  research on, 5
  in soups, 36
  in vegetables, decline of, 31
Nuts. *See also specific type*
  for bruises, <u>82</u>
  gallstones and, 188
  hives and, <u>242</u>
  for tinnitus, 346

O

Oatmeal
  for dry and itchy skin, 334
  for high cholesterol, 238–39
  for hives, 242
  for insect bites and stings, 250
  for poison ivy, oak, and sumac, 309
  for shingles, 328
  for sunburn, 344

Oats
for burns, 86
for fatigue, 169
for psoriasis, 318
Oat straw for warts, <u>367</u>
Oils. *See also specific type*
carotenoids and heated, 35, 37
constipation and, <u>119</u>
hemorrhoids and, <u>227</u>
Olive oil
for dandruff, 137
for dry and itchy skin, 333, 335
for heart disease, 219–20
for high cholesterol, 239
for laryngitis, 339–40
for psoriasis, 318
for rheumatoid arthritis, 324–25
for sore throat, 339–40
for sunburn, 341–42
for varicose veins, 362–63
Omega-3 fatty acids
in chia, <u>23</u>
in fish, 8, 51
in flaxseed, 8
in hempseed, 8
Omega-6 fatty acids and asthma, <u>49</u>
Onions
effects on
bad breath, 62, <u>63</u>
heartburn, <u>215</u>
garlic versus, <u>20</u>
importance of, 17
nutritional overview and eating tips,
18
in treating and preventing
asthma, 48, 50
bronchitis, 75
burns, 85
cataracts, 104
colds and flu, 107–8
coughs, 130–31
depression, 142
diabetes, 148
diarrhea, 154, 261
hay fever, 206
heart disease, 220
high blood pressure, 234
indigestion, 246
insect bites and stings, 249

intermittent claudication, 254–55
irritable bowel syndrome, 261
pneumonia, 306
poison ivy, oak, and sumac, 310
sinusitis, 330
Oral malodor, 62–66, <u>63</u>, <u>65–66</u>
Oranges
for cold sores, 115
for high cholesterol, 240
for shingles, 328–29
Oregano
for bad breath, 64
for bursitis, 92
for cold sores, 115
for depression, 143
for hives, 241
for nausea, 279
for osteoarthritis, 286
for pneumonia, 306
for sinusitis, 330–31
for toothaches, 349
Organic food, 32–33
Osteoarthritis, 281–87, <u>283</u>, <u>286</u>,
<u>287–88</u>
Osteoporosis, 288–97, <u>294</u>
Overweight, <u>59</u>, 297–300
Oxalate-rich foods, <u>187</u>
Oysters
for glaucoma, 194
for tinnitus, 346–47

P

PAD, 254
Pain
angina, 43–46, <u>44</u>, <u>45</u>
back, 57–61, <u>58</u>, <u>59</u>, <u>61–62</u>
ear, 161–63
fibromyalgia, 170–74, <u>173</u>,
<u>174–75</u>
head, 209–12, <u>211</u>, <u>213</u>
throat, 336–40, <u>338</u>, <u>340</u>
tooth, 347–50, <u>349</u>, <u>350–51</u>
Pansies for bruises, 82
Papayas
for bladder infections, 70
for burns, 87
for cold sores, 115

Pomegranates *(cont.)*
for sore throat, 338
for wrinkles, 370
Pork
for cold sores, 115
warts and, <u>365</u>
Potassium for kidney stones, 189
Potatoes
for bruises, 83
nutrients in, decline of, 31
for osteoporosis, 295–96
for sunburn, 342
Prebiotics, 154
Premenstrual dysphoric disorder (PMDD), 301–2
Premenstrual syndrome (PMS), 301–4
Prickly ash for toothaches, <u>350</u>
Prickly pears
for fungal infections, 202–3
for prostate enlargement, 315
Processed foods
in American diet, 10–11
diarrhea and, <u>151</u>, <u>153</u>
high blood pressure and, <u>234</u>
inflammation and, <u>90</u>
osteoarthritis and, <u>283</u>
Prostate cancer, 313
Prostate enlargement, 311–15
Prostate-specific antigens (PSAs), 312
Protein
animal, <u>283</u>
for osteoporosis, 291–92
for overweight, 300
psoriasis and, <u>317</u>
Prunes
for constipation, 120–21, 260
for diabetes, 150
for diverticulitis, 157
for hemorrhoids, 226
for irritable bowel syndrome, 260
for osteoporosis, 295
PSAs, 312
Psoriasis, 315–16, <u>317</u>, 318–19, <u>319–20</u>
Psyllium
for constipation, <u>123</u>
for diarrhea, <u>154</u>
for hemorrhoids, <u>231–32</u>
for irritable bowel syndrome, <u>262</u>

Pterostilbene, <u>6</u>
Pudding for dry mouth, 161
Pumpkin
for erection problems, 166
fresh versus canned, 35
for hay fever, 206
Pumpkin seeds
for insomnia, 253
for prostate enlargement, 312–13
Purines, <u>196</u>
Purslane
for heart disease, 224
magnesium in, 169
for premenstrual syndrome, 302
for psoriasis, 318
for yeast infection, 375
Pycnogenol for osteoarthritis, <u>287–88</u>

Q

Quercetin, 5, 8, 50, 104

R

RA, 320–26, <u>323</u>, <u>325</u>, <u>326</u>
Radishes
for gallstones, 186
for indigestion, 245
Raisins
for bad breath, 65
for constipation, 121, 260
for irritable bowel syndrome, 260
Ranolazine (Ranexa), 44
Rape seed oil for premenstrual syndrome, 302–3
Raspberries
for canker sores, 95
for nausea, 280
Red wine. *See also* Alcohol
for colds and flu, 111
for heart disease, 221–22
for rheumatoid arthritis, 325–26
Reishi mushroom for altitude sickness, 42–43
Repetitive stress injury, 96–101, <u>98</u>, <u>101</u>

U

V

Y

Yang, 3
Yeast infection, 372–76, <u>373</u>, <u>374</u>, <u>376</u>
Yegg formula, <u>359</u>
Yin, 3
Yogurt
    for bad breath, 63
    for bladder infections, 68–69
    for canker sores, 95
    for colds and flu, 110
    for dandruff, 137
    for dry mouth, 161
    for food allergies, 17 9–80
    for gingivitis, 191–92
    for premenstrual syndrome, 303

    for ulcers, 353
    for vaginitis, 358–59
    for yeast infection, 374–75

Z

Zanamivir (Relenza), 75
Zeaxanthin, 8–9
Zinc
    for hemorrhoids, 229
    for warts, 366
Zingibain, 59, 172
Zostrix, 58, 199
Zyflamend, <u>200</u>, 281